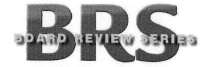

BOARD REVIEW SERIES

BRS Neuroanatomy

SEVENTH EDITION

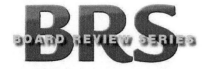

BRS Neuroanatomy

SEVENTH EDITION

Douglas J. Gould, PhD
Professor and Chair
Department of Foundational Medical Studies
Oakland University William Beaumont School of Medicine
Rochester, Michigan

*Author of **1st–4th** Editions:*
James D. Fix, PhD
(1931–2010)

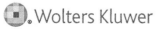. Wolters Kluwer

Philadelphia · Baltimore · New York · London
Buenos Aires · Hong Kong · Sydney · Tokyo

Acquisitions Editor: Crystal Taylor
Development Editor: Deborah Bordeaux
Freelance Development Editor: Maria McAvey
Editorial Coordinator: Priyanka Alagar
Marketing Manager: Danielle Klahr
Production Project Manager: Kirstin Johnson
Manager, Graphic Arts & Design: Stephen Druding
Art Director: Jennifer Clements
Manufacturing Coordinator: Margie Orzech
Prepress Vendor: S4Carlisle Publishing Services

Seventh Edition

9 8 7 6 5 4 3 2 1

Printed in the United States of America

Library of Congress Cataloging-in-Publication Data

ISBN-13: 978-1-975214-37-1

ISBN-10: 1-975214-37-4

Library of Congress Control Number: 2023912843

shop.lww.com

MPP0923

To Laurisa—my support and inspiration.
I would be lost without you.

Preface

BRS Neuroanatomy, seventh edition, is a concise review of human neuroanatomy intended for health professions students including medical and dental students preparing for their respective boards and other examinations. It presents the essentials of human neuroanatomy in a concise, tightly outlined, well-illustrated format. There are more than 650 questions with answers and explanations, some included at the end of each chapter and some in a comprehensive examination at the end of the book.

NEW TO THIS EDITION

- 20 new clinical correlates and 44 new clinical vignette-based practice questions
- Updated content and terminology referencing *Terminologia Anatomica* and UpToDate
- Expanded section on referred pain
- New section on the cranial nerve examination
- Updated glossary and expanded answer explanations in the chapters and comprehensive examinations

To the Student

Although this book is usable as a reference tool, to make the most of this book, work your way up the neuroaxis by starting at the beginning with the anatomy and blood supply, embryology and histology, and then proceeding up the spinal cord to higher centers. The illustrations, figures and tables, as well as their legends contain much board-relevant information that complement and inform the extensive question bank.

Acknowledgments

Special thanks to and in respectful memory of **Dr. James Fix**, for creating the first four editions of *BRS Neuroanatomy*—the foundation upon which all future editions are based. I thank my students and colleagues for their valuable input as the seventh edition was developed. I also thank the Wolters Kluwer staff and their associates for their contributions to this edition—Crystal Taylor, acquisitions editor; Deborah Bordeaux, development editor; Priyanka Alagar, editorial coordinator; and the student and faculty reviewers, who were invited by the publisher to provide valuable feedback and suggestions. Special thanks to Shannon Derthick for her contribution of the art for multiple new figures in Chapter 10.

Contents

5   NEUROHISTOLOGY   74

6   SPINAL CORD   90

7   TRACTS OF THE SPINAL CORD   102

8   LESIONS OF THE SPINAL CORD   116

Gross Anatomy of the Brain

I. INTRODUCTION

▨ the nervous system may be divided structurally or functionally:

▨ structural divisions include the central (brain + spinal cord) and peripheral (spinal and cranial nerves) nervous systems.

▨ functional divisions include the somatic and the visceral nervous systems.

▨ parts of both functional divisions are found throughout both structural divisions.

▨ somatic and visceral nervous systems can be further divided into motor and sensory components.

▨ somatic motor system includes voluntary and reflexive movement of skeletal muscle. Somatic sensory system provides specific and well-localized sensation from the body wall.

▨ visceral motor system—also known as the autonomic nervous system and can be divided into sympathetic and parasympathetic divisions (Chapter 20); innervates smooth and cardiac muscle. Visceral sensory system rides with visceral motor fibers and provides diffuse, nonspecific innervation, mainly stretch from hollow organs of the gut.

II. OVERVIEW

▨ part of the central nervous system (CNS) that lies within the cranial vault—the **encephalon**. Its surface is convoluted and exhibits **gyri** and **sulci**.

▨ consists of the **cerebrum** (cerebral hemispheres and diencephalon), the **brainstem** (midbrain, pons, and medulla), and the **cerebellum**.

▨ newborn brains weigh between 350 and 400 g.

▨ weight of average 20-year-old male brain is ~1,400 g, at 65 years old falls to 1,300 g; female brains weigh 100 to 150 g less on average.

▨ covered by three connective tissue membranes, the **meninges**.

▨ surrounded by **cerebrospinal fluid (CSF)** that provides support and protects the brain from trauma.

III. DIVISIONS OF THE BRAIN

The brain is divided into six postembryonic divisions: **telencephalon**, **diencephalon**, **mesencephalon**, **pons**, **medulla oblongata**, and **cerebellum**.

A. **Telencephalon**
- consists of the **cerebral hemispheres** and the **basal nuclei**. The cerebral hemispheres contain the **lateral ventricles**.
  1. **Cerebral hemispheres** (Figures 1.1 through 1.5)
     - separated by the longitudinal cerebral fissure and the falx cerebri.
     - interconnected by commissural fiber bundles (eg, corpus callosum).
     - consists of six lobes and the olfactory structures:
       a. **Frontal lobe** (see Figures 1.3 and 1.4)
          - involved with voluntary motor control, speech production, and high-order cognitive functions, such as future planning, attention, consciousness, problem-solving, emotions, and personality.
          - extends from the central sulcus to the frontal pole.
          - lies superior to the lateral sulcus and anterior to the central sulcus.
          - made up of the following gyri:
            (1) Precentral gyrus
            - consists of the primary motor area (area 4).
            - involved in voluntary movement of the contralateral face and body.

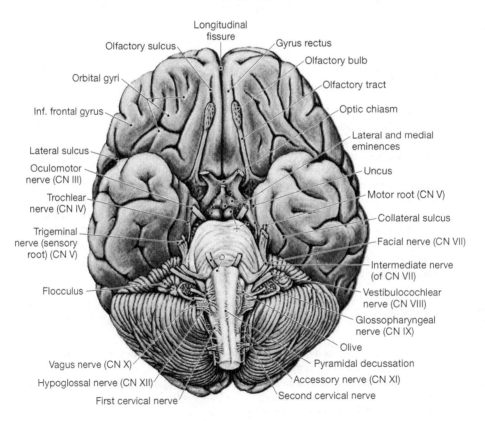

+ = Mammillary body; cerebral peduncle
o = Abducens nerve; pyramid of medulla

FIGURE 1.1. Base of the brain. (Adapted from Truex RC, Kellner CE. *Detailed Atlas of the Head and Neck.* Oxford University Press; 1958:34. Reproduced with permission of Oxford University Press (Books) through PLSclear.)

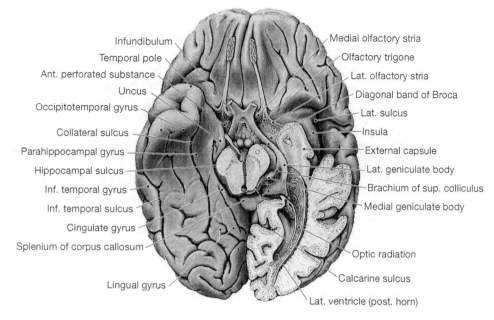

o = Optic tract
+ = Brachium of inf. colliculus

FIGURE 1.2. Inferior surface of the brain showing the principal gyri and sulci. The left hemisphere has been dissected to show the visual pathways and relation of the optic radiation to the lateral ventricle. (Adapted from Truex RC, Kellner CE. *Detailed Atlas of the Head and Neck.* Oxford University Press; 1958:46. Reproduced with permission of Oxford University Press (Books) through PLSclear.)

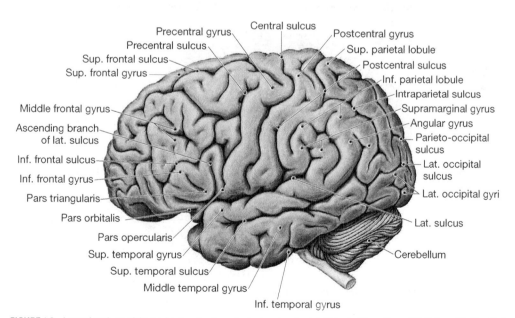

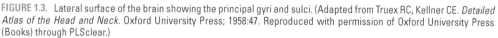

FIGURE 1.3. Lateral surface of the brain showing the principal gyri and sulci. (Adapted from Truex RC, Kellner CE. *Detailed Atlas of the Head and Neck.* Oxford University Press; 1958:47. Reproduced with permission of Oxford University Press (Books) through PLSclear.)

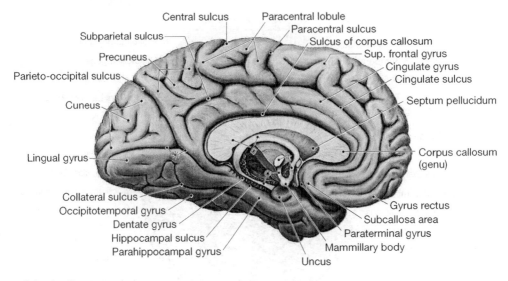

∗ = Calcarine fissure
◊ = Splenium of corpus callosum; body of fornix
+ = Interthalamic adhesion: ant. column of fornix
o = Fimbria of fornix; mammillothalamic tract

FIGURE 1.4. Medial surface of the brain showing the principal gyri and sulci. Parts of the thalamus and hypothalamus have been removed to show the fimbria and anterior column of the fornix and the mammillothalamic tract. (Adapted from Truex RC, Kellner CE. *Detailed Atlas of the Head and Neck*. Oxford University Press; 1958:49. Reproduced with permission of Oxford University Press (Books) through PLSclear.)

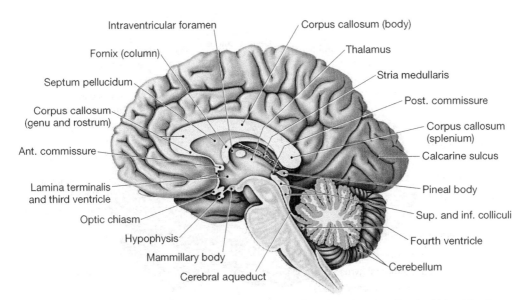

FIGURE 1.5. Midsagittal section of the brain and brainstem showing the structures surrounding the third and fourth ventricles. (Adapted with permission from Bear MF, Connors BW, Paradiso MA. *Neuroscience: Exploring the Brain*. 3rd ed. Lippincott Williams & Wilkins; 2007:207.)

(2) Superior frontal gyrus

- contains supplementary motor cortex on the medial surface (area 6) as well as the supplementary eye field.
- involved with impulse control and higher cognitive function, including memory.

(3) **Middle frontal gyrus**
- forms most of the frontal lobe.
- on the dominant side it is involved with language, on the nondominant side it is involved with orientation and attention.

(4) **Inferior frontal gyrus**
- contains the frontal eye field (area 8).
- contains the Broca speech area in the dominant hemisphere (areas 44 and 45).

(5) **Gyrus rectus and orbital gyri**

(6) **Anterior paracentral lobule**

b. **Parietal lobe (see Figures 1.3 through 1.5)**
- involved with sensory perception and integration.
- extends from the central sulcus to the occipital lobe and lies superior to the temporal lobe.
- contains the following lobules and gyri:

(1) **Postcentral gyrus**
- the primary somatosensory area of the cerebral cortex (areas 3, 1, and 2).
- of critical importance in localizing sensory stimuli.

(2) **Superior parietal lobule**
- comprises association areas involved in somatosensory functions (areas 5 and 7).

(3) **Inferior parietal lobule**
- **Supramarginal gyrus**
  a. interrelates somatosensory, auditory, and visual inputs (area 40).
- **Angular gyrus** (area 39)
  a. receives impulses from primary visual cortex.
  b. involved with the linkage between visual areas and the posterior language areas.

(4) **Precuneus**
- divided into an anterior region, involved with mental imagery and a posterior region, involved with memory retrieval.

(5) **Posterior paracentral lobule**
- involved with motor and sensory function of the lower limbs.

c. **Temporal lobe (see Figures 1.2 through 1.4)**
- involved with hearing and memory formation.
- extends from the temporal pole to the occipital lobe, lying inferior to the lateral sulcus.
- extends from the lateral sulcus to the collateral sulcus.
- contains the following gyri:

(1) **Transverse temporal gyri of Heschl (see Figure 1.6)**
- found within the lateral sulcus.
- contains the primary auditory areas of the cerebral cortex (areas 41 and 42).

(2) **Superior temporal gyrus**
- associated with auditory functions.
- contains the **Wernicke speech area** in the dominant hemisphere (area 22).
- contains the planum temporale on its superior (hidden) surface.

(3) **Middle temporal gyrus**

(4) **Inferior temporal gyrus**

(5) **Lateral occipitotemporal gyrus (fusiform gyrus)**

d. **Occipital lobe** (see Figures 1.3 through 1.5)
- involved with visual processing.
- lies posterior to a line connecting the parieto-occipital sulcus and the preoccipital notch.
- contains two structures that contain the visual cortex (areas 17, 18, and 19):

(1) **Cuneus**

(2) **Lingual gyrus**

e. **Insular lobe** (insula) (see Figure 1.2)
- involved with motor and sensory processing, and higher cognitive function, including emotions.
- lies within the lateral sulcus and is composed of short and long gyri.

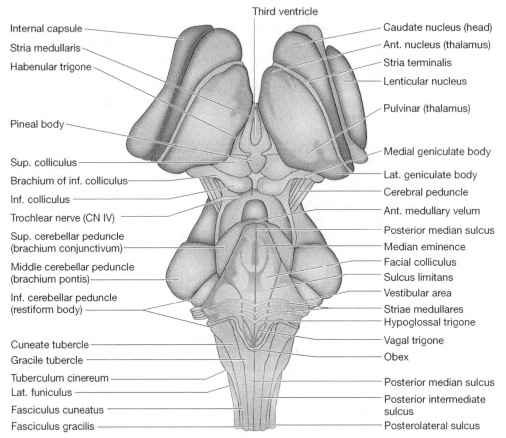

Third ventricle

Internal capsule

Stria medullaris

Habenular trigone

Pineal body

Sup. colliculus

Brachium of inf. colliculus

Inf. colliculus

Trochlear nerve (CN IV)

Sup. cerebellar peduncle
(brachium conjunctivum)

Middle cerebellar peduncle
(brachium pontis)

Inf. cerebellar peduncle
(restiform body)

Cuneate tubercle

Gracile tubercle

Tuberculum cinereum

Lat. funiculus

Fasciculus cuneatus

Fasciculus gracilis

Caudate nucleus (head)

Ant. nucleus (thalamus)

Stria terminalis

Lenticular nucleus

Pulvinar (thalamus)

Medial geniculate body

Lat. geniculate body

Cerebral peduncle

Ant. medullary velum

Posterior median sulcus

Median eminence

Facial colliculus

Sulcus limitans

Vestibular area

Striae medullares

Hypoglossal trigone

Vagal trigone

Obex

Posterior median sulcus

Posterior intermediate
sulcus

Posterolateral sulcus

FIGURE 1.6. Posterior surface anatomy of the brainstem. The cerebellum has been removed to show the three cerebellar peduncles and the floor of the fourth ventricle (rhomboid fossa). (Adapted with permission from Truex RC, Carpenter MB. *Human Neuroanatomy.* 6th ed. Williams & Wilkins; 1969:31.)

    f. Limbic lobe (see Figures 1.4 and 22.1B)
- involved with memory consolidation and emotional response.
- a C-shaped collection of structures found on the medial hemispheric surface that encircles the corpus callosum and the lateral aspect of the midbrain.
- includes the following structures:
  - **(1) Paraterminal gyrus and subcallosal area (see Figure 1.4)**
  - **(2) Cingulate gyrus**
  - **(3) Parahippocampal gyrus**[1]
    - terminates in the **uncus**.
  - **(4) Hippocampal formation** (see Figures 1.2 and 1.4)
    - connected to the hypothalamus and septal area via the fornix.
    - includes three structures:
      - **a. Dentate gyrus** (see Figure 1.4)
      - **b. Hippocampus**
      - **c. Subiculum** (see Figure 17.5)

   g. Olfactory structures (see Figure 1.2)
- found on the orbital surface of the brain and include the following:
  - **(1) Olfactory bulb and tract**
    - an outpouching of the telencephalon.
  - **(2) Olfactory bulb**
    - receives the olfactory nerve (CN I).

---

[1]Some authorities include the parahippocampal gyrus as a temporal lobe structure.

(3) **Olfactory trigone and striae**
(4) **Anterior perforated substance**
   ▧ created by penetrating striate arteries.
(5) **Diagonal band of Broca** (see Figure 1.2)
   ▧ interconnects the amygdaloid nucleus and the septal area.
2. **Basal nuclei (ganglia)** (Figure 1.7; see Figures 1.6 and 18.1)
   ▧ constitute the subcortical nuclei of the telencephalon.
   ▧ include the following structures:
   a. **(Corpus) Striatum: Caudate nucleus + putamen**
   b. **Lentiform nucleus: Globus pallidus + putamen**
   c. **Subthalamic nucleus**
   ▧ part of the diencephalon that functions with the basal nuclei.
3. **Lateral ventricles** (see Figure 2.4)
   ▧ ependyma-lined cavities of the cerebral hemispheres.
   ▧ contain **CSF** and **choroid plexus**.
   ▧ communicate with the third ventricle via the two interventricular foramina (of Monro) (see Figure 2.3).
   ▧ separated from each other by the septum pellucidum.
4. **Cerebral cortex**
   ▧ consists of a thin layer or mantle of gray matter.
   ▧ covers the surface of each cerebral hemisphere.
   ▧ folded into gyri (elevations), which are separated by sulci (depressions), which serve to increase the cortical surface area.

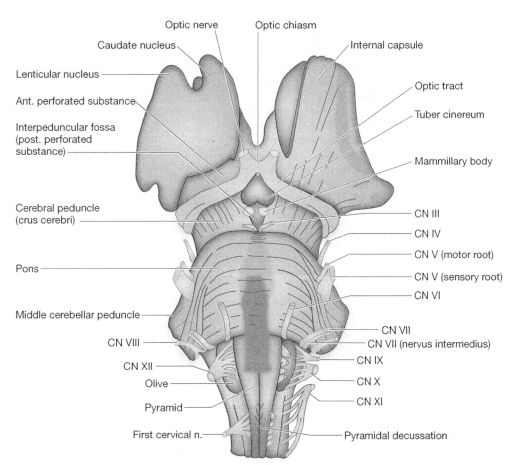

FIGURE 1.7. Anterior surface anatomy of the brainstem. (Adapted with permission from Truex RC, Carpenter MB. *Human Neuroanatomy*. 6th ed. Williams & Wilkins; 1969:31.)

5. White matter
- includes the cerebral commissures and the internal capsule.
  - **a. Cerebral commissures** (see Figures 1.4 and 1.5)
    - interconnect the cerebral hemispheres.
      - **(1) Corpus callosum**
        - the largest commissure of the brain.
        - interconnects the two hemispheres.
        - has four parts—from anterior to posterior:
          - **a. Rostrum**
          - **b. Genu**
          - **c. Body** and
          - **d. Splenium**
      - **(2) Anterior commissure**
        - located in the midsagittal section between the lamina terminalis and the columns of the fornix.
        - interconnects the olfactory bulbs with the middle and inferior temporal lobes.
      - **(3) Hippocampal commissure (commissure of the fornix)**
        - located between the fornices and inferior to the splenium of the corpus callosum.
  - **b. Internal capsule** (see Figures 1.6, 1.7, and 13.3)
    - consists of the white matter located between the basal nuclei and the thalamus.
    - has five parts:
      - **(1) Anterior limb**
        - located between the caudate nucleus and putamen.
        - contains a mixture of ascending and descending fibers.
      - **(2) Genu**
        - located between the anterior and posterior limbs.
        - contains corticobulbar fibers.
      - **(3) Posterior limb**
        - located between the thalamus and lentiform nucleus.
        - made up primarily of corticospinal fibers.
      - **(4) Retrolenticular portion**
        - located posterior to the lentiform nucleus.
        - contains the optic radiations.
      - **(5) Sublenticular portion**
        - located inferior to the lentiform nucleus.
        - contains the auditory radiations.

B. Diencephalon (see Figures 1.5 and 1.6)
- located between the telencephalon and the mesencephalon and between the interventricular foramina and the posterior commissure.
- receives the optic nerve (CN II).
- consists of the epithalamus, thalamus, hypothalamus, subthalamus, and the third ventricle and its associated structures.
  - **1. Epithalamus** (see Figures 1.5 and 1.6)
    - **Pineal body** (epiphysis cerebri)
    - **Habenular trigone** (see Figure 1.6)
    - **Medullary stria of the thalamus**
    - **Posterior commissure**
      - **a.** mediates the consensual reaction of the pupillary light reflex.
    - **Tela choroidea and choroid plexus of the third ventricle**
  - **2. (Dorsal) Thalamus** (see Figure 1.6)
    - separated from the hypothalamus by the **hypothalamic sulcus**.
    - **Pulvinar**
    - **Medial geniculate body (auditory system)**
    - **Lateral geniculate body (visual system)**
    - **Interthalamic adhesion (massa intermedia)**

3. **Hypothalamus** (see Figures 1.1, 1.2, and 1.6)
   - **Optic chiasm**
   - **Mammillary bodies**
   - **Infundibulum**
   - **Tuber cinereum**
4. **Subthalamus (ventral thalamus)**
   - lies inferior to the thalamus and lateral to the hypothalamus.
     a. **Subthalamic nucleus**
     b. **Zona incerta and fields of Forel**
5. **Third ventricle and associated structures** (see Figure 1.5)
   - **Lamina terminalis**
     a. results from closure of the cranial neuropore.
   - **Tela choroidea**
   - **Choroid plexus**
   - **Interventricular foramina (of Monro)**
     a. interconnect the lateral ventricles and the third ventricle.
   - Optic recess
   - Infundibular recess
   - Suprapineal recess
   - Pineal recess

C. **Mesencephalon (midbrain) (see Figure 1.6)**
   - located between the diencephalon and the pons.
   - extends from the posterior commissure to the frenulum of the superior medullary velum.
   - contains the **cerebral aqueduct** interconnecting the third and fourth ventricles.
   1. **Anterior surface**
      - **Cerebral peduncle**
      - **Interpeduncular fossa**
        a. **Oculomotor nerve (CN III)**
        b. **Posterior perforated substance**
           - created by the penetrating branches of the posterior cerebral and posterior communicating arteries.
   2. **Posterior surface**
      - **Superior colliculus (visual system)**
      - **Inferior colliculus (auditory system)**
      - **Trochlear nerve (CN IV)**
        a. the only cranial nerve to exit the brainstem from the posterior aspect.

D. **Pons (see Figures 1.1 and 1.7)**
   - located between the midbrain and the medulla.
   - extends from the inferior pontine sulcus to the superior pontine sulcus.
   1. **Anterior surface**
      - **Base of the pons**
      - **Cranial nerves**
        a. **Trigeminal nerve (CN V)**
        b. **Abducens nerve (CN VI)**
        c. **Facial nerve (CN VII)**
        d. **Vestibulocochlear nerve (CN VIII)**
   2. **Posterior surface (rhomboid fossa)**
      - **Locus ceruleus**
        a. contains the largest collection of norepinephrinergic neurons in the CNS.
      - **Facial colliculus**
        a. contains the abducens nucleus and internal genu of the facial nerve.
      - **Sulcus limitans**
        a. separates the embryonic alar and basal plates.
      - **Striae medullares of the rhomboid fossa**
        a. divides the rhomboid fossa into the superior pontine portion and the inferior medullary portion.

E. Medulla oblongata (myelencephalon) (see Figures 1.1 and 1.7)
- located between the pons and the spinal cord.
- extends from the first cervical nerve (C1) to the inferior pontine sulcus (also called the ponto-bulbar sulcus).
  1. **Anterior surface**
     - **Pyramid**
       a. contains descending tracts.
     - **Olive**
       a. contains the inferior olivary nucleus.
     - **Cranial nerves**
       a. **Glossopharyngeal nerve (CN IX)**
       b. **Vagal nerve (CN X)**
       c. **Accessory nerve (CN XI)**[2]
       d. **Hypoglossal nerve (CN XII)**
  2. **Posterior surface**
     - **Gracile** and **Cuneate tubercles**
     - contains the gracile and cuneate nuclei, respectively.
     - **Rhomboid fossa** (see Figure 1.6)
       a. **Striae medullares of the rhomboid fossa**
       b. **Vagal trigone**
       c. **Hypoglossal trigone**
       d. **Sulcus limitans**
       e. **Area postrema (vomiting center)**

F. Cerebellum (see Figures 1.1 and 1.5)
- located in the posterior cranial fossa.
- attached to the brainstem by three cerebellar peduncles.
- forms the roof of the fourth ventricle.
- separated from the occipital and temporal lobes by the **tentorium cerebelli**.
- consists of **folia** and **fissures** on its surface.
- contains the following surface structures/parts:
  1. **Hemispheres**
     - made up of two lateral lobes.
  2. **Vermis**
     - a midline structure.
  3. **Flocculus and vermal nodulus**
     - form the flocculonodular lobe.
  4. **Tonsil**
     - a rounded lobule on the inferior surface of each cerebellar hemisphere.
     - with increased intracranial pressure, it can herniate through the foramen magnum.
  5. **Superior cerebellar peduncle** (see Figure 1.6)
     - connects the cerebellum to the pons and the midbrain.
  6. **Middle cerebellar peduncle** (see Figure 1.6)
     - connects the cerebellum to the pons.
  7. **Inferior cerebellar peduncle** (see Figure 1.6)
     - connects the cerebellum to the pons and the medulla.
  8. **Anterior lobe**
     - lies anterior to the primary fissure.
  9. **Posterior lobe**
     - located between the primary and the posterolateral fissures.
  10. **Flocculonodular lobe**
     - lies posterior to the posterolateral fissure.

---

[2]CN XI's fibers ascend from the cervical spinal cord (C1-C4), although the nerve appears to emerge from the medulla.

IV. ATLAS OF THE BRAIN AND BRAINSTEM (Figures 1.8 through 1.12)

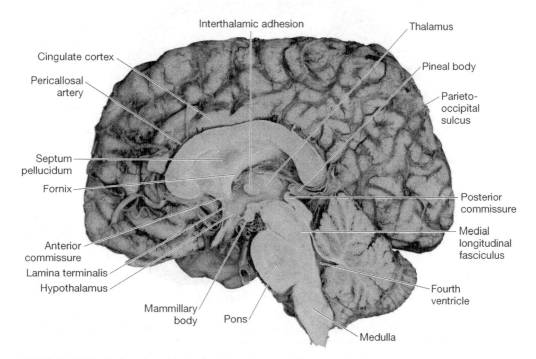

FIGURE 1.8. Midsagittal section of the brain with meninges and blood vessels intact. Note the cerebral veins in the subarachnoid space and the prominent pineal body, interthalamic adhesion, and intact septum pellucidum. (Courtesy of D. Schlegel, A. Luedtke, and A. Perez-Chavez.)

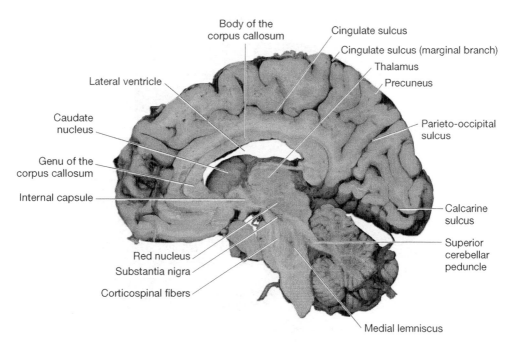

FIGURE 1.9. Parasagittal section through the red nucleus, medial lemniscus, and substantia nigra. The corticospinal fibers can be traced inferiorly from the crus cerebri through the medulla. The substantia nigra is easily seen in the medulla. (Courtesy of D. Schlegel, A. Luedtke, and A. Perez-Chavez.)

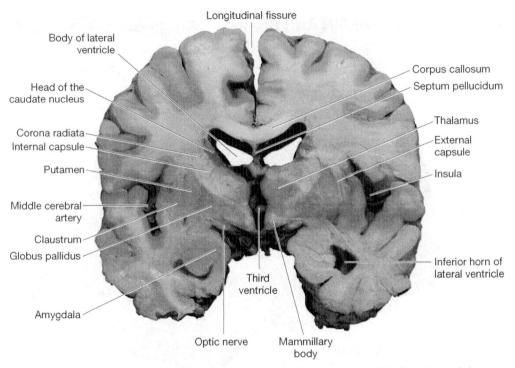

Longitudinal fissure

Body of lateral ventricle

Corpus callosum

Septum pellucidum

Head of the caudate nucleus

Thalamus

Corona radiata
Internal capsule

External capsule

Putamen

Insula

Middle cerebral artery

Claustrum
Globus pallidus

Inferior horn of lateral ventricle

Third ventricle

Amygdala

Optic nerve   Mammillary body

FIGURE 1.10. Coronal section through the amygdala and basal nuclei. Note the passage of the internal capsule between the basal nuclei and the thalamus. (Courtesy of D. Schlegel, A. Luedtke, and A. Perez-Chavez.)

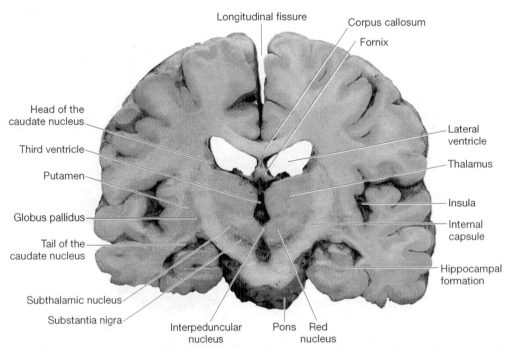

Longitudinal fissure   Corpus callosum

Fornix

Head of the caudate nucleus

Lateral ventricle

Third ventricle

Thalamus

Putamen

Insula

Globus pallidus

Internal capsule

Tail of the caudate nucleus

Hippocampal formation

Subthalamic nucleus

Substantia nigra

Interpeduncular nucleus   Pons   Red nucleus

FIGURE 1.11. Coronal section through the substantia nigra, red nucleus, and hippocampal formation. Note the fornix and the head and tail of the caudate. (Courtesy of D. Schlegel, A. Luedtke, and A. Perez-Chavez.)

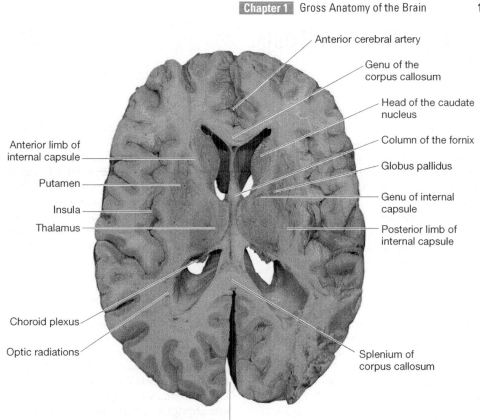

Anterior cerebral artery

Genu of the
corpus callosum

Head of the caudate
nucleus

Column of the fornix

Globus pallidus

Genu of internal
capsule

Posterior limb of
internal capsule

Anterior limb of
internal capsule

Putamen

Insula

Thalamus

Choroid plexus

Optic radiations

Splenium of
corpus callosum

Longitudinal fissure

FIGURE 1.12. Transverse section through the basal nuclei and thalamus. Note the anterior and posterior limbs of the internal capsule with the genu clearly visible. (Courtesy of D. Schlegel, A. Luedtke, and A. Perez-Chavez.)

Review Test

1. A 50-year-old woman presents to her primary care provider for a visit several months after suffering a stroke of one of the thalamogeniculate arteries (branches of the posterior cerebral artery). The stroke affected her diencephalon. Which of the following structures is part of the diencephalon?

(A) Caudate nucleus
(B) Cerebral hemispheres
(C) Globus pallidus
(D) Internal capsule
(E) Thalamus

2. A 75-year-old man presents to his primary care provider for evaluation of his advanced dementia. Testing has revealed significant cell loss in his hippocampal formation. The hippocampal formation is part of which lobe?

(A) Frontal
(B) Insular
(C) Limbic
(D) Occipital
(E) Parietal

3. A 30-year-old woman presents to her primary care provider with a primary complaint of worsening blurred vision. On evaluation, imaging is ordered that reveals a tumor compressing the posterior aspect of the midbrain. Which cranial nerve that exits the posterior aspect of the brainstem is most likely affected?

(A) CN I
(B) CN II
(C) CN III
(D) CN IV
(E) CN VI

4. An older adult patient presents to his audiologist for a hearing evaluation. In explaining the anatomy of the auditory system, the audiologist explains that the primary auditory cortex (Heschl gyrus) receives input from which gyrus/structure?

(A) Angular gyrus
(B) Globus pallidus
(C) Medial geniculate nucleus
(D) Pulvinar
(E) Supramarginal gyrus

5. A 35-year-old woman is hit by a car while crossing the street. She is taken by ambulance to the emergency department for treatment of her obviously damaged lower limb. During the evaluation, it becomes apparent that she has also sustained a traumatic injury to her head, in the region of the temporal bone. An injury to the underlying cerebral cortex in this region would most likely produce which of the following deficits?

(A) Hearing
(B) Smell
(C) Somatic sense
(D) Taste
(E) Vision

6. A 75-year-old woman presents to her primary care physician with a chief complaint of a chronic headache. Imaging reveals a large tumor growing in the anterior-most aspect of the longitudinal fissure. This tumor will most likely affect which part of the brain first?

(A) Anterior commissure
(B) Cerebellum
(C) Frontal lobe
(D) Midbrain
(E) Thalamus

Questions 7 to 11

Match the descriptions in items 7 to 11 with the appropriate lettered structure shown in the T_1-weighted MRI of the coronal section of the brain.

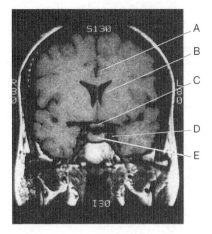

7. Lies within the cavernous sinus

8. Lies within the sella turcica

9. Is part of the striatum

10. Is part of the limbic lobe

11. Lies within a cistern

Questions 12 to 16

Match the structure or description in items 12 to 16 with the appropriate lettered structure shown in the stained section of the brain.

12. Has reciprocal connections between the hippocampal formation and the septal nuclei

13. Largest nucleus of the diencephalon

14. Internal capsule

15. Cingulate gyrus

16. Caudate nucleus

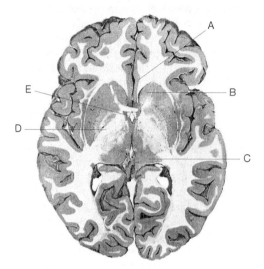

Adapted with permission from Roberts M, Hanaway J, Morest DK. *Atlas of the Human Brain in Section.* 2nd ed. Lea & Febiger; 1987:51.

Answers and Explanations

1. **E.** The (dorsal) thalamus, along with the epithalamus, hypothalamus, and subthalamus, forms the diencephalon. The caudate nucleus and globus pallidus, along with the putamen, are parts of the basal nuclei. The cerebral hemispheres are part of the telencephalon, along with the basal nuclei. The internal capsule is a large white matter tract conveying fibers between the cerebral cortex and lower centers; it is found between the diencephalon and basal nuclei.

2. **C.** The hippocampus is part of the limbic lobe/system and plays a role in memory consolidation. The hippocampus is one of the first regions damaged in Alzheimer disease. The frontal lobe may also be greatly impacted as part of dementia, but the hippocampus is not part of it. The occipital, parietal, and insular lobes may be impacted in dementia as well, but the hippocampal formation is not found in those lobes.

3. **D.** The trochlear nerve (CN IV) is the only cranial nerve to exit the brainstem from the dorsal/posterior aspect; it exits from the posterior aspect of the midbrain. Cranial nerve I is actually a series of nerves, the filia olfactoria—that pass through the cribriform plate to enter the olfactory bulb. Cranial nerve II is an outpocketing of the diencephalon and is not connected to the brainstem. Cranial nerve III (midbrain) and cranial nerve VI (midbrain/pons junction) both leave the brainstem anteriorly.

4. **C.** Primary auditory cortex (areas 41 and 42) is found in the transverse gyrus of Heschl and receives input from the medial geniculate nucleus. The parietal lobe includes the angular gyrus that receives visual impulses (area 39) and the supramarginal gyrus that interrelates somatosensory, auditory, and visual inputs (area 40). Destruction of the angular and supramarginal gyri on the dominant (usually left) side gives rise to Gerstmann syndrome, whose symptoms include agraphia, acalculia, finger agnosia, and left-right disorientation. The globus pallidus is the primary output (along with the substantia nigra pars reticulata) of the basal nuclei; it is not involved with hearing and does not project to the transverse gyrus of Heschl. Pulvinar is concerned with the integration of visual, auditory, and somesthetic inputs.

5. **A.** Primary auditory cortex lies on the superior temporal gyrus, deep to the temporal bone; therefore, an injury here would have the greatest impact on hearing. The sense of smell is widely distributed in the cortex, primarily on the ventral surface of the brain. Somatic sensation is located primarily deep to the parietal bone on the parietal lobe. Taste is found in the insula and parts of the frontal lobe, deep to the frontal bone. Vision is located posteriorly, deep to the occipital bone and as such would not be as impacted as the underlying temporal lobe structures.

6. **C.** The tumor is growing in between the two frontal lobes and would affect them first. The anterior commissure may be affected as the tumor continues to grow posteriorly, but it is a deep structure and not in the anterior-most region of the anterior cranial fossa. The cerebellum is in the posterior cranial fossa, far from this lesion. The midbrain is a deep structure in the middle of the brain, as is the thalamus.

7. **D.** The carotid artery lies within the cavernous sinus, in association with CN III, CN IV, CN V$_1$, CN V$_2$, and CN VI; aneurysms of the internal carotid artery and tumors of the cavernous sinus may cause cranial nerve palsies.

8. **E.** The hypophysis (pituitary gland) lies within the hypophyseal fossa of the sella turcica; common tumors in this region are pituitary adenomas, craniopharyngiomas, and meningiomas.

9. **B.** The caudate nucleus and putamen are parts of the (corpus) striatum. In Huntington disease, there is loss of neurons in the caudate nucleus, whereas in Parkinson disease there is loss of neurons in the substantia nigra.

10. **A.** The cingulate gyrus is part of the limbic lobe; lesions may result in akinesia, mutism, apathy, and indifference to pain.

11. **C.** The optic chiasm lies within the chiasmatic cistern.

12. **E.** The fornix contains fibers from the hippocampal formation and septal nuclei. The fornix projects into the mammillary nuclei of the hypothalamus.

13. **C.** The pulvinar is the largest nucleus of the thalamus. It has reciprocal connections with the association cortex of the occipital, parietal, and posterior lobes and is concerned with the integration of visual, auditory, and somesthetic inputs.

14. **D.** The posterior limb of the internal capsule lies between the lentiform nucleus (putamen and globus pallidus) and the thalamus. It contains the corticospinal tract and is perfused by the lateral striate arteries (branches of the middle cerebral artery) and the anterior choroidal artery.

15. **A.** The cingulate gyrus contains the cingulum, a fiber bundle that interconnects the hippocampal formation with the septal nucleus. Bilateral destruction of the cingulate gyrus causes loss of inhibition as well as dulling of the emotions. However, memory is unaffected. Lesions of the anterior cingulate gyri cause placidity; cingulectomy is used to treat severe anxiety and depression.

16. **B.** The caudate and the putamen comprise the (corpus) striatum, part of the basal nuclei. In Huntington disease, there is atrophy of the striatum caused by a mutation in the Huntington gene, resulting in choreiform movements.

2 Meninges and Cerebrospinal Fluid

Objectives

- Describe the location and identifying characteristics of the dura mater, arachnoid, and pia mater.
- Identify the meningeal spaces and include a description of what is found in each and whether the spaces are real or potential.
- List the major cisterns of the subarachnoid space and describe the location of each.
- Identify the ventricles and list the subdivisions and characteristics of each.
- Describe the origin and movement of cerebrospinal fluid through the ventricular system and the route it takes to the systemic circulation.
- Describe hydrocephalus and meningitis.
- List the circumventricular organs and describe their significance.

I. MENINGES

- comprise three connective tissue membranes that invest the spinal cord and brain.
- consist of the **pia mater** and the **arachnoid** (together known as the leptomeninges) and the **dura mater** (pachymeninx).

A. Pia mater
- a delicate, vascular layer of connective tissue.
- closely covers the surface of the brain and spinal cord.
- connected to the arachnoid by arachnoid trabeculae.
  1. **Denticulate ligaments** (see Figure 2.1)
     - consist of a lateral flattened band of pial tissue on each side of the spinal cord.
     - adhere to the spinal dura mater with 21 pairs of tooth-like extensions.
  2. **Filum terminale** (Figure 2.2)
     - consists of an extension of the pia mater.
     - extends from the conus medullaris to the end of the dural sac (interna) and from the dural sac to the coccyx (externa), known as the **coccygeal ligament**.

B. Arachnoid
- a delicate, nonvascular connective tissue membrane between the dura mater and the pia mater.
  1. **Arachnoid granulations**
     - accumulations of arachnoid villi (formed of evaginations of arachnoid through the meningeal layer of dura mater).

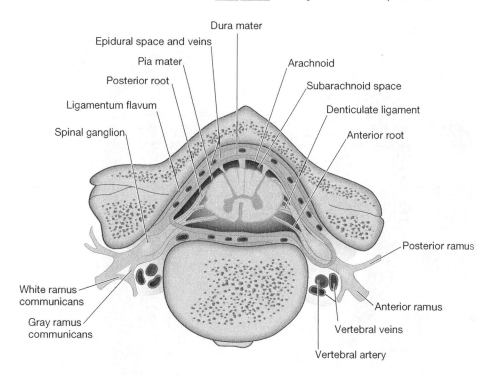

FIGURE 2.1. Cross-section of the spinal cord and its meningeal investments. The subarachnoid, subdural, and epidural spaces are visible. The anterior and posterior longitudinal ligaments are seen but are not labeled. (Adapted with permission from Carpenter MB, Sutin J. *Human Neuroanatomy.* 8th ed. Williams & Wilkins; 1983:9.)

▦ enter the venous dural sinuses and facilitate the one-way flow of cerebrospinal fluid (**CSF**) from the subarachnoid space into the venous circulation.

▦ found in large numbers along the **superior sagittal sinus** but are associated with all dural sinuses.

C. Dura mater

▦ the outer layer of the meninges, consisting of dense connective tissue.

▦ the supratentorial dura is innervated by the trigeminal nerve; the dura of the posterior cranial fossa is innervated by the vagal and upper spinal nerves.

▦ in multiple areas the dura mater divides into two parts: a periosteal layer and a meningeal layer.

▦ the meningeal layer of dura mater forms reflections that invaginate to support and protect parts of the brain; the reflections also form the walls of the dural venous sinuses.

1. Falx cerebri

▦ lies between the cerebral hemispheres in the longitudinal cerebral fissure.

▦ contains the superior and inferior sagittal sinuses between its layers.

2. Tentorium cerebelli (Figure 2.3)

▦ divides the cranial vault into supra- and infratentorial compartments.

▦ separates the temporal and occipital lobes from the cerebellum and infratentorial brainstem.

▦ contains the **tentorial incisure**, or notch, through which the brainstem passes.

3. Diaphragma sellae

▦ forms the roof of the **hypophyseal fossa**.

▦ contains an aperture through which the **hypophyseal stalk** (infundibulum) passes.

4. Dural sinuses (see Figure 2.3)

▦ endothelium-lined, valveless venous channels found in the attached edge of the dural folds.

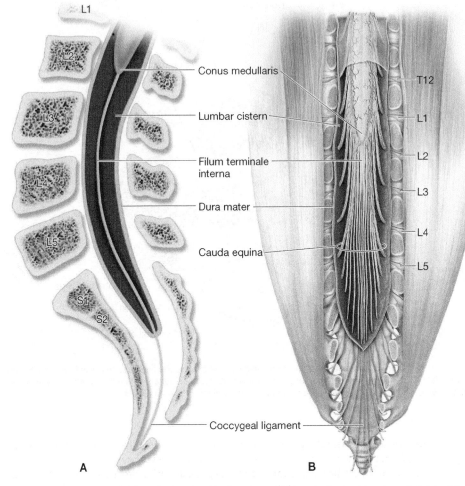

FIGURE 2.2. The caudal part of the spinal cord and lumbar cistern. **(A)** Longitudinal section through the caudal vertebral column and canal showing the conus medullaris and the lumbar cistern. Lumbar puncture is made between the spinous processes of L3 and L4 (or L4 and L5). **(B)** Posterior view of the cauda equina and spinal nerves. The adult spinal cord terminates at the L1-L2 vertebral level. (Adapted with permission from Carpenter MB, Sutin J. *Human Neuroanatomy*. 8th ed. Williams & Wilkins; 1983:8.)

D. Meningeal spaces (see Figures 2.1 through 2.3)

1. Spinal epidural space
- located between the spinal dura mater and the vertebral periosteum.
- contains loose areolar tissue, venous plexuses, and lymphatics.
- can be injected with a local anesthetic to produce a paravertebral nerve block.

2. Cranial epidural space
- a *potential* space between the dura mater and the bones of the cranial vault.
- contains the meningeal arteries and veins.

3. Subdural space
- a *potential* space between the dura mater and the arachnoid.
- intracranially transmits cerebral veins to the venous lacunae of the superior sagittal sinus. Laceration of these "bridging veins" results in **subdural hemorrhage** (hematoma).

4. Subarachnoid space
- located between the pia mater and the arachnoid.
- contains **CSF**.

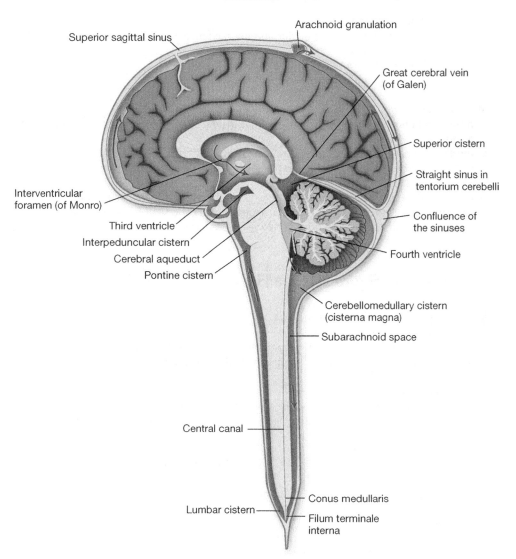

FIGURE 2.3. The subarachnoid spaces and cisterns of the brain and spinal cord. Cerebrospinal fluid is produced in the choroid plexuses of the ventricles, exits the fourth ventricle, circulates in the subarachnoid space, and enters the superior sagittal sinus via the arachnoid granulations. Red arrows indicate the direction of CSF flow. (Adapted with permission from Noback CR, Strominger NL, Demarest RJ. *The Human Nervous System.* 4th ed. Williams & Wilkins; 1991:68.)

- surrounds the entire brain and spinal cord.
- extends, in the adult, below the conus medullaris to the level of the second sacral verte-bra as the **lumbar cistern** (see Figure 2.2A).
5. **Subarachnoid cisterns** (see Figure 2.3)
   - dilations of the subarachnoid space, which contain CSF.
   - named after the structures over which they lie (eg, pontine, chiasmatic, and interpedun-cular cisterns).
   a. **Cerebellopontine angle cistern**
      - receives CSF from the fourth ventricle via the lateral foramina (of Luschka).
      - contains the facial nerve (**CN VII**) and the vestibulocochlear nerve (**CN VIII**).
   b. **Cerebellomedullary cistern (cisterna magna)**
      - located in the midline between the cerebellum and the medulla.
      - receives CSF from the fourth ventricle via the median foramen (of Magendie).
      - can be tapped for CSF (suboccipital tap).

 c. **Ambient cistern**
- interconnects the superior and interpeduncular cisterns; contains the trochlear nerve (**CN IV**).

 d. **Superior cistern**
- overlies the midbrain tectum.

E. Meningiomas
- most common type of primary central nervous system (CNS) tumor; account for one-third of all primary CNS tumors.
- mostly benign, slow-growing, well-demarcated tumors.
- 90% are found in the brain (anterior cranial fossa—parasagittal, 25%; convexity, 20%; and basal, 40%) and 10% are found in the spinal cord.
- histologically characterized by a whorling pattern and calcified **psammoma bodies**.
- commonly linked to antecedent radiation exposure and abnormal chromosome 22.
- occur most commonly in older adults (>60 years), and occur in women twice as much as men.

II. VENTRICLES (Figure 2.4; See Figure 2.3)

- lined with ependyma and contain CSF.
- all ventricles contain choroid plexus.
- communicate with the subarachnoid space via three foramina in the fourth ventricle.
- consist of four fluid-filled communicating cavities within the brain.

A. Lateral ventricles
- the two ventricles are located within the cerebral hemispheres.
- communicate with the third ventricle via the **interventricular foramen (of Monro)**.
- consist of five parts:
    1. **Frontal (anterior) horn**
        - located in the frontal lobe; its lateral wall is formed by the head of the caudate nucleus.
    2. **Body**
        - located in the medial part of the frontal and parietal lobes.
        - communicates with the third ventricle via the interventricular foramina.
    3. **Temporal (inferior) horn**
        - located in the medial part of the temporal lobe.
    4. **Occipital (posterior) horn** (see Figure 1.2)
        - located in the parietal and occipital lobes.
    5. **Trigone (atrium)**
        - found at the junction of the body, occipital horn, and temporal horn.
        - contains the **glomus**, a large tuft of choroid plexus, which is calcified in adults, making it a useful radiologic landmark.

B. Third ventricle (see Figures 1.5, 2.3, and 2.4)
- a slit-like vertical midline cavity of the diencephalon.
- communicates with the lateral ventricles via the interventricular foramina and with the fourth ventricle via the cerebral aqueduct.

C. Cerebral aqueduct (of Sylvius)
- lies in the midbrain.
- connects the third ventricle with the fourth ventricle.
- lacks choroid plexus.
- blockage (aqueductal stenosis) leads to hydrocephalus.

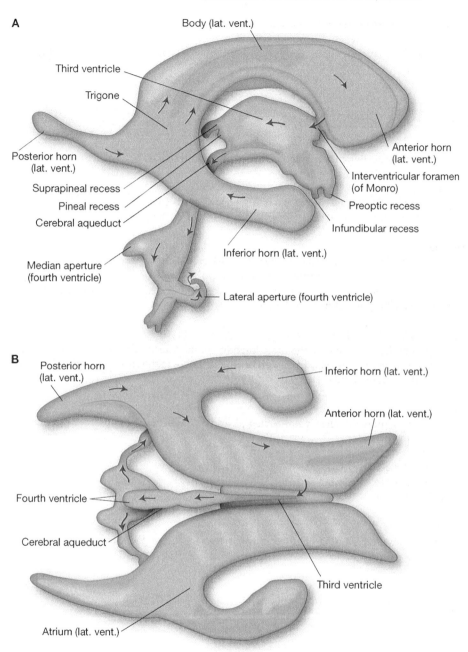

A

Body (lat. vent.)

Third ventricle

Trigone

Posterior horn
(lat. vent.)

Suprapineal recess

Pineal recess

Cerebral aqueduct

Median aperture
(fourth ventricle)

Anterior horn
(lat. vent.)

Interventricular foramen
(of Monro)

Preoptic recess

Infundibular recess

Inferior horn (lat. vent.)

Lateral aperture (fourth ventricle)

B

Posterior horn
(lat. vent.)

Inferior horn (lat. vent.)

Anterior horn (lat. vent.)

Fourth ventricle

Cerebral aqueduct

Third ventricle

Atrium (lat. vent.)

FIGURE 2.4. The ventricular system of the brain. The red arrows indicate the direction of cerebrospinal fluid flow. **(A)** Lateral aspect. **(B)** Dorsal aspect. (Adapted with permission from Carpenter MB, Sutin J. *Human Neuroanatomy*. 8th ed. Williams & Wilkins; 1983:44.)

D. **Fourth ventricle (see Figures 1.5, 2.3, and 2.4)**
- lies between the cerebellum and the brainstem.
- expresses CSF into the subarachnoid space via the two lateral foramina and the single median foramen.

III. CEREBROSPINAL FLUID

- a clear, colorless, acellular fluid found in the subarachnoid space and ventricles.

A. **Formation**
- produced by the **choroid plexus** at a rate of 500 to 700 mL/d.
- total CSF volume is ~140 mL.

B. **Function**
- supports and cushions the CNS against concussive injury.
- transports hormones and hormone-releasing factors.
- removes metabolic waste products through absorption; the sites of greatest absorption are the **arachnoid villi/granulations** (see Figure 2.3).

C. **Circulation (see Figure 2.3)**
- flows from the ventricles via the three foramina of the fourth ventricle into the subarachnoid space and over the convexity of the cerebral hemisphere to the superior sagittal sinus, where it enters the venous circulation.

D. **Composition**
- contains not more than five lymphocytes/µL and is usually sterile.
- other **normal values** are:
  1. **pH:** 7.35
  2. **Specific gravity:** 1.007
  3. **Glucose:** 66% of plasma glucose
  4. **Total protein:** <45 mg/dL in the lumbar cistern

E. **Normal pressure**
- is 80 to 180 mm H_2O (CSF) in the lumbar cistern when the patient is in a lateral recumbent position.

IV. HYDROCEPHALUS

- dilation of the cerebral ventricles (ventriculomegaly).
- characterized by excessive accumulation of CSF in the ventricles or subarachnoid space.

A. **Noncommunicating (obstructive) hydrocephalus**
- results from obstruction within the ventricular system (eg, congenital aqueductal stenosis).
- most common form in children.
- associated with increased intracranial pressure.

B. **Communicating hydrocephalus**
- results from blockage within the subarachnoid space (eg, adhesions after meningitis).
- associated with increased intracranial pressure.

C. **Hydrocephalus ex vacuo**
- enlargement of the ventricular system and subarachnoid space.

  ▨ results from reduced brain tissue volume.
  ▨ no increase in intracranial pressure.

D. Pseudotumor cerebri (idiopathic intracranial hypertension)
  ▨ results from increased resistance to CSF outflow at the arachnoid villi.
  ▨ characterized by papilledema, elevated CSF pressure, and deteriorating vision, that is, symptoms mimic those from a brain tumor.
  ▨ typically occurs in women with obesity between 20 and 50 years old.

CLINICAL CORRELATES Normal pressure hydrocephalus occurs when CSF is not absorbed by the arachnoid villi, causing ventricular enlargement. It is characterized by the triad of progressive dementia, ataxic gait, and urinary incontinence (**wacky, wobbly, and wet**). It typically occurs in older adults, often secondary to posttraumatic meningeal hemorrhage.

V. MENINGITIS

  ▨ an inflammation of the pia-arachnoid.
  ▨ defined by elevated white blood cell levels in the CSF.

A. Bacterial (pyogenic) meningitis
  ▨ occurs most often in infants (1-2 months old), >70% of cases are in children younger than 5 years of age.
  ▨ ~1.2 million new cases annually.
  ▨ characterized clinically by fever, headache, and nuchal rigidity.
  ▨ may result in cranial nerve palsies (CN III, CN IV, CN VI, and CN VIII) and hydrocephalus.
  1. **Globally, the three causes:**
     ▨ *Streptococcus pneumoniae*
     ▨ *Neisseria meningitidis*
     ▨ *Haemophilus influenzae*
  2. **CSF findings** (Table 2.1)
     ▨ Numerous neutrophils
     ▨ Decreased glucose level
     ▨ Elevated protein level

B. Viral (lymphocytic) meningitis
  ▨ also called aseptic meningitis.
  ▨ most common type of meningitis.

---

table 2.1 Properties of CSF in Subarachnoid Hemorrhage, Bacterial Meningitis, and Viral Encephalitis

CSF	Normal	Subarachnoid Hemorrhage	Bacterial Meningitis	Viral Encephalitis
Color	Clear	Bloody	Cloudy	Clear or cloudy
Cell count (per mm^3)	<5 lymphocytes	Red blood cells present (~5 x 10^6/mm^3)	>1,000 PML	25-500 lymphocytes
Protein	<45 mg/dL	Normal to slightly elevated	Elevated (<100 mg/dL)	Slightly elevated (>100 mg/dL)
Glucose (~66% of blood [80-120 mg/dL])	45 mg/dL	Normal	Reduced normal	

In infants: cell counts <10 cells/mm^3; protein = 20 to 170 mg/dL.
CSF, cerebrospinal fluid; PML, polymorphonuclear leukocytes.

■ characterized by fever, headache, lethargy, and nuchal rigidity.

1. **Viruses isolated include the following:**
   ■ Mumps
   ■ Measles
   ■ Influenza
   ■ Arboviruses (eg, West Nile virus)
   ■ Nonpolio enterovirus: most common
   ■ Herpes simplex
2. **CSF findings**
   ■ Numerous lymphocytes
   ■ Normal glucose
   ■ Normal to slightly increased protein

VI. HERNIATION (Figures 2.5 through 2.8)

A. **Transtentorial (uncal) herniation**
   ■ protrusion of the brain through the tentorial incisure.

B. **Transforaminal (tonsillar) herniation**
   ■ protrusion of the brainstem and cerebellum through the foramen magnum.

C. **Subfalcine herniation**
   ■ herniation below the falx cerebri.

VII. CIRCUMVENTRICULAR ORGANS

■ chemosensitive areas that monitor the concentrations of circulating hormones in the blood and CSF.
■ located in the periphery of the third ventricle; the **area postrema** is found on the floor of the fourth ventricle.

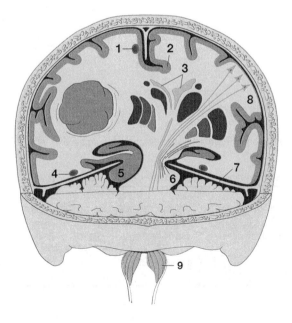

FIGURE 2.5. Coronal section of a tumor in the supratentorial compartment. (1) Anterior cerebral artery; (2) subfalcial herniation; (3) shifting of ventricles; (4) posterior cerebral artery (compression results in contralateral hemianopia); (5) uncal (transtentorial) herniation; (6) Kernohan notch, with damaged corticospinal and corticobulbar fibers; (7) tentorium cerebelli; (8) pyramidal cells that give rise to the corticospinal tract; (9) tonsillar (transforaminal) herniation, which damages vital medullary centers. (Adapted with permission from Leech RW, Shuman RM. *Neuropathology.* Harper & Row; 1982:16.)

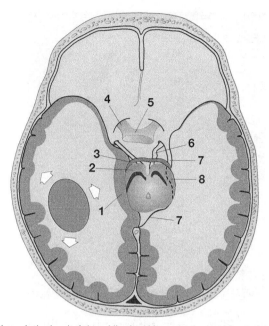

FIGURE 2.6. Axial section through the level of the midbrain with a space-occupying lesion (arrows indicate pressure being exerted on nearby tissues). The left oculomotor nerve is being stretched (dilated pupil). The left posterior cerebral artery is compressed, resulting in a contralateral hemianopia. The right crus cerebri is compressed (Kernohan notch) by the free edge of the tentorial incisure, resulting in hemiparesis ipsilateral to the lesion. The caudal displacement of the brainstem may cause rupture of the branches of the basilar artery. Hemorrhage into the midbrain and rostral pontine tegmentum (Duret hemorrhages) may be fatal. (1) Parahippocampal gyrus; (2) crus cerebri; (3) posterior cerebral artery; (4) optic nerve; (5) optic chiasma; (6) oculomotor nerve; (7) free edge of tentorium; (8) Kernohan notch. (Adapted with permission from Leech RW, Shuman RM. *Neuropathology.* Harper & Row; 1982:19.)

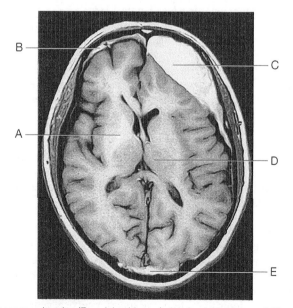

FIGURE 2.7. Magnetic resonance imaging (T_1-weighted image) showing brain trauma. Epidural hematomas may cross dural attachments. Subdural hematomas do not cross dural attachments. **(A)** Internal capsule; **(B)** subdural hematoma; **(C)** subdural hematomas; **(D)** thalamus; **(E)** epidural hematoma. (Adapted with permission from Fix JD. *High-Yield Neuro-anatomy.* 3rd ed. Lippincott Williams & Wilkins; 2005:27.)

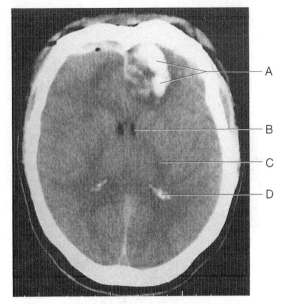

FIGURE 2.8. Computed tomography scan (axial section) showing an intraparenchymal hemorrhage in the left frontal lobe. **(A)** Intraparenchymal hemorrhage; **(B)** lateral ventricle; **(C)** internal capsule; **(D)** calcified glomus in the trigone region of the lateral ventricle. (Adapted with permission from Fix JD. *High-Yield Neuroanatomy.* 3rd ed. Lippincott Williams & Wilkins; 2005:27.)

■ highly vascularized with fenestrated capillaries and no blood-brain barrier (the subcommissural organ is an exception).
■ include the following structures:

A. Organum vasculosum of the lamina terminalis
■ considered to be a vascular outlet for luteinizing hormone–releasing hormone and somatostatin.

B. Median eminence of the tuber cinereum (see Figure 1.1)
■ contains neurons that elaborate releasing and inhibiting hormones into the hypophyseal portal system.

C. Subfornical organ
■ located on the inferior surface of the fornix at the level of the interventricular foramina.
■ contains neurons that project to the supraoptic nuclei and the organum vasculosum.
■ a central receptor site for angiotensin II.

D. Subcommissural organ
■ located below the posterior commissure at the junction of the third ventricle and the cerebral aqueduct.
■ composed of specialized ependymal cells, glial elements, and a capillary bed containing non-fenestrated endothelial cells.

E. Pineal body (see Figures 1.5 and 1.6)
■ contains **calcareous granules**, in **brain sand** or acervulus cerebri, which are seen on x-ray and computed tomography (CT); calcification occurs after 16 years of age.
■ contains **pinealocytes** (epiphyseal cells) and is highly vascular, with fenestrated capillaries.
■ derived from the diencephalon.
■ innervated by postganglionic fibers from the superior cervical ganglion of the autonomic nervous system.
■ synthesizes serotonin and melatonin.
■ **Pinealomas** may result in dorsal midbrain (Parinaud) syndrome (see Figure 12.3A).

F. Area postrema (Figure 2.9)

- consists of two small subependymal oval areas on either side of the fourth ventricle, rostral to the obex.
- contains modified neurons and astrocyte-like cells surrounded by fenestrated capillaries.
- considered to be a chemoreceptor zone that triggers vomiting in response to circulating emetic substances.
- plays a role in food intake and cardiovascular regulation.

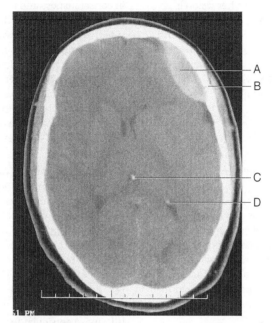

FIGURE 2.9. Computed tomography scan (axial section) showing an epidural hematoma and a skull fracture. The epidural hematoma has a classic biconvex, or lentiform, shape. **(A)** Epidural hematoma; **(B)** skull fracture; **(C)** calcified pineal gland; **(D)** calcified glomus in the trigone region of the lateral ventricle.

Review Test

1. A 25-year-old woman complains of headaches of 4 months' duration. She is obese and has bilateral papilledema, and her vision is deteriorating. Her opening CSF pressure is elevated; other CSF findings are normal. CT and magnetic resonance imaging (MRI) scans are normal. These signs are due to the result of impairment of CSF egress. At which of the following loci is obstruction most likely?

(A) Arachnoid villi
(B) Cerebral aqueduct
(C) Foramen of Luschka (lateral)
(D) Foramen of Magendie (median)
(E) Foramen of Monro (interventricular)

2. A newborn is brought to the pediatrician by his mother for a routine wellness check. During the physical examination, the physician notes papilledema through the ophthalmoscope. Seeking the cause of the increased intracranial pressure, imaging is ordered. A diagnosis of hydrocephalus is eventually made. What is the most likely form of hydrocephalus in the young patient?

(A) Communicating
(B) Hydrocephalus ex vacuo
(C) Noncommunicating
(D) Normal pressure
(E) Pseudomotor cerebri

3. A 75-year-old man is involved in a motor vehicle accident while returning from a trip to the grocery store. The airbags deployed, but his head was jarred violently against the airbags and the head rest. He is released after a brief evaluation at the hospital. Over the next few hours, he develops a headache and slurred speech and reports blurred vision to his wife. Symptoms persist over the next few days, with increasing confusion and drowsiness. His wife decides to take him back for evaluation 1 week after the accident, as he has developed severe nausea and vomiting. Based on the patient, symptoms, and timeline, what is the most likely type of injury the man has sustained?

(A) Meningioma
(B) Normal pressure hydrocephalus
(C) Subdural hematoma
(D) Transtentorial herniation
(E) Viral meningitis

4. A 50-year-old woman is brought to the emergency department by her husband for lapses in consciousness and movement disturbances. Examination reveals a dilated pupil on the right side that is directed down and out; the contralateral pupil exhibits no indirect pupillary response. There is weakness over the entire left side of the body. Her husband describes an intermittent, but progressively worsening stuporous state. Imaging reveals a supratentorial space-occupying lesion on the right. What is the initial diagnosis of the cause of the symptoms in this patient?

(A) Hydrocephalus ex vacuo
(B) Subfalcial herniation
(C) Transforaminal (tonsillar) herniation
(D) Transtentorial (uncal) herniation
(E) Viral (lymphocytic) meningitis

5. Which part of the ventricular system contains the choroid plexus?

(A) Cerebral aqueduct
(B) Frontal horn of the lateral ventricle
(C) Interventricular foramen
(D) Occipital horn
(E) Third ventricle

6. Choose the normal quantity of daily CSF production.

(A) 300 mL
(B) 400 mL
(C) 500 mL
(D) 600 mL
(E) 700 mL

7. Which one of the following tumors contains cellular whorls and psammoma bodies?

(A) Acoustic schwannoma
(B) Astrocytoma
(C) Glioblastoma multiforme
(D) Meningioma
(E) Oligodendroglioma

Questions 8 to 12

Match each structure or description in items 8 to 12 with the appropriate lettered structure shown in the T_1-weighted MRI of a coronal section of the brain.

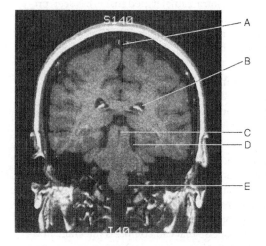

Questions 13 to 17

Match each structure or description in items 13 to 17 with the appropriate lettered structure shown on the T_1-weighted MRI of a midsagittal section of the brain.

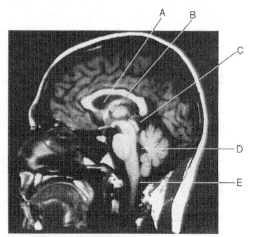

8. Olive

9. It contains the trochlear nerve (CN IV).

10. Its stenosis results in hydrocephalus.

11. Contains a calcified glomus

12. Receives CSF from the arachnoid villi

13. Superior cistern

14. Blockage results in hydrocephalus.

15. Lateral ventricle

16. Contains the two lateral foramina of Luschka

17. Receives CSF via the median foramen (of Magendie)

Answers and Explanations

1. **A.** This condition, called pseudotumor cerebri (benign intracranial hypertension), is seen primarily in young women who are obese. It is linked to an excessive amount of CSF. Blockage of the cerebral aqueduct (most common), lateral or median foramina of the fourth ventricle, or the interventricular foramina lead to noncommunicating hydrocephalus, which is most common in children and produces symptoms of increased intracranial pressure.

2. **C.** Noncommunicating hydrocephalus is the most common form in newborns. Communicating hydrocephalus may also be seen in newborns, but may also result from infection, hemorrhage, or meningitis. Hydrocephalus ex vacuo does not lead to increased intracranial pressure. Pseudomotor cerebri typically occurs in women who are obese and of childbearing age. Normal pressure hydrocephalus is normally seen in older adults.

3. **C.** Subdural hematomas are caused by tearing/shearing injuries of the cerebral or bridging veins. Such injuries are more common in the older adults, as the brain shrinks, the veins are stretched, and their walls are pulled thin. As subdural hematomas are venous injuries, they may be slow to develop with progressively worsening symptoms over a period of time. A meningioma is a brain tumor and its effects would be relatively slowly developing and unrelated to the accident. Normal pressure hydrocephalus is an abnormal buildup of CSF that can compress the brain; however, it would be unrelated to the accident. Transtentorial herniation involves a space-occupying lesion that forces part of the deep structures of the brain through the tentorial incisure; this patient's symptoms are initially cortical in nature and would not be produced by compression of deep structures. Viral meningitis initially presents as flu-like symptoms, including a fever and is unrelated to the accident.

4. **D.** A tumor in the right supratentorial compartment may cause herniation of the uncus through the tentorial incisure, compressing the midbrain. The first signs would likely be compression of CN III, causing the ipsilateral pupillary effects and eye position. Further compression would impinge upon the right corticospinal tract, causing left hemiplegia. The loss of consciousness results from compression of the ascending reticular activation system, which may eventually lead to coma. Hydrocephalus ex vacuo typically occurs in older patients and leads to a different sequelae of symptoms, for example, fatigue, personality changes, and memory lapses. Subfalcial herniation involves herniation of the cingulate gyrus and produces symptoms such as slowed pulse, headache, high blood pressure, and in more severe cases loss of consciousness and brainstem activity. Tonsillar herniation produces motor deficits, not stupor. Viral meningitis initially presents as flu-like symptoms, including a fever, not eye movement deficits.

5. **E.** The third ventricle contains choroid plexus, as do the other three ventricles; the frontal and occipital horns and the cerebral aqueduct are devoid of choroid plexus; the interventricular foramen has no choroid plexus of significance.

6. **C.** The choroid plexus produces CSF at a rate of ~500 mL/d.

7. **D.** Meningiomas contain cellular whorls and calcified psammoma bodies. Astrocytomas type II have near normal cellularity, little nuclear pleomorphism, no endothelial proliferation, and no necrosis. Acoustic schwannomas are benign tumors arising from Schwann cells. Oligodendrogliomas show calcification in 50% of cases—cells look like fried eggs (perinuclear halos). Glioblastoma multiforme represents 55% of gliomas, is malignant and rapidly fatal, and is the most common primary brain tumor.

8. **E.** The olive is a prominent surface structure of the medulla, under which lie the olivary nuclei.

9. **D.** The ambient cisterns contain the trochlear nerves (CN IV); they are expansions of the subarachnoid space lateral to the crus cerebri on either side of the midbrain.

10. C. Stenosis of the cerebral aqueduct prevents CSF from entering the fourth ventricle; this results in a noncommunicating hydrocephalus.

11. B. The trigone of the lateral ventricle contains a large tuft of choroid plexus called the glomus. It is often calcified and highly visible in CT imaging.

12. A. The superior sagittal sinus receives CSF via the arachnoid granulations/villi.

13. C. The superior (quadrigeminal) cistern overlies the dorsal/posterior aspect of the midbrain.

14. B. Blockage of the interventricular foramen (of Monro) (eg, due to a colloid cyst of the third ventricle) results in hydrocephalus.

15. A. The lateral ventricle is seen between the corpus callosum and the fornix.

16. D. The fourth ventricle contains the two lateral foramina (of Luschka), which drain into the cerebellopontine angle cisterns. The other foramen of the fourth ventricle, the median foramen (of Magendie), empties into the cerebellomedullary cistern (cisterna magna).

17. E. The cerebellomedullary cistern (cisterna magna) receives CSF via the median foramen (of Magendie).

3 Blood Supply of the Central Nervous System

Objectives

■ List the major branches of the vertebral and internal carotid arteries and indicate the regions/structures that each artery supplies.
■ Describe the cerebral arterial circle (of Willis).
■ List the major deep cerebral veins.
■ Identify the dural venous sinuses and include a description of their drainage patterns and the location of each sinus.
■ Describe the various types of intracranial hemorrhage.

I. ARTERIES OF THE SPINAL CORD

■ arise from the vertebral and segmental arteries.

A. Vertebral artery (Figure 3.1)

■ paired branches of the subclavian artery.
■ gives rise to the anterior spinal artery and 25% of the time, gives rise to the posterior spinal artery.

1. Anterior spinal artery

■ supplies the anterior two-thirds of the spinal cord, including the anterior and lateral horns and anterior and lateral funiculi.
■ supplies the pyramids, medial lemniscus, and intra-axial fibers of the hypoglossal nerve (CN XII) in the medulla.

2. Posterior spinal arteries

■ supply the posterior third of the spinal cord, including the posterior horns and columns.
■ supply the gracile and cuneate fasciculi and nuclei in the medulla.

B. Segmental arteries

■ arise from the aorta, vertebral arteries, and common iliac arteries as medullary arteries, which anastomose with the anterior and posterior spinal arteries.
■ provide the main blood supply to the spinal cord at thoracic and lumbar levels where the spinal arteries become inconsistent. Typically, the second lumbar artery gives rise to a large anterior medullary artery, the **artery of Adamkiewicz**. Its origin varies from T12 to L4, and it usually arises on the left side.

C. Anterior cord (anterior spinal artery) syndrome

■ caused by lesion of the anterior spinal arteries or the artery of Adamkiewicz.
■ affects the anterior two-thirds of the spinal cord.

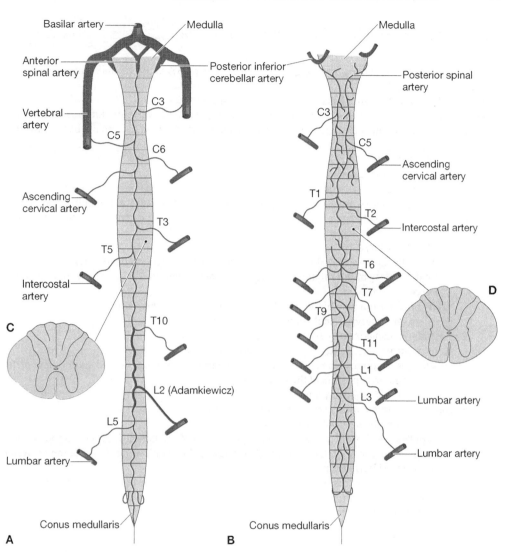

FIGURE 3.1. Arterial blood supply of the spinal cord. **(A)** Anterior surface, **(B)** posterior surface, **(C)** occlusion of the anterior spinal artery resulting in infarction of the anterior two-thirds of the spinal cord, and **(D)** occlusion of the posterior spinal arteries resulting in infarction of the posterior columns. Note the large lumbar feeder artery of Adamkiewicz, whose origin varies from segments T12 to L4. (Adapted with permission from Parent A. *Carpenter's Human Neuroanatomy*. 9th ed. Lippincott Williams & Wilkins; 1995:94.)

- leads to bilateral loss of motor function from loss of the corticospinal tracts and the anterior horns, bilateral loss of pain and temperature below the lesion from loss of the spinothalamic tracts, and sexual dysfunction and urinary and bowel incontinence from loss of descending autonomic tracts.

II. VENOUS DRAINAGE OF THE SPINAL CORD

- generally follows the arterial pattern.
- blood passes from spinal veins within the subarachnoid space to the epidural internal venous plexus before draining into intracranial, cervical, thoracic, intercostal, or abdominal veins.
- conducted by valveless veins that permit bidirectional flow, depending on the existing pressure gradients and body position.
- potential pathway for transmission of infectious agents and tumor cells.

III. ARTERIES OF THE BRAIN (Figures 3.2 through 3.6)

▓ provide the brain with 20% of the oxygen used by the body; 15% of the cardiac output goes to the brain.

▓ normal blood flow of 50 mL/100 g of brain tissue per minute.

▓ consist of two pairs of vessels—the **internal carotid arteries** and the **vertebral arteries**. At the junction between the medulla and the pons, the two vertebral arteries fuse to form the **basilar artery**.

A. Internal carotid artery

▓ enters the cranium via the carotid canal of the temporal bone.

▓ lies within the cavernous sinus as the carotid siphon.

▓ supplies tributaries to the dura mater, hypophysis, tympanic cavity, and trigeminal ganglion.

▓ provides branches to the optic nerve, optic chiasm, hypothalamus, and genu of the internal capsule.

▓ gives the following branches:

1. **Ophthalmic artery**
   ▓ enters the apex of the orbit via the optic canal with the optic nerve (CN II).
   ▓ **Central artery of the retina**: a branch of the **ophthalmic artery** that runs within the optic nerve.
      ▓ provides the only blood supply to the inner aspect of the retina.
      ▓ an end artery; its **occlusion results in blindness**.

2. **Posterior communicating artery** (see Figures 3.2 and 3.6)
   ▓ joins the posterior and the middle cerebral arteries.
   ▓ supplies the optic chiasm and tract, hypothalamus, subthalamus, and anterior half of the ventral/inferior portion of the thalamus.
   ▓ a common site of berry aneurysms.

3. **Anterior choroidal artery** (see Figures 3.2 and 3.6)
   ▓ arises from the internal carotid artery.
   ▓ supplies the choroid plexus of the temporal horn of the lateral ventricle, hippocampus, amygdala, optic tract, lateral geniculate body, globus pallidus, and part of the posterior limb of the internal capsule.
   ▓ supplies the proximal portion of the optic radiations as they leave the lateral geniculate body.

4. **Anterior cerebral artery** (see Figure 3.3)
   ▓ divided into five surgical segments (A1-A5) from origin to termination (see Figures 3.9 and 3.13).
   ▓ together with the middle cerebral artery is one of the terminal branches of the internal carotid artery.
   ▓ supplies the medial surface of the frontal and parietal lobes and the corpus callosum.
   ▓ supplies part of the striatum and the anterior limb of the internal capsule via the **medial striate artery (of Heubner)** (see Figure 3.2).
   ▓ supplies the leg and foot area of the motor and sensory cortices (paracentral lobule) (see Figure 22.2).

5. **Anterior communicating artery**
   ▓ connects the two anterior cerebral arteries.
   ▓ the commonest site of berry aneurysms.

6. **Middle cerebral artery** (see Figures 3.3 and 3.5)
   ▓ divided into four surgical segments (M1-M4) from origin to termination as it passes laterally through the Sylvian fissure to the lateral surface of the cerebral hemispheres (see Figures 3.7, 3.8, and 3.13).
   ▓ together with the anterior cerebral artery is one of the terminal branches of the internal carotid artery.
   ▓ supplies the lateral convexity of the cerebral hemisphere and insula.
   ▓ supplies the trunk, arm, and face areas of the motor and sensory cortices (see Figure 22.2).
   ▓ supplies Broca and Wernicke speech areas.
   ▓ supplies the striatum, pallidum, and anterior and posterior limbs of the internal capsule via the **lateral striate arteries**.

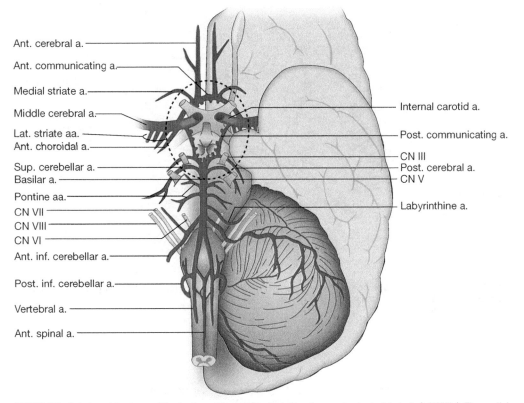

Ant. cerebral a.
Ant. communicating a.
Medial striate a.
Middle cerebral a.
Lat. striate aa.
Ant. choroidal a.
Sup. cerebellar a.
Basilar a.
Pontine aa.
CN VII
CN VIII
CN VI
Ant. inf. cerebellar a.
Post. inf. cerebellar a.
Vertebral a.
Ant. spinal a.

Internal carotid a.
Post. communicating a.
CN III
Post. cerebral a.
CN V
Labyrinthine a.

FIGURE 3.2. Arteries of the base of the brain and brainstem, including the cerebral arterial circle (of Willis). The medial and lateral striate arteries and the anterior choroidal artery supply the basal nuclei and internal capsule.

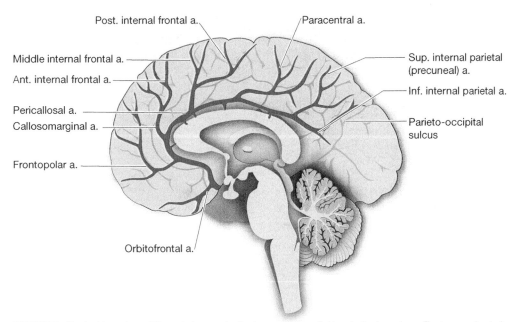

Post. internal frontal a.
Paracentral a.
Middle internal frontal a.
Ant. internal frontal a.
Pericallosal a.
Callosomarginal a.
Frontopolar a.
Orbitofrontal a.

Sup. internal parietal (precuneal) a.
Inf. internal parietal a.
Parieto-occipital sulcus

FIGURE 3.3. Cortical branches of the anterior cerebral artery on the medial hemispheric surface. The temporal pole is supplied by the middle cerebral artery; the occipital lobe is supplied by the posterior cerebral artery. Areas shaded in pink are supplied by branches of the anterior cerebral artery.

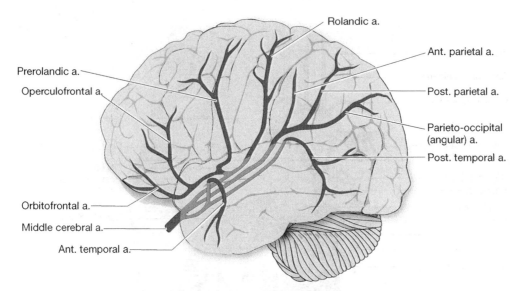

FIGURE 3.4. Cortical branches of the middle cerebral artery. The unshaded area represents the terminal territories of the anterior and posterior cerebral arteries.

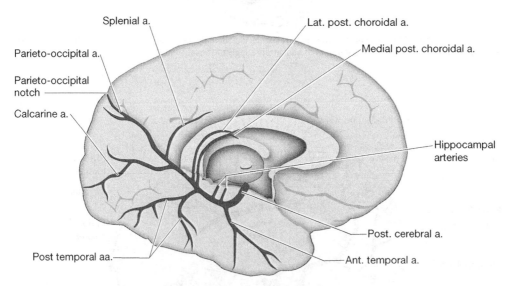

FIGURE 3.5. Cortical branches of the posterior cerebral artery. The splenium of the corpus callosum is supplied by the callosal branch of the posterior cerebral artery.

Medial

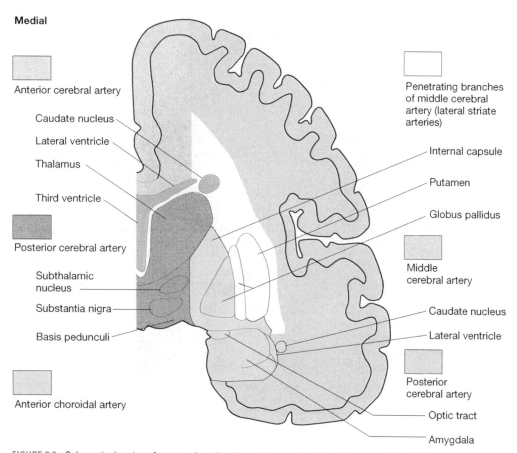

Anterior cerebral artery

Caudate nucleus

Lateral ventricle

Thalamus

Third ventricle

Posterior cerebral artery

Subthalamic nucleus

Substantia nigra

Basis pedunculi

Anterior choroidal artery

Penetrating branches of middle cerebral artery (lateral striate arteries)

Internal capsule

Putamen

Globus pallidus

Middle cerebral artery

Caudate nucleus

Lateral ventricle

Posterior cerebral artery

Optic tract

Amygdala

FIGURE 3.6. Schematic drawing of a coronal section through the cerebral hemisphere at the level of the internal capsule and thalamus, showing the major vascular territories. (Modified with permission from Fix JD. *High-Yield Neuroanatomy.* 3rd ed. Lippincott Williams & Wilkins; 2005:31.)

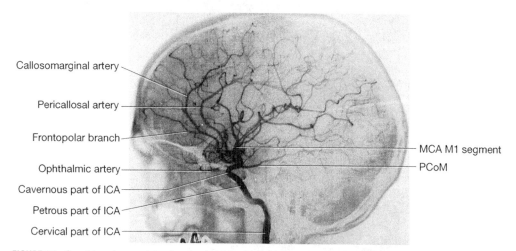

Callosomarginal artery

Pericallosal artery

Frontopolar branch

Ophthalmic artery

Cavernous part of ICA

Petrous part of ICA

Cervical part of ICA

MCA M1 segment

PCoM

FIGURE 3.7. Carotid angiogram, lateral projection. Identify the cortical branches of the anterior cerebral artery, internal cerebral artery (ICA), and middle cerebral artery (MCA). PCoM, posterior communicating artery. (Modified with permission from Fix JD. *High-Yield Neuroanatomy.* 3rd ed. Lippincott Williams & Wilkins; 2005:36.)

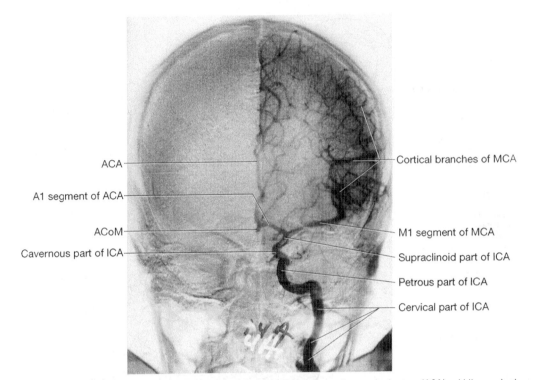

ACA

A1 segment of ACA

ACoM

Cavernous part of ICA

Cortical branches of MCA

M1 segment of MCA

Supraclinoid part of ICA

Petrous part of ICA

Cervical part of ICA

FIGURE 3.8. Carotid angiogram, anteroposterior projection. Identify the anterior cerebral artery (ACA), middle cerebral artery (MCA), and internal carotid artery (ICA). ACoM, anterior communicating artery. (Adapted with permission from Fix JD. *High-Yield Neuroanatomy*. 3rd ed. Lippincott Williams & Wilkins; 2005:37.)

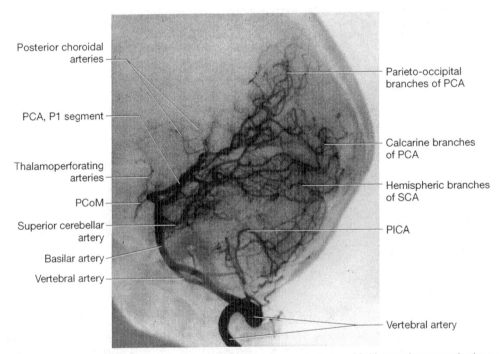

Posterior choroidal arteries

PCA, P1 segment

Thalamoperforating arteries

PCoM

Superior cerebellar artery

Basilar artery

Vertebral artery

Parieto-occipital branches of PCA

Calcarine branches of PCA

Hemispheric branches of SCA

PICA

Vertebral artery

FIGURE 3.9. Vertebral angiogram, lateral projection. PCA, posterior cerebral artery; PCoM, posterior communicating artery; PICA, posterior inferior cerebellar artery; SCA, superior cerebellar artery. (Adapted with permission from Fix JD. *High-Yield Neuroanatomy*. 3rd ed. Lippincott Williams & Wilkins; 2005:37.)

B. **Vertebral artery (see Figure 3.1)**
   - paired branches of the subclavian artery.
   - join to form the basilar artery.
   1. **Anterior spinal artery**
      - supplies anterior two-thirds of the spinal cord.
   2. **Posterior inferior cerebellar artery**
      - gives rise to the posterior spinal artery 75% of the time.
      - supplies the dorsolateral zone of the medulla.
      - supplies the inferior surface of the cerebellum and the choroid plexus of the fourth ventricle.
      - supplies the medial and inferior vestibular nuclei, inferior cerebellar peduncle, nucleus ambiguus, intra-axial fibers of the glossopharyngeal nerve (CN IX) and the vagal nerve (CN X), spinothalamic tract, and spinal trigeminal nucleus and tract.
      - supplies the hypothalamospinal tract to the ciliospinal center (of Budge) at T1-T2—damage which leads to Horner syndrome.

C. **Basilar artery (see Figure 3.1)**
   - formed by the joining of the two vertebral arteries.
   1. **Pontine arteries**
      - include penetrating and short circumferential branches.
      - supply corticospinal tracts and the intra-axial fibers of the abducens nerve (CN VI).
   2. **Labyrinthine artery**
      - supplies the inner ear.
   3. **Anterior inferior cerebellar artery**
      - supplies the inferior surface of the cerebellum.
      - supplies the facial motor nucleus and intra-axial fibers of the facial nerve, spinal trigeminal nucleus and tract, vestibular nuclei, cochlear nuclei, intra-axial fibers of the vestibulocochlear nerve, spinothalamic tract, and inferior and middle cerebellar peduncles.
      - gives rise to the labyrinthine artery in 85% of the population.
      - supplies the hypothalamospinal tract—damage to which leads to Horner syndrome.
   4. **Superior cerebellar artery**
      - supplies the superior surface of the cerebellum and the deep cerebellar nuclei.
      - supplies the rostral and lateral pons, including the superior cerebellar peduncle and spinothalamic tract.
   5. **Posterior cerebral artery** (see Figure 3.5)
      - divided into four surgical segments (P1-P4) from origin to termination (see Figure 3.9).
      - the terminal branches of the basilar artery.
      - provides the major blood supply to the midbrain.
      - supplies the posterior half of the thalamus and the medial and lateral geniculate bodies.
      - supplies the occipital lobe, visual cortex, and inferior surface of the temporal lobe, including the hippocampal formation.
      - gives rise to the lateral and medial **posterior choroidal arteries** that supply the dorsal thalamus, pineal body, and choroid plexus of the third and lateral ventricles.

IV. CEREBRAL ARTERIAL CIRCLE (OF WILLIS) (See Figure 3.2)

- formed by the anterior communicating, anterior cerebral, internal carotid, posterior communicating, and posterior cerebral arteries.
- gives off penetrating arteries to supply the inferior aspect, hypothalamus, subthalamus, thalamus, and the midbrain.

V. MENINGEAL ARTERIES

- supply the intracranial dura mater.
- usually arise from branches of the external carotid artery.

A. Anterior meningeal arteries
- arise from the anterior and posterior ethmoidal arteries.
- supply the dura mater of the anterior cranial fossa.

B. Middle meningeal artery
- a branch of the **maxillary artery**.
- enters the cranium via the **foramen spinosum**.
- lies within the dura mater, forming a groove on the internal surface of the temporal and parietal bones.
- supplies most of the dura mater.
- laceration results in **epidural hemorrhage** (hematoma).

C. Posterior meningeal arteries
- branches of the ascending pharyngeal, vertebral, and occipital arteries.
- supply the dura mater of the posterior cranial fossa.

VI. VEINS OF THE BRAIN

- devoid of valves and lie along the surface.
- drain the cortex and subcortical tissue.
- terminate in the dural sinuses.

A. Superficial cerebral veins
- drain into the superior sagittal sinus (bridging veins).
- laceration of these vessels results in subdural hemorrhage (hematoma).

B. Deep cerebral veins
- drain the deep subcortical structures of the cerebral hemispheres: **septal area, thalamus,** and **basal nuclei.**
  1. **Internal cerebral veins**
     - drain the following vessels:
       a. **Septal vein**
       b. **Thalamostriate vein**
       c. **Terminal vein**
       d. **Venous angle**
          - the point where the septal and the thalamostriate veins meet.
          - a useful neuroradiologic landmark, as it indicates the location of the interventricular foramen (of Monro).
  2. **Great cerebral vein (of Galen)**
     - receives blood from the internal cerebral veins and drains into the straight sinus.

VII. VENOUS DURAL SINUSES (Figure 3.10)

- endothelium-lined valveless channels whose walls are formed by the periosteal and meningeal layers of dura mater.
- collect blood from the superficial and deep cerebral veins.
- receive arachnoid granulations and absorb cerebrospinal fluid.

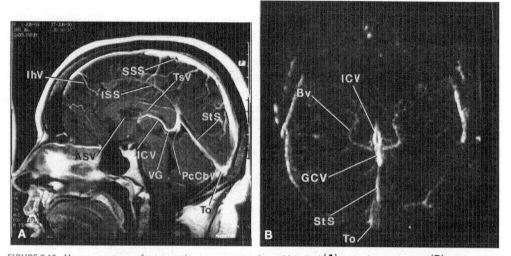

FIGURE 3.10. Venous anatomy of a magnetic resonance section; midsagittal **(A)** and submental vertex **(B)**. ASV, anterior septal vein; Bv, basal vein; GCV, great cerebral vein; ICV, internal cerebral vein; IhV, interhemispheric veins; ISS, inferior sagittal sinus; PcCbV, precentral cerebellar vein; SSS, superior sagittal sinus; StS, straight sinus; To, torcula; TsV, thalamostriate vein; VG, vein of anterior pontomesencephalic veins. (Adapted with permission from Grossman CB. *Magnetic Resonance Imaging and Computed Tomography of the Head and Spine.* 2nd ed. Lippincott Williams & Wilkins; 1996:124.)

A. Superior sagittal sinus (see Figure 2.3)
- extends from the foramen cecum to the internal occipital protuberance and typically terminates in the right transverse sinus.
- receives blood from the superficial cerebral veins, diploic veins, and emissary veins.
- receives most arachnoid granulations.

B. Inferior sagittal sinus
- courses in the inferior (free) edge of the falx cerebri.
- joins the great cerebral vein to form the straight sinus.

C. Straight sinus
- formed by the junction of the great cerebral vein and the inferior sagittal sinus.
- terminates at the internal occipital protuberance and usually drains into the left transverse sinus.
- drains the superior surface of the cerebellum.

D. Left and right transverse sinuses
- originate at the confluence of the sinuses and course anterolaterally along the edge of the tentorium cerebelli to become the sigmoid sinus at the point where the superior petrosal sinuses join.

E. Occipital sinus
- found in the attached edge of the falx cerebelli.

F. Confluence of the sinuses (torcula)
- lies at the internal occipital protuberance.
- formed by the union of the superior sagittal, straight, occipital, and transverse sinuses.

G. Sigmoid sinus
- a continuation of the transverse sinus at the point where the superior petrosal sinus joins the transverse sinus.
- passes inferiorly and medially into the jugular foramen to become the internal jugular vein.

H. Sphenoparietal sinus
- lies along the lesser wing of the sphenoid bone and drains into the cavernous sinus.

I. Superior petrosal sinus
- extends from the cavernous sinus to the junction of the transverse and sigmoid sinus.
- receives tributaries from the pons, medulla, cerebellum, and inner ear.

J. Inferior petrosal sinus
- passes between the glossopharyngeal (CN IX) and vagal (CN X) nerves and drains into the internal jugular vein after exiting the skull via the jugular foramen.
- drains the inferior portion of the cerebellum.
- drains the cavernous sinus and clival plexus into the internal jugular vein.

K. Cavernous sinus (see Figure 11.5)
- surrounds the sella turcica and the body of the sphenoid bone.
- contains, *within the sinus*, the internal carotid artery, its periarterial plexus, and the abducens nerve (CN VI).
- contains, *within the lateral wall of the sinus*, the oculomotor nerve (CN III), the trochlear nerve (CN IV), the ophthalmic nerve (CN V-1), and the maxillary branches (CN V-2) of the trigeminal nerve (CN V).
- communicates anteriorly with the superior and inferior ophthalmic veins.

VIII. ANGIOGRAPHY

A. Carotid angiography (Figures 3.7 and 3.8)

B. Vertebral angiography (Figures 3.9 and 3.11)

C. Cerebral veins and dural sinuses (Figure 3.12)

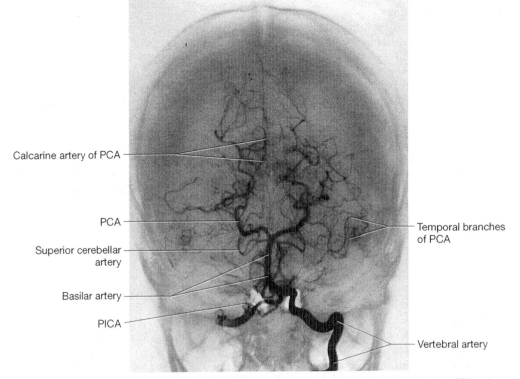

FIGURE 3.11. Vertebral angiogram, anteroposterior projection. Occlusion of the posterior cerebral artery (PCA; calcarine artery) results in a contralateral homonymous hemianopia, with macular sparing. PICA, posterior inferior cerebellar artery. (Adapted with permission from Fix JD. *High-Yield Neuroanatomy.* 3rd ed. Lippincott Williams & Wilkins; 2005:38.)

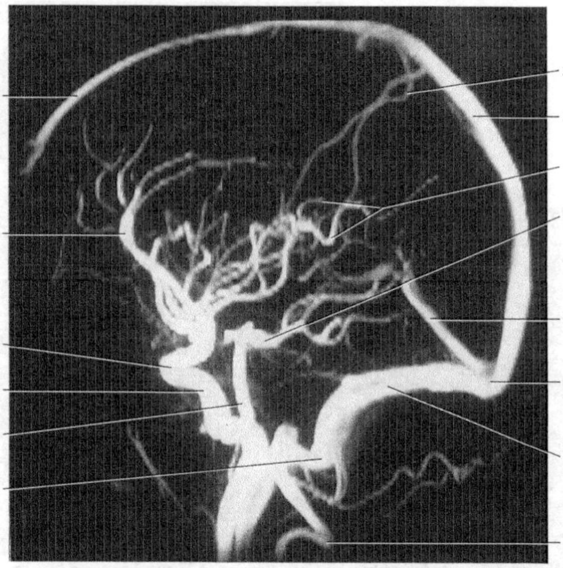

FIGURE 3.12. Magnetic resonance angiogram—lateral projection—showing the major venous sinuses and arteries. Note the bridging veins entering the superior sagittal sinus. ICA, internal carotid artery; MCA, middle cerebral artery; PCA, posterior cerebral artery. (Adapted with permission from Fix JD. *High-Yield Neuroanatomy.* 3rd ed. Lippincott Williams & Wilkins; 2005:32.)

IX. INTRACRANIAL HEMORRHAGE

A. Aneurysms

- circumscribed dilations (ectasias) of an artery.
   1. **Berry (saccular) aneurysms** (Figure 3.13)
      - typically develop at arterial bifurcations. The **cerebral arterial circle** contains 60% of aneurysms; 30% arise from the middle cerebral artery; and the remaining 10% are found in the vertebrobasilar system.
      - of the anterior communicating artery may pressure the optic chiasm and cause a **bitemporal lower quadrantanopia.**
      - of the posterior communicating artery may cause an **oculomotor nerve palsy.**
      - rupture is a common cause of nontraumatic **subarachnoid hemorrhage.**
   2. **Microaneurysms (Charcot-Bouchard aneurysms)**
      - found in small arteries, most frequently within the territory of the middle cerebral artery (eg, the lenticulostriate arteries).
      - rupture occurs most frequently in the basal nuclei and is the commonest cause of nontraumatic **intraparenchymal hemorrhage.**

CLINICAL CORRELATES The escape of blood from a ruptured blood vessel is a **hematoma** or **hemorrhage.** In the cranial vault, a **subdural hematoma** (Figure 3.14) results from the rupture of superior cerebral veins, the "bridging" veins that drain into the superior sagittal sinus. Subdural hematomas are often caused by sudden deceleration of the head, whereas an **epidural hematoma** (Figure 3.15) typically results from rupture of the middle meningeal artery (or a branch) that lies between the dura mater and the inner table of the skull. Epidural hematomas are typically caused by trauma.

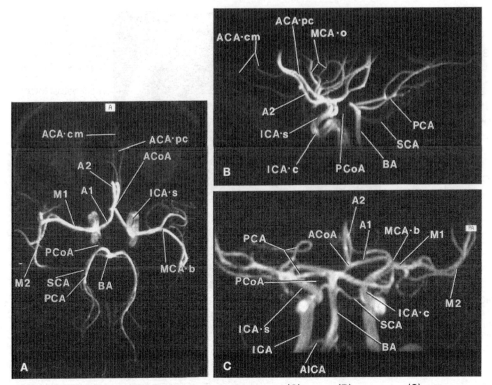

FIGURE 3.13. Arterial anatomy of a magnetic resonance section: axial **(A)**, sagittal **(B)**, and coronal **(C)**. ACAcm, anterior cerebral artery, callosal marginal branch; A2 and A1, branches of the anterior cerebral artery; ACApc, pericallosal branch of the anterior cerebral artery; ACoA, anterior communicating artery; M1 and M2, segments of the middle cerebral artery (MCA); BA, basilar artery; ICAc, internal cerebral artery callosal branch; ICAs, internal carotid artery siphon; MCAb, bifurcation; MCAo, middle cerebral artery occipital branch; PAC, posterior cerebral artery; PCoA, posterior communicating artery; SCA, superior cerebellar artery. (Adapted with permission from Grossman CB. *Magnetic Resonance Imaging and Computed Tomography of the Head and Spine.* 2nd ed. Lippincott Williams & Wilkins; 1996:124.)

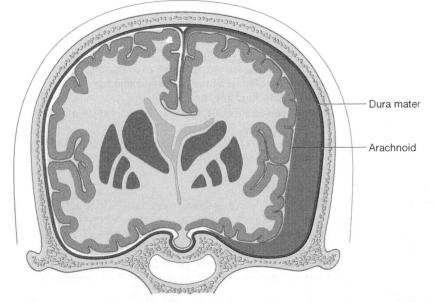

FIGURE 3.14. Subdural hematomas result from lacerated bridging veins. They are frequently accompanied by traumatic subarachnoid hemorrhages and cortical contusions. The hematoma extends over the crest of the convexity into the interhemispheric fissure but does not cross the dural attachment of the falx cerebri; the clot can be crescent shaped, biconvex, or multiloculated. Subdural hematomas are more common than epidural hematomas. (Adapted from Osburn AG, Tong KA. *Handbook of Neuroradiology: Brain and Skull.* 2nd ed. Mosby; 1996:192. Copyright © 1996 Elsevier. With permission.)

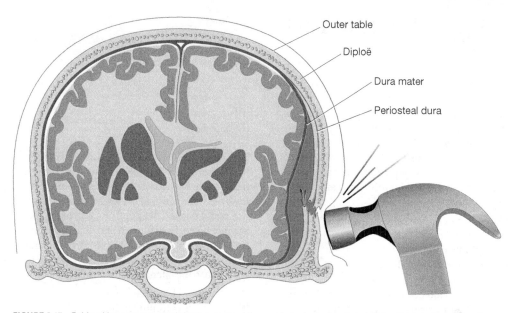

Outer table

Diploë

Dura mater

Periosteal dura

FIGURE 3.15. Epidural hematomas result from rupture of the meningeal arteries. Arterial bleeding into the epidural space forms a biconvex clot. A lucid interval is seen in up to 50% of cases. Skull fractures are typically found. Epidural hematomas seldom cross sutural lines. (Adapted from Osburn AG, Tong KA. *Handbook of Neuroradiology: Brain and Skull*. 2nd ed. Mosby; 1996:191. Copyright © 1996 Elsevier. With permission.)

Review Test

1. A 50-year-old woman with previously diagnosed hypertension presents to her primary care physician with a concern about recently developed numbness and weakness in her left leg and foot. Which of the following arteries' occlusion may account for this complaint?

(A) Anterior cerebral
(B) Anterior choroidal
(C) Internal carotid
(D) Middle cerebral
(E) Posterior cerebral

2. A 15-year-old boy is hit on the temple with a baseball and becomes unconscious. After about 10 min, he regains consciousness, but he soon becomes lethargic, and over the next 2 h, he becomes stuporous. His pupils are unequal. Intracranial hemorrhage is suspected. Which of the following arteries is most likely to be the source of the hemorrhage?

(A) Anterior cerebral
(B) Anterior communicating
(C) Basilar
(D) Middle cerebral
(E) Middle meningeal

3. Which artery supplies the corpus striatum (caudate + putamen) and anterior limb of the internal capsule via the medial striate artery (of Heubner)?

(A) Anterior cerebral
(B) Anterior choroidal
(C) Anterior communicating
(D) Middle cerebral
(E) Posterior communicating

4. Which artery supplies the cochlea?

(A) Anterior inferior cerebellar
(B) Labyrinthine
(C) Pontine
(D) Posterior cerebral
(E) Superior cerebellar

5. Which sinus drains the superior surface of the cerebellum?

(A) Inferior petrosal
(B) Inferior sagittal
(C) Sigmoid

(D) Sphenoparietal
(E) Straight

6. A 40-year-old woman had an excruciating headache. When she looked in the mirror, she noticed that her eyelid was drooping; when she lifted the eyelid, she saw that her eyeball was looking down and out and her pupil was very large. She complained of both blurred and double vision. A magnetic resonance angiogram showed an aneurysm of the cerebral arterial circle. Which artery gives rise to the offending aneurysm?

(A) Anterior choroidal
(B) Anterior communicating
(C) Vertebral
(D) Medial striate
(E) Posterior communicating

7. A 34-year-old woman was referred to a neurologist for recently developed headaches and visual disturbances. Patient interview reveals the use of oral contraceptives and describes obscurations, which are transient in both visual fields and worse with bad headaches. Examination reveals papilledema. CT and MRI appear normal. MR venography reveals a dural venous thrombus in the cavernous sinus. Which of the following systems is likely to be most affected by this thrombus?

(A) Autonomic nervous
(B) Limbic
(C) Olfactory
(D) Vestibular
(E) Visual

8. A 65-year-old man presents to the emergency department with a chief complaint of a sudden loss of vision in his right eye. Interview reveals that the patient is not in pain, is a heavy smoker, and has diabetes and hypertension. Examination reveals that the patient is unable to discern anything from his right eye; the left eye is normal. There are no other notable symptoms. In which artery is this patient's lesion?

(A) Anterior communicating
(B) Central artery of the retina
(C) Middle cerebral
(D) Ophthalmic
(E) Pontine

Questions 9 to 13

The response options for items 9 to 13 are the same. Select one answer for each item in the set.

(A) Anterior inferior cerebellar
(B) Anterior spinal
(C) Posterior cerebral
(D) Posterior inferior cerebellar
(E) Superior cerebellar

Match each of the following descriptions with the most appropriate artery from the list above.

9. Usually gives rise to the artery that supplies the inner ear

10. Supplies the facial nucleus and the spinal trigeminal nucleus and tract

11. Is the terminal branch of the basilar artery

12. Supplies the deep cerebellar nuclei

13. Supplies the nucleus ambiguus

Questions 14 to 18

Match the statements in items 14 to 18 with the appropriate lettered artery shown in the figure.

14. An aneurysm of this artery may cause a third nerve palsy.

15. Irrigates the posterior limb of the internal capsule

16. Occlusion of this artery results in a fluent receptive aphasia.

17. An aneurysm of this artery may result in Horner syndrome.

18. Occlusion of this artery results in infarction of the paracentral lobule with Babinski sign.

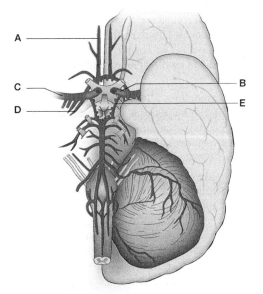

Answers and Explanations

1. **A.** The anterior cerebral artery perfuses the paracentral lobule, which contains the motor and sensory areas of the leg and foot. The anterior choroidal artery supplies deeper structures, including the optic radiations and parts of the diencephalon and basal nuclei. The internal carotid artery is one of the four major arteries that supply the brain. The middle cerebral artery does supply areas of sensory cortex, but it deals with the upper body and head, not the lower limbs. The posterior cerebral artery supplies much of the undersurface of the brain, occipital and temporal lobes.

2. **E.** Laceration of the middle meningeal artery gives rise to an epidural hematoma. Classic signs of an epidural hematoma are skull trauma, usually with fracture, and sequential progression from unconsciousness to lucidity to progressive coma to death owing to transtentorial herniation with ipsilateral third nerve palsy. The anterior cerebral artery is a deep structure, not commonly injured through trauma. The anterior communicating artery would not have such great effects on consciousness if injured, as it is primarily a connection between the two anterior cerebral arteries. The basilar artery would be difficult to injure from such an injury and if it is injured very quickly produces life-threatening symptoms owing to it supplying the brainstem with arterial blood. The middle cerebral artery may become injured through trauma, but would produce a different sequelae of motor and sensory deficits, initially evident as an issue with speech.

3. **A.** The anterior cerebral artery supplies part of the caudate nucleus and putamen and anterior limb of the internal capsule via the medial striate artery (of Heubner) (see Figure 3.2). The anterior choroidal artery supplies the posterior limb of the internal capsule and the globus pallidus of the basal nuclei. The anterior communicating artery connects the two anterior cerebral arteries; it does not supply the striatum. The middle cerebral artery does provide blood to the striatum, but it does so via branches—the lateral striate arteries. The posterior communicating arteries do not supply the striatum; they supply deep structures around the diencephalon.

4. **B.** The labyrinthine artery supplies the cochlea and the vestibular apparatus. In 15% of the population, it arises from the basilar artery; in the remaining 85% of the population, it arises from the anterior inferior cerebellar artery. The anterior inferior cerebellar artery does supply the cochlear nuclei (and multiple other structures), but not the cochlea itself. Pontine arteries supply the corticospinal tracts and intra-axial fibers of the abducens nerve. The posterior cerebral artery supplies much of the undersurface of the brain, occipital and temporal lobes. Superior cerebellar arteries supply the cerebellum and parts of the pons.

5. **E.** The straight sinus drains the superior surface of the cerebellum. It is formed by the great cerebral vein (of Galen) and the inferior sagittal sinus. The inferior petrosal sinus drains the cavernous sinus and part of the cerebellum. The inferior sagittal sinus joins the great cerebral vein to form the straight sinus. The sigmoid sinus is a continuation of the transverse sinus. The sphenoparietal sinus is connected to the cavernous sinus and is not involved in cerebellar circulation.

6. **E.** The posterior communicating artery may give rise to a berry aneurysm, which compresses the third cranial nerve, resulting in third nerve palsy. The medial striate artery (of Heubner) is a branch of the anterior cerebral artery. A communicating artery may harbor berry aneurysms that impinge on the optic chiasm causing a bitemporal lower quadrantanopia. Aneurysms of the vertebral artery are uncommon and would cause more widespread effects. The anterior choroidal artery is a branch of the internal carotid artery and irrigates the globus pallidus and posterior limb of the internal capsule.

7. **E.** A thrombus of the cavernous sinus (rare) may lead to progressively worsening symptoms—the most common of which is a headache. Dural venous thrombi are more common in women in their early 30s on oral contraceptives. The proximity of CN II to the cavernous sinus and CN III, IV, and VI within the sinus may result in worsening visual symptoms. The cavernous sinus lies

too far from the hypothalamus to impact the autonomic nervous system. The limbic and olfactory systems are widely distributed on the ventral surface of the brain and also unlikely to be impacted. In the vestibular system, the vestibular nuclei are brainstem structures and are too far removed from the cavernous sinus to be directly impacted.

8. **B.** The central artery of the retina is an end artery; blockage leads to blindness. The ophthalmic artery has a host of branches in addition to the central artery of the retina, which supply muscles, mucosa, and skin of the region and so may lead to other symptoms in addition to the blindness in this patient. Lesion of the anterior communicating artery would not produce blindness in one eye. Lesion of the middle cerebral would cause massive motor and sensory loss from the body, not blindness. Lesion of the ophthalmic artery would cause ischemia to all of the structures of the orbit; it may also produce blindness if the blockage occurs prior to branching of the central artery of the retina. Lesions of the pontine arteries often produce life-threatening symptoms because they irrigate the brainstem, a lesion here would not affect vision directly.

9. **A.** The anterior inferior cerebellar artery usually gives rise to the labyrinthine artery, which supplies the structures of the inner ear (ie, the cochlea and vestibular apparatus).

10. **A.** The facial motor nucleus and the spinal trigeminal nucleus and tract are supplied by the anterior inferior cerebellar artery.

11. **C.** The posterior cerebral artery is the terminal branch of the basilar artery.

12. **E.** The superior cerebellar artery supplies the superior surface of the cerebellum and the deep cerebellar nuclei (eg, dentate nucleus).

13. **D.** The posterior inferior cerebellar artery supplies the posterolateral medullary field, including nucleus ambiguus.

14. **E.** An aneurysm of the posterior communicating artery may cause a third nerve palsy, as the nerve passes very close to the artery.

15. **D.** The anterior choroidal artery irrigates the posterior limb of the internal capsule. The anterior limb is supplied primarily by the medial striate artery (of Heubner), a branch of the anterior cerebral artery.

16. **C.** Occlusion of the proximal stem of the left middle cerebral artery results in Wernicke aphasia—a fluent receptive aphasia.

17. **B.** An aneurysm of the internal carotid artery within the cavernous sinus can interrupt postganglionic sympathetic fibers, resulting in Horner syndrome.

18. **A.** The anterior cerebral artery perfuses the medial aspect of the hemisphere from the frontal pole to the parieto-occipital sulcus, including the paracentral lobule. The paracentral lobule gives rise to corticospinal fibers to the contralateral foot and leg. Destruction of these fibers results in the Babinski sign.

chapter 4

Development of the Nervous System

Objectives

■ Describe the development of the neural tube, including the stages of development and the adult derivatives of each vesicle.
■ Trace the lineage of the cells and layers of the neural tube wall.
■ Identify the derivatives of the neural crest.
■ Describe the development of the spinal cord and include a description of the alar and basal plates.
■ Describe the development of the brainstem and cerebellum as well as the general arrangement of motor versus sensory components and somatic versus visceral components.
■ Describe the development of the diencephalon.
■ Describe the development of the telencephalon and list the major adult derivatives.
■ Characterize major congenital malformations of the central nervous system.

I. OVERVIEW

A. Central nervous system (CNS)

■ begins to form in the third week of embryonic development as the **neural plate**—an ectodermal thickening. The neural plate develops into the **neural tube**, which gives rise to the brain and spinal cord.

B. Peripheral nervous system (PNS)

■ consists of spinal and cranial nerves and associated ganglia.
■ derived from three sources:

1. **Neural crest cells**
   ■ give rise to peripheral ganglia, Schwann cells, and afferent nerve fibers.
2. **Neural tube**
   ■ gives rise to all preganglionic autonomic fibers and all fibers that innervate skeletal muscles.
3. **Mesoderm**
   ■ gives rise to the dura mater and to connective tissue investments of peripheral nerve fibers (endoneurium, perineurium, and epineurium).

II. DEVELOPMENT OF THE NEURAL TUBE (Figures 4.1 and 4.2)

■ begins in the third week and is complete in the fourth week.

A. Neural plate

■ a thickened pear-shaped region of embryonic ectoderm between the primitive node and the oropharyngeal membrane.

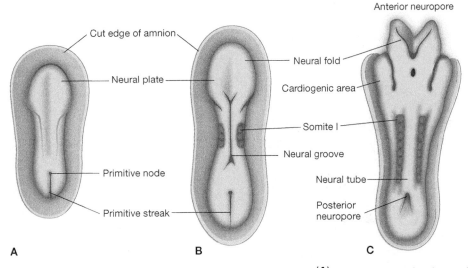

FIGURE 4.1. Diagrams illustrating the dorsal aspect of the human embryo. **(A)** Late presomite and early neural plate stage. **(B)** Early somite stage and neural groove stage. **(C)** Eight-somite stage and early neural tube stage. The anterior and posterior neuropores provide transitory communication between the neural tube and the amniotic cavity. (Adapted with permission from Carpenter MB, Sutin J. *Human Neuroanatomy.* 8th ed. Williams & Wilkins; 1983:63.)

B. Neural groove
- forms as the neural plate begins to grow and fold inward.
- flanked by parallel neural folds.
- deepens as the neural folds continue to expand and close over it.

C. Neural folds
- fuse in the midline beginning near the middle and proceed cranially and caudally to form the neural tube.
- the edges are the sites of neural crest cell differentiation.

D. Neural tube
- forms as the neural folds fuse in the midline and separate from the surface ectoderm.
- lies between the surface ectoderm and the notochord.
- gives rise to the CNS:
  1. **Cranial part** becomes the brain.
  2. **Caudal part** becomes the spinal cord.
  3. **Cavity** gives rise to the central canal of the spinal cord and ventricles of the brain.
  4. **Two transitory openings at either end of the neural tube** that connect the central canal with the amniotic cavity:
     - **Anterior neuropore**
       a. closes in the fourth week (~day 25) to become the **lamina terminalis**.
     - **Posterior neuropore**
       a. closes in the fourth week (~day 27).

III. NEURAL CREST (See Figure 4.2)

- forms near the edges of the neural folds.
- a group of multipotent migratory cells.

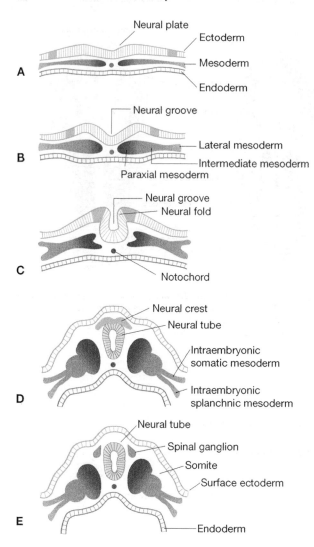

FIGURE 4.2. Schematic diagrams of transverse sections through embryos at various stages. **(A)** Neural plate stage. **(B)** Early neural groove stage. **(C)** Late neural groove stage. **(D)** Early neural tube and neural crest stage. **(E)** Neural tube and spinal ganglion stage. (Adapted with permission from Truex RC, Carpenter MB. *Human Neuroanatomy.* 6th ed. Williams & Wilkins; 1969:91.)

Derivatives

- Pseudounipolar cells of the spinal and cranial nerve ganglia.
- Schwann cells.
- Multipolar cells of the autonomic ganglia.
- Leptomeninges (pia-arachnoid cells).
- Chromaffin cells of the suprarenal medulla.
- Pigment cells (melanocytes).
- Odontoblasts (dentin-forming cells), dental papilla, and the dental follicle.
- Aorticopulmonary septum of the heart.
- Parafollicular cells (calcitonin-producing C-cells).
- Skeletal and connective tissue components of the pharyngeal arches.

IV. PLACODES

- localized thickenings of the cephalic surface ectoderm.
- give rise to cells that migrate into the underlying mesoderm and develop into the sensory receptive organs of the olfactory nerve (CN I) and the vestibulocochlear nerve (CN VIII).

A. Olfactory placodes
- differentiate into neurosensory cells that give rise to the **olfactory nerve** (**CN I**).
- induce the formation of the **olfactory bulbs**.

B. Otic placodes
- give rise to the following statoacoustic organs:
  1. **Organ of Corti** and **spiral ganglion**.
  2. **Cristae ampullares, maculae of the utricle** and **saccule**, and **vestibular ganglion**.
  3. **Vestibulocochlear nerve (CN VIII)**.

V. STAGES OF NEURAL TUBE DEVELOPMENT

A. Vesicle development
1. **Three primary brain vesicles** and associated flexures (Figure 4.3)
   - develop during the fourth week.
   - give rise to dilations of the primary brain vesicles and two curvatures.
   a. **Prosencephalon (forebrain)**
      - associated with the appearance of the **optic vesicles**.
      (1) **Telencephalon**
      (2) **Diencephalon**
   b. **Mesencephalon (midbrain)**
      - remains as the mesencephalon.
   c. **Rhombencephalon (hindbrain)**
      - gives rise to:
      (1) **Metencephalon**
         - forms the pons and cerebellum.
      (2) **Myelencephalon (medulla oblongata)**
   d. **Cephalic flexure (midbrain flexure)**
      - located between the prosencephalon and the rhombencephalon.
   e. **Cervical flexure**
      - located between the rhombencephalon and the future spinal cord.

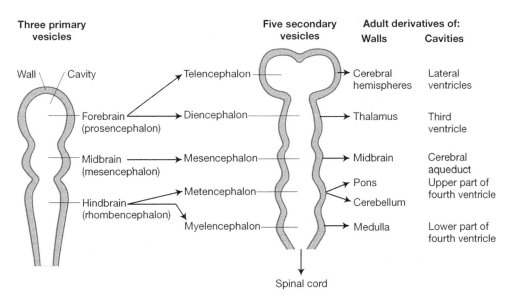

FIGURE 4.3. Diagrammatic sketches of the brain vesicles indicating the adult derivatives of their walls and cavities. (Adapted from Moore KL. *The Developing Human: Clinically Oriented Embryology.* 4th ed. WB Saunders; 1988:380. Copyright © 1988 Elsevier. With permission.)

2. **Five secondary brain vesicles** (with four ventricles) (see Figure 4.3)
   - become visible in the sixth week; the brain vesicles are visible as the primordia of the five major brain divisions:
   a. **Telencephalon**
      - lateral outpocketings form the **cerebral hemispheres**.
      - inferior outpocketings form the **olfactory bulbs**.
      - visible lateral ventricles.
   b. **Diencephalon**
      - third ventricle, optic chiasm and optic nerves, infundibulum, and mammillary eminences become visible.
   c. **Mesencephalon**
      - contains a large cavity that will become the **cerebral aqueduct**.
   d. **Metencephalon**
      - separated from the mesencephalon by the rhombencephalic isthmus.
      - separated from the myelencephalon by the pontine flexure.
      - contains **rhombic lips** on the dorsal surface that give rise to the cerebellum.
      - becomes the **pons** and the **cerebellum**.
      - contains the rostral half of the fourth ventricle.
   e. **Myelencephalon (medulla oblongata)**
      - lies between the pontine and cervical flexures.
      - becomes the medulla.
      - contains the **caudal half of the fourth ventricle**.

B. **Histogenesis**
   1. **Cells of the neural tube wall**
      - composed of neuroepithelial cells that give rise to the following:
      a. **Neuroblasts**
         - form the neurons of the CNS.
      b. **Glioblasts**
         - form the supporting cells of the CNS.
         (1) **Macroglia**
            - **Astroglia (astrocytes)**
               a. contain glial fibrillary acidic protein (**GFAP**), an astrocytic marker.
               b. surround blood capillaries with perivascular feet that contribute to the blood-brain barrier.
            - **Radial glial cells**
               a. of astrocytic lineage and **GFAP**-positive.
               b. provide guidance for migrating neuroblasts.
            - **Oligodendroglia (oligodendrocytes)**
               c. produce the myelin of the CNS.
         (2) **Ependymal cells**
            - ciliated.
            a. **Ependymocytes**
               - line the ventricles and the central canal.
            b. **Tanycytes**
               - located in the wall of the third ventricle.
               - transport substances from the cerebrospinal fluid (**CSF**) to the hypophyseal portal system.
            c. **Choroid plexus cells**
               - produce CSF.
               - form the blood-CSF barrier with the arachnoid membrane.
      c. **Microglia**
         - macrophages of the CNS.
         - arise from monocytes.
         - enter the developing nervous system in the third week with the developing blood vessels.

2. **Layers of the neural tube wall**
   ▪ **Neuroepithelial (ventricular) layer**
      a. the innermost layer.
      b. a monocellular layer of ependymal cells that lines the central canal and future brain ventricles.
   ▪ **Mantle (intermediate) layer**
      a. the middle layer.
      b. consists of neurons and glial cells.
      c. contains the developing **alar** and **basal plates**.
   ▪ **Marginal layer**
      a. the outermost layer.
      b. contains nerve fibers of neuroblasts of the mantle layer and glial cells.
      c. produces the **white matter of the spinal cord** through the myelination of growing axons.

VI. SPINAL CORD (MEDULLA SPINALIS) (Figure 4.4 and Table 4.1)

▪ develops from the neural tube caudal to the fourth pair of somites.

A. Alar and basal plates, sulcus limitans, and roof and floor plates (Figure 4.4)
   1. **Alar plate**
      ▪ a posterolateral thickening of the mantle layer of the neural tube.
      ▪ gives rise to second-order **sensory neuroblasts** of the posterior horn (general somatic afferent [GSA] and general visceral afferent [GVA] cell regions).
      ▪ receives axons from the spinal ganglion to become the posterior roots.
      ▪ becomes the **posterior horn** of the spinal cord.

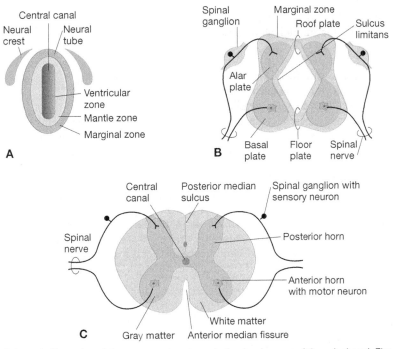

FIGURE 4.4. Schematic illustration of three successive stages in the development of the spinal cord. The neural crest gives rise to the spinal ganglia and the alar and basal plates give rise to the posterior and anterior horns, respectively. **(A)** Early cross-section through the neural tube. **(B)** Developing spinal cord cross-section. **(C)** Mature spinal cord cross-section. (Adapted with permission from Fix JD, Dudek RW. *BRS Embryology*. 3rd ed. Williams & Wilkins; 2005:67.)

table **4.1** Classification of the Nerve Fiber Types Found in the Body

Component		Abbreviation	Description
Somatic sensory	General somatic afferent	GSA	General sensation from skin and structures of head, neck, and body
Visceral sensory	General visceral afferent	GVA	Sensation from organs and blood vessels
Special sensory	Special somatic afferent	SSA	Vision, hearing, and balance
	Special visceral afferent	SVA	Smell and taste
Somatic motor	General somatic efferent	GSE	Muscles of head, neck and body wall, and extremities that develop from somites
Special motor	Special visceral efferent	SVE	Muscles of head, neck, and body wall that develop from pharyngeal arches
Visceral motor	General visceral efferent	GVE	Parasympathetic: smooth muscle, cardiac muscle, and glands

2. **Basal plate**
   - an anterolateral thickening of the mantle layer of the neural tube.
   - gives rise to the **motor neuroblasts** of the anterior and lateral horns (general somatic efferent [GSE] and general visceral efferent [GVE] cell regions). Axons from motor neuroblasts exit the spinal cord and form the anterior roots.
   - becomes the **anterior horn** of the spinal cord.
3. **Sulcus limitans**
   - a longitudinal groove in the lateral wall of the neural tube that appears during the fourth week.
   - separates the alar (sensory) and the basal (motor) plates.
   - disappears in the adult spinal cord but is retained in the rhomboid fossa of the brainstem.
   - extends from the spinal cord to the rostral midbrain.
4. **Roof plate**
   - the nonneural roof of the central canal.
5. **Floor plate**
   - the nonneural floor of the central canal.
   - contains the anterior white commissure.

B. **Myelination**
   - commences in the fourth fetal month in the spinal cord motor roots.
   1. **Oligodendrocytes accomplish myelination in the CNS**.
   2. **Schwann cells accomplish myelination in the PNS**.
   3. **Myelination** of the **corticospinal tracts** is not complete until the **end of the second postnatal year** (ie, when the corticospinal tracts become myelinated and functional).
   4. **Myelination of the association neocortex** extends into the **third decade**.

C. **Positional changes of the spinal cord**
   - Disparate growth results in the formation of the **cauda equina**, consisting of posterior and anterior roots (L3-Co) that descend inferior to the conus medullaris, and in the formation of the **filum terminale**, which anchors the spinal cord to the dura mater and coccyx.
   1. At **8 weeks**, the spinal cord extends the entire length of the vertebral canal.
   2. At **birth**, the **conus medullaris** extends to the level of the third lumbar vertebra (VL3).
   3. In **adults**, the conus medullaris terminates at the VL1-VL2 level.

VII. MEDULLA OBLONGATA (MYELENCEPHALON) (Figure 4.5 and Table 4.1)

   - develops from the caudal rhombencephalon.
   - contains the medullary pyramids (corticospinal tracts) in its base.

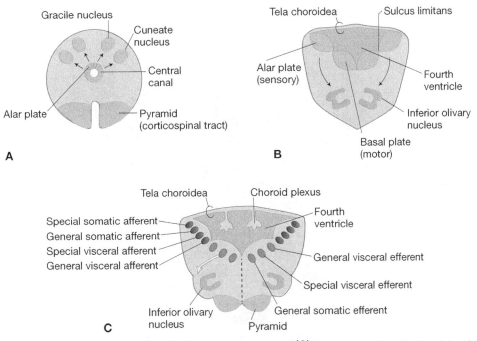

FIGURE 4.5. Schematic illustrations of the development of the medulla. **(A)** Transverse section of the caudal medulla showing the development of the gracile and cuneate nuclei from the alar plates. **(B)** Schematic sketch through the rostral (open) medulla showing the relationships of the alar and basal plates; the inferior olivary nucleus is derived from the alar plate. **(C)** A later stage of B shows the four sensory modalities of the alar plate and the three motor modalities of the basal plate; the yellow arrow indicates the lateral migration of the special visceral efferent column (CN IX and CN X); pyramids consist of motor fibers, the corticospinal tracts. (Adapted with permission from Fix JD, Dudek RW. *BRS Embryology*. 3rd ed. Williams & Wilkins; 2005:69.)

A. Alar (sensory) and basal (motor) plates

1. Closed (caudal) medulla

▪ **Alar plate sensory neuroblasts give rise to the following:**

a. **Posterior column nuclei** made up of the gracile and cuneate nuclei.

b. **Inferior olivary nuclei**—cerebellar relay nuclei.

c. **Solitary nucleus** forms the GVA (taste) and special visceral afferent (SVA) column.

d. **Spinal trigeminal nucleus** forms the GSA column.

e. **Cochlear and vestibular nuclei**

▪ form the special somatic afferent (SSA) column.

▪ lie in the medullopontine junction.

▪ **Basal plate motor neuroblasts give rise to the following:**

a. **Hypoglossal nucleus** forms **the GSE column**.

b. **Nucleus ambiguus** forms the special visceral efferent (SVE) column (CN IX and CN X).

c. **Dorsal motor nucleus of the vagus and the inferior salivatory nucleus of the glossopharyngeal nerve** form the GVE column.

2. Open (rostral) medulla (Figure 4.6; see Figure 4.5)

▪ extends from the **obex** to the **striae medullares** of the rhomboid fossa (see Figure 1.6).

▪ formation of the pontine flexure causes the lateral walls of the rostral medulla to open like a book and form the rhomboid fossa (the floor of the fourth ventricle).

a. **Alar plate**

▪ lies lateral to the sulcus limitans.

▪ its sensory neuroblasts give rise to the following:

(1) Solitary nucleus

▪ forms the GVA and SVA columns.

(2) Cochlear and vestibular nuclei

▪ form the special SSA column.

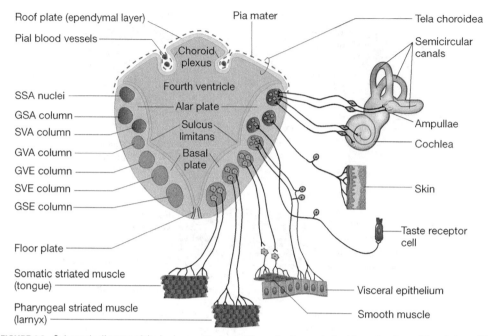

Roof plate (ependymal layer)
Pial blood vessels
Pia mater
Choroid plexus
Tela choroidea
Semicircular canals
Fourth ventricle
SSA nuclei
GSA column
SVA column
GVA column
GVE column
SVE column
GSE column
Alar plate
Sulcus limitans
Basal plate
Ampullae
Cochlea
Skin
Taste receptor cell
Floor plate
Somatic striated muscle (tongue)
Pharyngeal striated muscle (larnyx)
Visceral epithelium
Smooth muscle

FIGURE 4.6. Schematic diagram of the brainstem illustrating the cell columns derived from the alar and basal plates. The seven cranial nerve modalities are shown. GSA, general somatic afferent; GVA, general visceral afferent; GVE, general visceral efferent; SSA, special somatic afferent; SSE, special somatic efferent; SVA, special visceral afferent; SVE, special visceral efferent. (Adapted with permission from Fix JD, Dudek RW. *BRS Embryology*. 3rd ed. Williams & Wilkins; 2005:69.)

      (3) Spinal trigeminal nucleus
          ▓ forms the GSA column.
    b. Basal plate
       ▓ lies medial to the sulcus limitans.
       ▓ its motor neuroblasts give rise to the following:
         (1) Hypoglossal nucleus
             ▓ forms the GSE column.
         (2) Nucleus ambiguus
             ▓ forms the SVE column.
         (3) Dorsal motor nucleus of the vagus and the inferior salivatory nucleus of the glossopharyngeal nerve
             ▓ form the GVE column.

B. Roof plate
   ▓ forms the caudal roof of the fourth ventricle.
   ▓ the **tela choroidea**, a monolayer of ependymal cells covered with pia mater.
   ▓ invaginated by pial vessels to form the **choroid plexus of the fourth ventricle**.

VIII. METENCEPHALON (Figure 4.7 and Table 4.1; See Figure 4.3)

   ▓ develops from the rostral division of the rhombencephalon.
   ▓ gives rise to the pons and the cerebellum.

A. Pons
    1. Alar plate sensory neuroblasts give rise to the following:
       ▓ **Solitary nucleus**—forms the GVA and the SVA (taste) columns of CN VII.
       ▓ **Cochlear and vestibular nuclei**—form the SSA column of CN VIII.

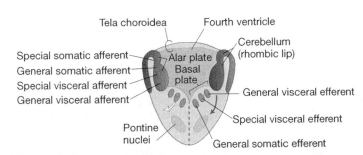

FIGURE 4.7. Schematic illustration (transverse section) of the development of the pons and cerebellum. The alar plate (rhombic lip) gives rise to the cerebellum, the four sensory cell columns, and the pontine nuclei. The basal plate gives rise to the three motor columns. The base of the pons contains the corticospinal tracts, which originate from the motor strip of the cerebral cortex. The yellow arrow indicates the lateral migration of the special visceral efferent column (CN V and CN VII). The blue arrow indicates the medial movement of visceral efferent columns. (Adapted with permission from Fix JD, Dudek RW. *BRS Embryology.* 3rd ed. Williams & Wilkins; 2005:71.)

- **Spinal and principal trigeminal nuclei**—form the GSA column of CN V.
- **Pontine nuclei**—consist of cerebellar relay nuclei (pontine gray).
2. **Basal plate motor neuroblasts give rise to the following:**
   - **Abducens nucleus**—forms the GSE column.
   - **Facial and trigeminal motor nuclei of CN VII and CN V**—form the SVE column.
   - **Superior salivatory nucleus**—forms the GVE column of CN VII.
3. **Base of the pons contains:**
   - pontine nuclei from the alar plate.
   - corticobulbar, corticospinal, and corticopontine fibers.
   - pontocerebellar fibers that are axons of neurons found in the pontine nuclei.

B. **Cerebellum**
   - formed by the **rhombic lips**, which are the thickened alar plates of the mantle layer. The **rostral** part of the cerebellum is derived from the **caudal mesencephalon**.
   - the **cerebellar anlage (primordium)**.
   1. **Vermis.**
   2. **Cerebellar hemispheres**.
   3. **Cerebellar cortex (molecular layer, Purkinje cell layer, and granular [internal] cell layer) and four pairs of deep cerebellar nuclei** formed by cell migration from the ventricular zone into the marginal layer.
   4. **External granular layer (EGL)**
      - a germinal layer on the surface of the cerebellum, present from week 8 of development to the end of the second postnatal year.
      - gives rise only to granule cells, not to basket (inner stellate) or stellate (outer stellate) neurons.
      - persistent cell nests can give rise to a neoplasm, **medulloblastoma** (see Chapter 19 VI E 2).
      - sensitive to antiviral agents that block DNA synthesis.
   5. **Folia and fissures**

IX. MESENCEPHALON (MIDBRAIN) (Figure 4.8 and Table 4.1; See Figure 4.3)

- develops from the walls of the mesencephalic vesicle.
- contains the **cerebral aqueduct** that develops from the mesencephalic cavity.

A. **Alar plate sensory neuroblasts**
   - form the cell layers of the superior colliculi and the nuclei of the inferior colliculi.

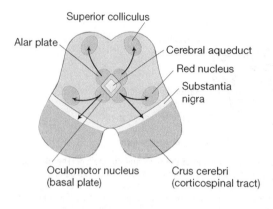

FIGURE 4.8. Schematic illustration (transverse section) of the development of the midbrain. The alar plate gives rise to the layers of the superior colliculus and the nuclei of the inferior colliculus. The basal plate gives rise to the oculomotor and trochlear nuclei, the substantia nigra, and the red nucleus. The cerebral peduncles contain the descending corticospinal tracts. (Adapted with permission from Fix JD, Dudek RW. *BRS Embryology*. 3rd ed. Williams & Wilkins; 2005:71.)

B. Basal plate motor neuroblasts
- give rise to the:
  1. **Trochlear and oculomotor nuclei of CN IV and III** that form the GSE column.
  2. **Accessory oculomotor nucleus of CN III** that forms the most rostral cell group of the GVE column.
  3. **Red nucleus and substantia nigra**.

C. Basis pedunculi (crus cerebri)
- contains corticobulbar, corticospinal, and corticopontine fibers from the cerebral cortex.

X. DEVELOPMENT OF THE DIENCEPHALON, OPTIC STRUCTURES, AND HYPOPHYSIS

A. Diencephalon (see Figure 4.3)
- develops from the **caudal part of the prosencephalon**, within the walls of the primitive third ventricle.
  1. **Epithalamus**
     - develops from the embryonic roof plate and posterior aspects of the alar plates.
     - gives rise to the **pineal body** (epiphysis) and the habenular nuclei.
     - gives rise to the habenular and posterior commissures.
     - gives rise to the **tela choroidea** and **choroid plexus of the third ventricle** from the roof plate and the pia mater.
  2. **Thalamus**
     - an alar plate derivative.
     - includes the **metathalamus** that includes the lateral geniculate body (visual system) and the medial geniculate body (auditory system).
  3. **Hypothalamus**
     - develops inferior to the hypothalamic sulcus from the alar plate and floor plates.
     - gives rise to hypothalamic nuclei, including the **mammillary bodies**, and to the **neurohypophysis**.
  4. **Subthalamus**
     - an alar plate derivative located inferior to the thalamus and lateral to the hypothalamus.
     - includes the **subthalamic nucleus, zona incerta**, and **lenticular and thalamic fasciculi**.
     - contains subthalamic neuroblasts that migrate into the telencephalon and form the **globus pallidus** (pallidum).

B. Optic vesicles, cups, and stalks (see Figure 4.3)
- derivatives of diencephalic vesicle walls.
- give rise to the retina, optic nerve, optic chiasm, and optic tract.

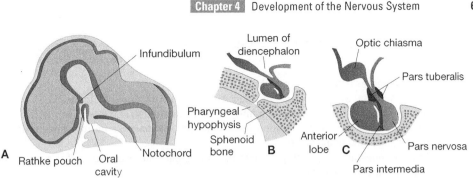

FIGURE 4.9. Schematic drawings illustrating the development of the hypophysis (pituitary gland). **(A)** Midsagittal section through the 6-week-old embryo showing Rathke pouch as a dorsal outpocketing of the oral cavity and the infundibulum as a thickening in the floor of the hypothalamus. **(B)** and **(C)** Development at 11 weeks and 16 weeks, respectively. The anterior lobe, the pars tuberalis, and the pars intermedia are derived from Rathke pouch. (Adapted with permission from Sadler TW. *Langman's Medical Embryology*. 10th ed. Lippincott Williams & Wilkins; 2006:301.)

C. Hypophysis (pituitary gland) (Figure 4.9)

1. Anterior lobe (adenohypophysis)

  ▧ develops from **Rathke pouch**, an ectodermal diverticulum of the primitive oral cavity (**stomodeum**). A craniopharyngioma is a benign suprasellar epithelial tumor that may arise from remnants of Rathke pouch (Figure 4.10).

  ▧ includes the pars tuberalis, pars intermedia, and pars distalis.

2. Posterior lobe (neurohypophysis)

  ▧ develops from a ventral evagination of the hypothalamus.

  ▧ includes the median eminence, infundibular stem, and pars nervosa.

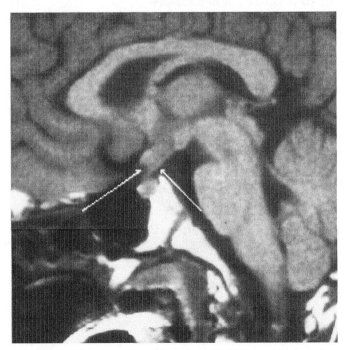

FIGURE 4.10. Midsagittal section of T_1-weighted magnetic resonance image through the brainstem and diencephalon. A craniopharyngioma (arrows) lies suprasellar in the midline, compressing the optic chiasm and hypothalamus. (Adapted with permission from Fix JD. *High-Yield Neuroanatomy*. 3rd ed. Lippincott Williams & Wilkins; 2005:45.)

XI. DEVELOPMENT OF THE TELENCEPHALON

A. Cerebral hemispheres (Figure 4.11; see Figure 4.3)
- develop as **bilateral evaginations** of the lateral walls of the **prosencephalic vesicle**.
- contain the **cerebral cortex, cerebral white matter, basal nuclei,** and **lateral ventricles**.
- are interconnected by three commissures: the **corpus callosum, anterior commissure,** and **hippocampal (fornix) commissure**.
- continuous hemispheric growth gives rise to frontal, parietal, occipital, and temporal lobes, which overlie the insula and posterior brainstem.

B. Cerebral cortex (pallium)
- formed by prosencephalic neuroblasts that migrate from the mantle layer into the marginal layer and give rise to cortical cell layers.
- classified phylogenetically as:
  1. **Neocortex** (isocortex), six-layered cortex
     - separated from the paleocortex by the **rhinal sulcus**, a continuation of the collateral sulcus.
     - represents 90% of the cortical mantle.
  2. **Allocortex**, a three-layered cortex, including the following:
     - **Paleocortex** (olfactory cortex)
     - **Archicortex** (hippocampal cortex)

C. Corpus striatum (see Figure 4.11)
- appears in the fifth week as a bulging eminence on the floor of the lateral telencephalic vesicle.
- gives rise to the caudate nucleus, putamen, amygdaloid nucleus, and claustrum. The neurons of the **globus pallidus** originate in the subthalamus; they migrate into the telencephalic white matter and become the medial segments of the lentiform nucleus.
- divided into the caudate nucleus and the lentiform nucleus by corticofugal and corticopetal fibers; these fibers make up the **internal capsule**.

D. Commissures
- fiber bundles that interconnect the two cerebral hemispheres.
  1. **Anterior commissure**
     - the first commissure to appear.
     - interconnects the olfactory structures and the middle and inferior temporal gyri.

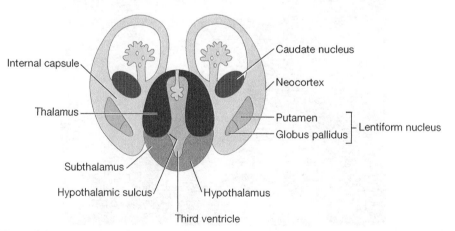

FIGURE 4.11. Schematic illustration (transverse section) of the development of the forebrain. The cerebral cortex and basal nuclei are shown. The alar plate of the diencephalon gives rise to the thalamus and the hypothalamus. Cells from the subthalamus give rise to the globus pallidus. (Adapted with permission from Fix JD, Dudek RW. *BRS Embryology*. 2nd ed. Williams & Wilkins; 1998:90.)

2. **Hippocampal commissure (fornical commissure)**
   - the second commissure to appear.
   - interconnects the two hippocampi.
3. **Corpus callosum**
   - appears between weeks 12 and 22 of development.
   - the third commissure to appear.
   - the largest commissure of the brain, which interconnects the corresponding neocortical areas of the two cerebral hemispheres.
   - does *not* project commissural fibers from the visual cortex (area 17) or the hand area of the motor or sensory strips (areas 1, 2, 3, and 4).

E. **Gyri and sulci (fissures)**
   - In the fourth month, no gyri or sulci are present; the brain is smooth or **lissencephalic**.
   - At the eighth month, all major gyri and sulci are present; the brain is convoluted or **gyrencephalic**.

XII. CONGENITAL MALFORMATIONS OF THE CENTRAL NERVOUS SYSTEM

- result from failure of the neural tube to close or separate from the surface ectoderm (eg, spina bifida).
- result from failure of the vertebral arches to fuse.
- result from failure of midline cleavage of the embryonic forebrain (eg, holoprosencephaly).

A. **Neural tube defects (eg, spina bifida and anencephaly)**
   - can be detected prenatally by screening for **high alpha-fetoprotein levels** in the amniotic fluid or in the maternal serum (**low alpha-fetoprotein levels** are found in **Down syndrome**) and subsequently confirmed through ultrasound.
   1. **Spina bifida** (Figure 4.12)
      - usually occurs in the sacrolumbar region.
      - results from failure of the **posterior neuropore** to close.
      - includes the following variations:

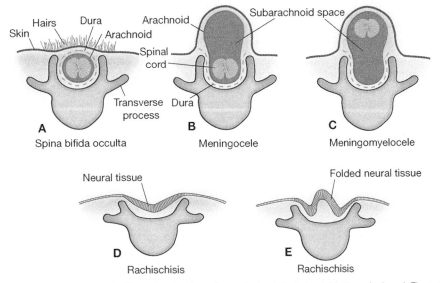

FIGURE 4.12. Schematic drawings illustrating a variety of neural tube defects involving the spinal cord. The term *spina bifida* applies to all of the defects because the bony arch of one or more vertebrae has failed to fuse posteriorly to the spinal cord. (Adapted with permission from Sadler TW. *Langman's Medical Embryology.* 10th ed. Lippincott Williams & Wilkins; 2006:294.)

a. **Spina bifida occulta**
   - a defect in the vertebral arches.
   - the least severe type of spina bifida.
   - occurs in ~10% of the population.
   - often indicated by a tuft of hair over the defect.

b. **Spina bifida cystica**
   - the major form of **dysraphism**.
   - most often localized in lumbar and lumbosacral regions.

   (1) Spina bifida with meningocele
   - occurs when the meninges project through a vertebral defect forming a sac filled with CSF.
   - exists with the spinal cord remaining in its normal position.

   (2) Spina bifida with meningomyelocele
   - occurs when the meninges and spinal cord project through a vertebral defect and forms a sac.
   - is the commonest variation of spina bifida cystica (80%-90%).
   - is usually present in Chiari malformation (See Figure 4.14).

   (3) Spina bifida with myeloschisis
   - the most severe type of spina bifida.
   - results in an open neural tube that lies on the surface of the back.

CLINICAL CORRELATES   Failure of the **anterior neuropore** to close results in **anencephaly** (meroanencephaly), which leads to failure of the brain and skull to properly develop. A rudimentary brainstem is usually present. Anencephaly occurs once in every 1,000 births.

B. **Ossification defects of the occipital bone (Figure 4.13)**
   - also called **cranium bifidum**.
   - occurs once in every 2,000 births.
   - **Encephaloceles** occur in the occiput (75%) and in the sinciput (25%).
   - include the following variations:
     1. **Cranial meningocele**
     2. **Meningoencephalocele**
     3. **Meningohydroencephalocele**

C. **Chiari malformation (Figures 4.14 and 4.15)**
   - a cerebellomedullary malformation where the caudal vermis, cerebellar tonsils, and medulla herniate through the foramen magnum and result in obstructive hydrocephalus.
   - frequently associated with spina bifida (meningomyelocele) and platybasia (flattening of the skull base), with malformation of the occipitovertebral joint.
   - affected children may have dysphonia, laryngeal stridor, and respiratory arrest (involvement of CN X).
   - occurs once in every 1,000 births.

D. **Dandy-Walker syndrome (Figure 4.16)**
   - consists of a huge **cyst of the posterior fossa** associated with atresia of the outlet foramina of the fourth ventricle.
   - associated with dilation of the fourth ventricle, **agenesis of the cerebellar vermis**, occipital meningocele, and frequently agenesis of the splenium of the corpus callosum.

E. **Fetal alcohol syndrome**
   - includes the following clinical characteristics: (1) growth retardation, (2) CNS abnormalities, and (3) facial dysmorphisms—short palpebral fissures, thin vermilion border, and a smooth philtrum.
   - occurs in 0.5 to 2 per 1,000 births.

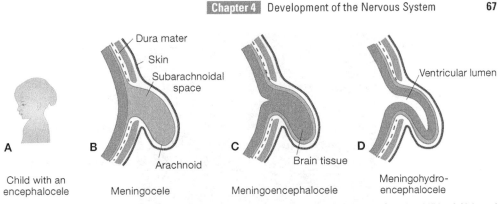

FIGURE 4.13. Schematic drawings illustrating the various types of occipital encephaloceles (cranium bifidum). (Adapted with permission from Sadler TW. *Langman's Medical Embryology.* 10th ed. Lippincott Williams & Wilkins; 2006:308.)

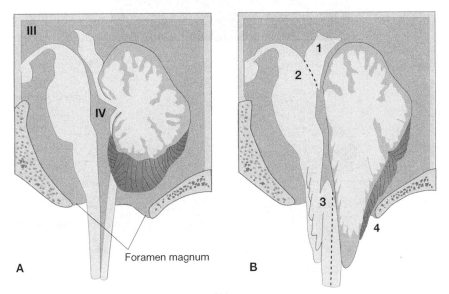

FIGURE 4.14. Chiari malformation, midsagittal section. **(A)** Normal cerebellum, fourth ventricle (IV), and brainstem. **(B)** Abnormal cerebellum, fourth ventricle, and brainstem showing the common congenital anomalies: (1) breaking of the tectal plate, (2) aqueductal stenosis, (3) kinking and transforaminal herniation of the medulla into the vertebral canal, and (4) herniation and unrolling of the cerebellar vermis into the vertebral canal. An accompanying meningomyelocele is common. (Adapted with permission from Fix JD. *High-Yield Neuroanatomy.* 3rd ed. Lippincott Williams & Wilkins; 2005:46.)

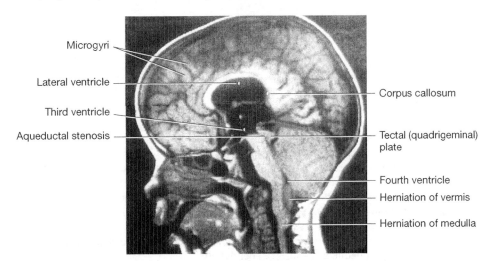

FIGURE 4.15. Chiari malformation, midsagittal section, T_2-weighted magnetic resonance imaging.

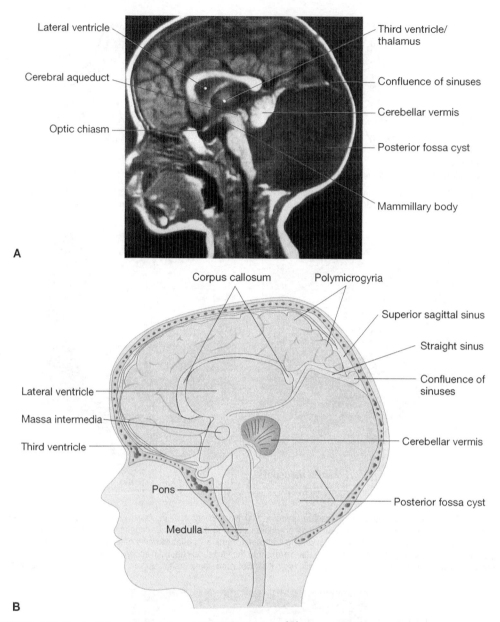

FIGURE 4.16. Dandy-Walker malformation, midsagittal section. **(A)** T$_2$-weighted magnetic resonance imaging. **(B)** Diagram. An enormous dilation of the fourth ventricle results from the failure of the median and lateral foramina to open. This condition is associated with occipital meningocele, elevation of the confluence of the sinuses (torcular herophili), agenesis of the cerebellar vermis, and splenium of the corpus callosum. (Adapted from Fix JD. *High-Yield Embryology.* 3rd ed. Williams & Wilkins; 2005:46.)

F. Hydrocephalus (Figure 4.17 and Chapter 2 IV)

▨ a dilation of the ventricles owing to an excess of CSF.

▨ typically results from blockage of CSF circulation (eg, aqueductal stenosis). **Aqueductal stenosis** is the commonest cause of congenital hydrocephalus; it may be transmitted by an X-linked trait or may be caused by **cytomegalovirus** infection or **toxoplasmosis**.

1. **Communicating hydrocephalus** results from impaired absorption in the subarachnoid space (eg, meningitis).
2. **Noncommunicating (obstructive) hydrocephalus** results from obstruction within the ventricle system (eg, aqueductal stenosis or ependymitis).

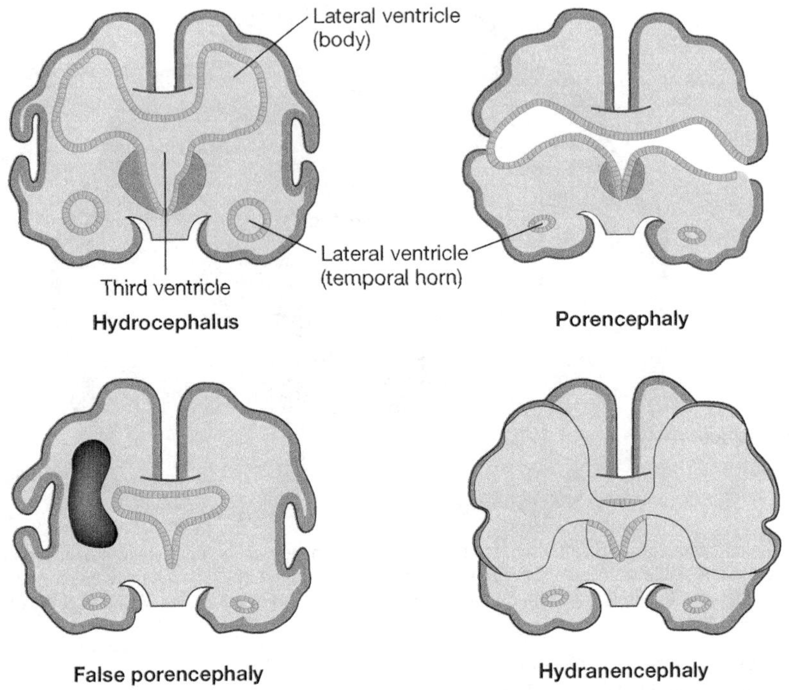

FIGURE 4.17. Cystic malformations of the prosencephalon (forebrain). Note the ependymal lining of these cysts. In hydranencephaly, the cyst is lined by glia and leptomeninges. In false porencephaly, the cyst is lined by glia. (Adapted with permission from Dudek RW, Fix JD. *BRS Embryology.* 2nd ed. Williams & Wilkins; 1998:98.)

G. Holoprosencephaly (Figure 4.18)

- results from failure of midline cleavage (diverticularization) of the embryonic forebrain. The telencephalon contains a single ventricular cavity.
- characterized by the absence of olfactory bulbs and tracts (**arhinencephaly**) and, commonly, midfacial defects.
- seen in trisomy 13 (**Patau syndrome**).
- may result from alcohol abuse during pregnancy, especially in the first 4 weeks.
- the most severe manifestation of **fetal alcohol syndrome**.
- in extreme forms (alobar and semilobar), it results in the absence of corpus callosum and septum pellucidum.
- occurs a little over once in every 10,000 births.

H. Polyhydramnios

- an excess of amniotic fluid.
- may result from decreased fetal swallowing of amniotic fluid (eg, esophageal atresia) or an increase in fetal urine production.
- occurs in 1% to 2% of pregnancies.

I. Hydranencephaly (see Figure 4.17)

- a congenital absence of the cerebral hemispheres that are replaced by immensely dilated ventricles.
- most likely results from bilateral hemispheric infarction secondary to occlusion of the carotid arteries in utero.
- cerebellum, thalami, and basal nuclei are preserved.

J. Porencephaly (see Figure 4.17)

- fluid-filled cystic cavitation of the prosencephalon. The cavity is lined with white matter and communicates with the lateral ventricle.

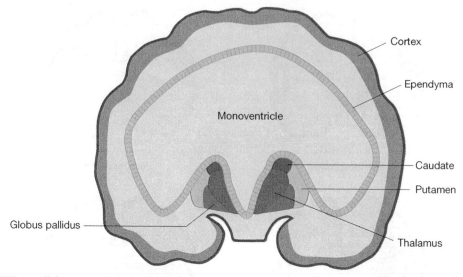

FIGURE 4.18. Holoprosencephaly results from failure of midline cleavage of the embryonic prosencephalon. The telencephalon contains a single ventricular cavity. It may result from alcohol abuse, especially during the first 4 weeks of pregnancy. (Adapted with permission from Dudek RW, Fix JD. *BRS Embryology*. 2nd ed. Williams & Wilkins; 1998:99.)

- called schizencephaly when lined with gray matter.
- most likely caused by fetal stroke or infection.

K. False porencephaly (see Figure 4.17)
- a malformation consisting of cystic cavities that are lined with glia and do not communicate with the lateral ventricle.

L. Tethered spinal cord (filum terminale syndrome)
- results from a thick, short filum terminale.
- often coincident with spina bifida.
- leads to weakness and sensory deficits in the lower extremity and a neurogenic bladder.

Review Test

1. A 17-year-old girl presents to her primary care physician for evaluation, suspecting that she became pregnant some months prior. She is referred to an OB-GYN, who determines that she is in her third trimester. An ultrasound reveals an absence of the brain and calvaria. What is the diagnosis of this malformation?

(A) Anencephaly
(B) Chiari malformation
(C) Holoprosencephaly
(D) Meningoencephalocele
(E) Spina bifida occulta

2. A 28-year-old woman presents to her OB-GYN for routine evaluation of her pregnancy. Patient history is unremarkable, except that she had a difficult time conceiving and had been trying for several years. Sonogram of the fetus reveals a large cyst in the posterior cranial fossa with enlargement of the fourth ventricle. The tentorium cerebelli is displaced superiorly. Further imaging reveals agenesis of the cerebellar vermis. What is the diagnosis of this malformation?

(A) Chiari malformation
(B) Cranial meningocele
(C) Dandy-Walker syndrome
(D) Porencephaly
(E) Spina bifida cystica

3. The neural retina is derived from the

(A) alar plate.
(B) choroids.
(C) neural crest.
(D) neural tube.
(E) telencephalic vesicle wall.

4. At which vertebral level is the conus medullaris found at birth?

(A) VT12
(B) VL1
(C) VL3
(D) VS1
(E) VS4

5. Caudal herniation of the cerebellar tonsils and medulla through the foramen magnum is called

(A) Chiari syndrome.
(B) cranium bifidum.
(C) Dandy-Walker syndrome.
(D) Down syndrome.
(E) myeloschisis.

6. A newborn has multiple congenital defects owing to dysgenesis of the neural crest. Which of the following cells is most likely to be spared?

(A) Geniculate ganglion cells
(B) Melanocytes
(C) Motor neurons
(D) Parafollicular cells
(E) Spinal ganglion cells

Questions 7 to 11

Match the statements in items 7 to 11 with the appropriate lettered structure shown in the figure.

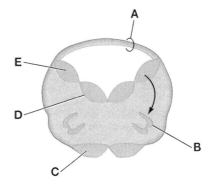

7. Is derived from the telencephalon

8. Gives rise to the choroid plexus

9. Is derived from the alar plate

10. Gives rise to motor neurons that innervate the tongue

11. Gives rise to the solitary nucleus

Questions 12 to 16

Match the statements in items 12 to 16 with the appropriate lettered structure shown in the figure.

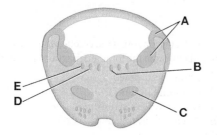

12. Innervates the lateral rectus

13. Gives rise to a parasympathetic nucleus

14. Gives rise to the cerebellum

15. Is derived from the alar plate

16. Gives rise to motor neurons that migrate into the lateral pontine tegmentum

Answers and Explanations

1. **A.** Anencephaly is caused by failure of the anterior neuropore to close, leading to the absence of brain and calvaria superior to the orbits. It is diagnosed with high accuracy using ultrasound. Chiari malformation involves deviation of the cerebellum, not the brain per se. Holoprosencephaly is a condition where the prosencephalon fails to develop, the forebrain, but other parts of the brain and skull may develop appropriately. The other anomalies listed are not related to lack of a brain or calvaria. Meningoencephalocele is related to the meninges and spina bifida occulta to the spinal cord.

2. **C.** Dandy-Walker syndrome is a genetic malformation that is most prevalent in individuals that have difficulty conceiving. It is accurately diagnosed with sonography that shows cystic dilation in the fourth ventricle, displaced cerebellar tentorium, and agenesis of the cerebellar vermis. Chiari malformation involves herniation of the cerebellum, and it is typically displaced inferiorly, not superiorly. Cranial meningocele would not cause cerebellar agenesis. Porencephaly refers to the development of cysts in the brain, typically multiple and unlikely to cause displacement of the tentorium. Spina bifida cystica involves the spinal cord, not the brain.

3. **D.** The retina is derived from the neural tube, which gives rise to the entire CNS. It develops as an outpocketing of the diencephalon. The alar plate is involved with spinal cord development, specifically the sensory-oriented structures posterior to the sulcus limitans. The choroid is the middle (vascular) tunic of the eye in the adult; it is separate from and external to the retina. Neural crest gives rise to a large number of structures, including ganglia, Schwann cells, and even the aorticopulmonary septum. The telencephalic vesicle wall forms the cerebral hemispheres and olfactory bulbs.

4. **C.** At birth, the conus medullaris extends to VL3, and in the adult, it extends to the VL1-VL2 interspace. At 8 weeks, the spinal cord extends the entire length of the vertebral canal.

5. **A.** Chiari syndrome is a cerebellomedullary malformation where the inferior vermis and medulla herniate through the foramen magnum and result in communicating hydrocephalus. Chiari syndrome is frequently associated with spina bifida. Cranium bifidum is an ossification defect of the occipital bone, which leads to encephaloceles. Dandy-Walker syndrome involves the formation of a large cyst in the posterior cranial fossa and cerebellar agenesis. Myeloschisis involves failure of the neural tube to properly close and does not involve cranial structures.

6. **C.** Motor neurons develop from the neural tube, more specifically from the basal plate. All other options are derivatives of the neural crest.

7. **C.** The corticospinal tract (pyramid) has its origin in the neocortex of the telencephalon.

8. **A.** The tela choroidea gives rise to the choroid plexus.

9. **B.** The inferior olivary nucleus is derived from the alar plate of the developing medulla.

10. **D.** The basal plate gives rise to the hypoglossal nucleus, which provides motor innervation to the tongue.

11. **E.** The alar plate gives rise to the solitary nucleus.

12. **B.** The GSE column innervates the lateral rectus.

13. **E.** The GVE column gives rise to the superior salivatory nucleus of CN VII. This parasympathetic nucleus innervates the lacrimal, the sublingual, and the submandibular glands and also the palatine and nasal glands.

14. **A.** The cerebellum is derived from the alar plate. The alar plate gives rise to the rhombic lip, which becomes the cerebellum.

15. **C.** The pontine nuclei are derived from the alar plate.

16. **D.** The SVE column gives rise to motor neurons that migrate into the lateral pontine tegmentum and become the facial nucleus, CN VII.

Objectives

- Classify neurons according to their morphology.
- Recognize unique structural and functional characteristics of neurons.
- List the various types of neuroglia and include a description of each along with a description of the various types of gliomas.
- Describe the processes of nerve cell degeneration and regeneration.
- List the types of axonal transport and the mechanisms associated with each type.
- Describe the types of peripheral nervous system receptors and include characteristics such as adaption level, modality, and fiber types associated with each.

I. OVERVIEW

- consists of neurons and glial cells.
- cells develop from ectoderm (neural tube and neural crest), microglia are of mesodermal origin.

II. NEURONS

- electrically excitable.
- limited capacity for cell division.
- capacity to *receive* impulses from receptor organs or other neurons.
- capacity to *transmit* impulses to other neurons or effector organs.
- consist of a **cell body** and its processes, **dendrites**, and an **axon**.

A. Classification of neurons (Figure 5.1)

- according to **number of processes** (unipolar, bipolar, or multipolar), **axonal length, function**, and **neurotransmitter**.
  1. Processes
     - **Unipolar or pseudounipolar neurons**
       a. sensory neurons in the posterior root and cranial nerve (CN) ganglia and in the mesencephalic nucleus midbrain.
     - **Bipolar neurons**
       a. located in the vestibular and cochlear ganglia of the vestibulocochlear nerve (CN VIII), the retina, and the olfactory epithelium (CN I).

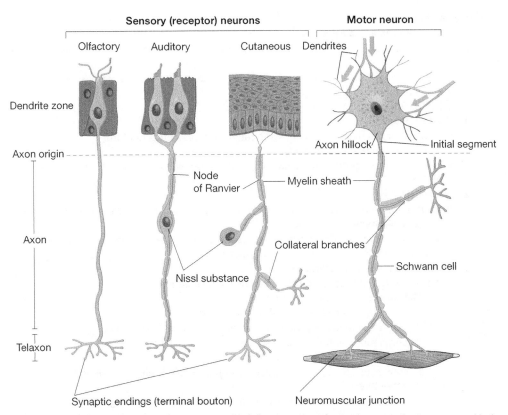

FIGURE 5.1. Types of nerve cells. Olfactory neurons are bipolar and unmyelinated, whereas auditory neurons are bipolar and myelinated. Spinal ganglion cells (cutaneous) are pseudounipolar and myelinated and motor neurons are multipolar and myelinated. Arrows indicate input via axons of other neurons. Nerve cells are characterized by the presence of Nissl substance and rough endoplasmic reticulum. (Adapted with permission from Carpenter MB, Sutin J. *Human Neuroanatomy.* 8th ed. Williams & Wilkins; 1983:92.)

> **Multipolar neurons**
>   **a.** possess one axon and multiple dendrites.
>   **b.** the largest population of nerve cells in the nervous system.
>   **c.** include motor neurons, interneurons, pyramidal cells of the cerebral cortex, and Purkinje cells of the cerebellar cortex.
>
> **2. Axonal length**
> > **Golgi type I neurons**
> >   **a.** long axons (eg, giant pyramidal cells of Betz of the motor cortex).
> > **Golgi type II neurons**
> >   **a.** short axons (eg, interneurons).
>
> **3. Function**
> > **Motor neurons**
> >   **a.** conduct impulses to muscles, glands, and blood vessels.
> >   **b.** found in the anterior horn of the spinal cord.
> > **Sensory neurons**
> >   **a.** receive stimuli from the external and internal environment (eg, spinal ganglion cells).
> > **Interneurons**
> >   **a.** intercalated or internuncial neurons that interconnect motor or sensory neurons within the central nervous system (CNS).
>
> **4. Neurotransmitter (discussed in Chapter 21)**

B. Nerve cell body

- also called the **soma** or **perikaryon**.
- contains the organelles found in other cells, including a large nucleus and a prominent nucleolus.
- has receptor molecules on its plasmalemmal surface that confer sensitivity to various neurotransmitters.
- contains the following structures/specializations:

1. Nissl substance
- consists of rosettes of polysomes and rough endoplasmic reticulum.
- plays a role in **protein synthesis**.
- abundant throughout cytoplasm and dendrites but is *not* found in the axon hillock or in the axon.

2. Lysosomes
- membrane-bound dense bodies that contain hydrolytic enzymes and are involved in the process of **intracellular digestion**.
- a genetic defect in the synthesis of lysosomal enzymes results in a storage disease (eg, Tay-Sachs disease [GM_2 gangliosidosis]).

3. Filamentous protein structures
- form an internal support framework—the **cytoskeleton**:
  - **a. Microtubules** (25 nm in diameter)
    - found in the cell body, dendrites, and axons.
    - play a role in the **development** and **maintenance** of cell shape.
    - play a role in intracellular transport.
  - **b. Neurofilaments** (10 nm in diameter)
    - consist of spiral protein threads that play a role in **developing** and **regenerating nerve fibers**.
    - degenerate in Alzheimer disease to form **neurofibrillary tangles**.
    - contain a neurofilament protein that is exclusive to neurons and their precursors.
  - **c. Microfilaments** (5 nm in diameter)
    - composed of **actin**.
    - found in the tips of growing axons.
    - facilitate movement of plasma membrane and growth of nerve cell processes.

4. Inclusion bodies
  - **a. Lipofuscin (lipochrome) granules**
    - pigment granules:
    - common pigmented inclusions of cytoplasm that accumulate with aging.
    - considered to be residual bodies derived from lysosomes.
  - **b. Neuromelanin (melanin)**
    - blackish pigment in the neurons of substantia nigra and locus ceruleus.
    - disappears from the substantia nigra and the locus ceruleus in Parkinson disease.
  - **c. Lewy bodies**
    - eosinophilic intracytoplasmic inclusion bodies found in the substantia nigra in patients with Parkinson disease.

5. Dendrites
- processes that extend from the cell body.
- contain cytoplasm similar in composition to that of the cell body; however, no Golgi apparatus is present.
- conduct in a decremental fashion and capable of generating action potentials.
- receive synaptic input and transmit toward the cell body.

6. Axons
- typically arise from the cell body.
- originate from the axon hillock, which lacks Nissl substance.
- give rise to collateral branches.
- myelinated or unmyelinated.
- **generate, propagate, and transmit action potentials**.
- end distally in terminal boutons in synapses with neurons, muscle cells, and glands.

t a b l e **5.1**	Classification of Nerve Fibers		
Fibers	Diameter (mm)ª	Conduction Velocity (m/s)	Function
Sensory axons			
Ia (A-α)	12-20	70-120	Proprioception and muscle spindles
Ib (A-α)	12-20	70-120	Proprioception and Golgi tendon organs
II (A-β)	5-12	30-70	Touch, pressure, and vibration
III (A-δ)	2-5	12-30	Touch, pressure, fast pain, and temperature
IV (C)	0.5-1	0.5-2	Slow pain and temperature, unmyelinated fibers
Motor axons			
Alpha (A-α)	12-20	15-120	Alpha motor neurons of anterior horn (innervate extrafusal muscle fibers)
Gamma (A-γ)	2-10	10-45	Gamma motor neurons of anterior horn (innervate intrafusal muscle fibers)
Preganglionic autonomic fibers (B)	<3	3-15	Myelinated preganglionic autonomic fibers
Postganglionic autonomic fibers (C)	1	2	Unmyelinated postganglionic autonomic fibers

ªMyelin sheath included if present.

7. **Nerve fibers** (Table 5.1)
   - consist of axons, dendrites, and their glial investments.
   - classified by function, fiber size, and conduction velocity.
8. **Myelin sheath**
   - formed in the peripheral nervous system (PNS) by Schwann cells.
   - formed in the CNS by oligodendrocytes.
   - interrupted by the nodes of Ranvier.
   - consists of wrappings of the Schwann cell or oligodendrocyte plasma membrane around nerve fibers.
   - speeds impulses along the nerve fiber via saltatory conduction.
9. **Synapses**
   - the **sites of functional contact** of a nerve cell with another nerve cell, an effector cell, or a sensory receptor cell.
   - consist of presynaptic membrane, synaptic cleft, and postsynaptic membrane.
   - classified by the site of contact (eg, axosomatic, axodendritic, or axoaxonic).
   - also classified as chemical or electrical:
     a. **Chemical synapses**
        - use neurotransmitters.
     b. **Electrical synapses (ephapses)**
        - consist of gap junctions.
        - allow ions to pass from cell to cell.

III. NEUROGLIA

- non-neuronal cells of the CNS and the PNS.
- arise from the neural tube and neural crest.
- capable of cell division.
- classified as **macroglia** (**astrocytes** and **oligodendrocytes**), **microglia**, and **ependyma**. Schwann cells are classified as peripheral neuroglia.

A. Astrocytes
- the largest glial cells.
- consist of **fibrous astrocytes** that are found mainly in white matter and **protoplasmic astrocytes** that are found mainly in gray matter.

■ play a role in the metabolism of certain neurotransmitters (gamma-aminobutyric acid, serotonin, and glutamate).
■ buffer the potassium concentration of the extracellular space.
■ contain glial filaments and glycogen granules as their most characteristic cytoplasmic components.
■ form glial scars in damaged areas of the brain—**gliosis**.
■ contain or give rise to the following structures:

1. Astrocytic end feet
■ the processes that form the external glial limiting membrane (interface between pia mater and the CNS) and the internal glial limiting membrane (interface between the ependyma and the CNS).

a. Perivascular end feet
■ surround capillaries.
■ contribute to the blood-brain barrier.

b. Perineuronal end feet
■ surround neurons.

2. Glial filaments
■ contain **glial fibrillary acidic protein (GFAP)**, a marker for astrocytes.

3. Glycogen granules
■ accumulations of polysaccharide.

B. Oligodendrocytes
■ small glial cells with few short processes.
■ lack glial filaments and glycogen granules.
■ myelin-forming cells of the CNS; one oligodendrocyte can myelinate the internodal parts of numerous axons.

1. Interfascicular oligodendrocytes
■ found in white matter.

2. Satellite cells
■ found in gray matter.

C. Microglia
■ arise from monocytes that enter the CNS from the blood.
■ activated by inflammatory and degenerative processes.
■ are macrophages that are migratory and phagocytic.

D. Ependymal cells
■ line the central canal of the spinal cord and ventricles of the brain.
■ possess cilia.
■ include the choroid epithelial cells of the choroid plexus and tanycytes of the third ventricle; the choroid plexus cells produce cerebrospinal fluid (CSF) and are interconnected by tight junctions that contribute to the **blood-CSF barrier**.

E. Schwann cells (neurolemmal cells)
■ derivatives of the neural crest.
■ myelin-forming cells of the PNS; a Schwann cell myelinates only one internode.
■ invest unmyelinated axons of the PNS.
■ function in regeneration and remyelination of severed axons in the PNS (Figure 5.2).
■ separated from each other by the **node of Ranvier**.

F. Tumors (gliomas) (Figure 5.3)
■ derived from astrocytes, oligodendrocytes, or ependymocytes.
■ result from proliferation of glioblasts—embryonic precursors.
■ represent the majority of malignant brain tumors.

1. Astrocytomas (see Figure 5.3)
■ most commonly found in the white matter of the cerebral hemisphere in middle and late life.
■ astrocytomas of the cerebellum are the commonest intracranial tumor in children.
■ commonest type of brain cancer.

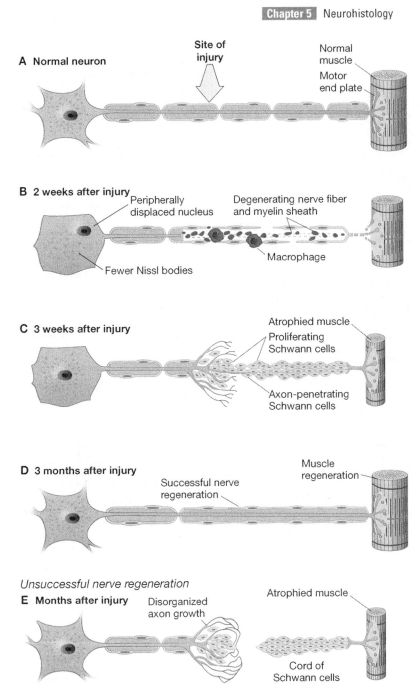

A Normal neuron

Site of injury

Normal muscle

Motor end plate

B 2 weeks after injury

Peripherally displaced nucleus

Degenerating nerve fiber and myelin sheath

Macrophage

Fewer Nissl bodies

C 3 weeks after injury

Atrophied muscle

Proliferating Schwann cells

Axon-penetrating Schwann cells

D 3 months after injury

Muscle regeneration

Successful nerve regeneration

Unsuccessful nerve regeneration

E Months after injury

Disorganized axon growth

Atrophied muscle

Cord of Schwann cells

FIGURE 5.2. Wallerian (anterograde) degeneration and regeneration of a peripheral nerve fiber.

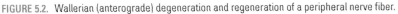

CLINICAL CORRELATES   **Astrocytomas** arise from **astroblasts**; they may be benign or malignant. **Benign astrocytomas** are slow-growing infiltrative neoplasms. They represent ~25% of primary intracranial tumors and frequently become malignant. **Malignant astrocytomas** (glioblastoma multiforme) are rapidly growing, fatal astrocytic tumors. They occur twice as frequently in men as in women and are the commonest primary brain tumors.

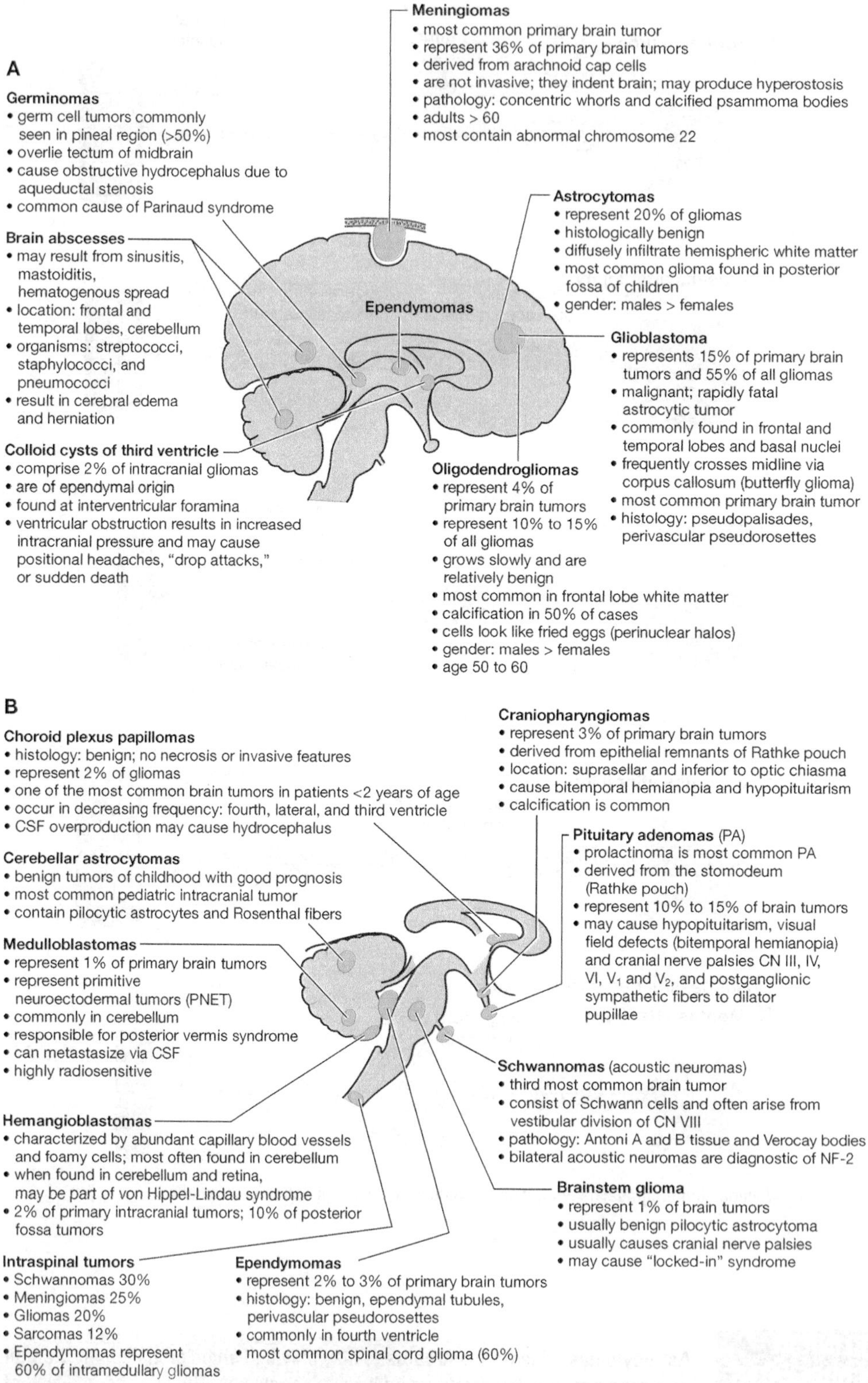

A

Germinomas
- germ cell tumors commonly seen in pineal region (>50%)
- overlie tectum of midbrain
- cause obstructive hydrocephalus due to aqueductal stenosis
- common cause of Parinaud syndrome

Brain abscesses
- may result from sinusitis, mastoiditis, hematogenous spread
- location: frontal and temporal lobes, cerebellum
- organisms: streptococci, staphylococci, and pneumococci
- result in cerebral edema and herniation

Colloid cysts of third ventricle
- comprise 2% of intracranial gliomas
- are of ependymal origin
- found at interventricular foramina
- ventricular obstruction results in increased intracranial pressure and may cause positional headaches, "drop attacks," or sudden death

Meningiomas
- most common primary brain tumor
- represent 36% of primary brain tumors
- derived from arachnoid cap cells
- are not invasive; they indent brain; may produce hyperostosis
- pathology: concentric whorls and calcified psammoma bodies
- adults > 60
- most contain abnormal chromosome 22

Ependymomas

Astrocytomas
- represent 20% of gliomas
- histologically benign
- diffusely infiltrate hemispheric white matter
- most common glioma found in posterior fossa of children
- gender: males > females

Glioblastoma
- represents 15% of primary brain tumors and 55% of all gliomas
- malignant; rapidly fatal astrocytic tumor
- commonly found in frontal and temporal lobes and basal nuclei
- frequently crosses midline via corpus callosum (butterfly glioma)
- most common primary brain tumor
- histology: pseudopalisades, perivascular pseudorosettes

Oligodendrogliomas
- represent 4% of primary brain tumors
- represent 10% to 15% of all gliomas
- grows slowly and are relatively benign
- most common in frontal lobe white matter
- calcification in 50% of cases
- cells look like fried eggs (perinuclear halos)
- gender: males > females
- age 50 to 60

B

Choroid plexus papillomas
- histology: benign; no necrosis or invasive features
- represent 2% of gliomas
- one of the most common brain tumors in patients <2 years of age
- occur in decreasing frequency: fourth, lateral, and third ventricle
- CSF overproduction may cause hydrocephalus

Cerebellar astrocytomas
- benign tumors of childhood with good prognosis
- most common pediatric intracranial tumor
- contain pilocytic astrocytes and Rosenthal fibers

Medulloblastomas
- represent 1% of primary brain tumors
- represent primitive neuroectodermal tumors (PNET)
- commonly in cerebellum
- responsible for posterior vermis syndrome
- can metastasize via CSF
- highly radiosensitive

Hemangioblastomas
- characterized by abundant capillary blood vessels and foamy cells; most often found in cerebellum
- when found in cerebellum and retina, may be part of von Hippel-Lindau syndrome
- 2% of primary intracranial tumors; 10% of posterior fossa tumors

Intraspinal tumors
- Schwannomas 30%
- Meningiomas 25%
- Gliomas 20%
- Sarcomas 12%
- Ependymomas represent 60% of intramedullary gliomas

Ependymomas
- represent 2% to 3% of primary brain tumors
- histology: benign, ependymal tubules, perivascular pseudorosettes
- commonly in fourth ventricle
- most common spinal cord glioma (60%)

Craniopharyngiomas
- represent 3% of primary brain tumors
- derived from epithelial remnants of Rathke pouch
- location: suprasellar and inferior to optic chiasma
- cause bitemporal hemianopia and hypopituitarism
- calcification is common

Pituitary adenomas (PA)
- prolactinoma is most common PA
- derived from the stomodeum (Rathke pouch)
- represent 10% to 15% of brain tumors
- may cause hypopituitarism, visual field defects (bitemporal hemianopia) and cranial nerve palsies CN III, IV, VI, V_1 and V_2, and postganglionic sympathetic fibers to dilator pupillae

Schwannomas (acoustic neuromas)
- third most common brain tumor
- consist of Schwann cells and often arise from vestibular division of CN VIII
- pathology: Antoni A and B tissue and Verocay bodies
- bilateral acoustic neuromas are diagnostic of NF-2

Brainstem glioma
- represent 1% of brain tumors
- usually benign pilocytic astrocytoma
- usually causes cranial nerve palsies
- may cause "locked-in" syndrome

FIGURE 5.3. Tumors of the central nervous system. **(A)** Supratentorial tumors. **(B)** Infratentorial tumors (posterior fossa) and intraspinal tumors. In children, 70% of tumors are infratentorial. In adults, 70% of tumors are supratentorial. CN, cranial nerve; CSF, cerebrospinal fluid. (Adapted with permission from Fix JD. *High-Yield Neuroanatomy.* 3rd ed. Lippincott Williams & Wilkins; 2005:52.)

1. **Oligodendrogliomas** (see Figure 5.3)
   - slow-growing, benign tumors.
   - occur mainly in adults.
   - most frequently found in the cerebral hemisphere.
   - may arise from **oligodendroblasts**, embryonic precursors.
   - usually well-circumscribed and are frequently calcified.
   - may change and become glioblastomas.
2. **Ependymomas** (see Figure 5.3)
   - slow-growing, benign circumscribed neoplasms typically found within the ventricles.
   - the commonest gliomas found in the spinal cord, most frequently in the lumbosacral segments.
   - arise from **ependymal cells**.
3. **Schwannomas** (see Figure 5.3)
   - benign tumors of peripheral nerves.
   - account for 6% of primary intracranial tumors.
   - occur twice as frequently in females as in males.
   - arise from **Schwann cells**.
4. **Meningiomas** (see Figure 5.3)
   - slow-growing tumors of mesenchymal origin.
   - account for 15% of primary intracranial tumors.
   - supratentorial in 90% of cases.
   - have a female-to-male ratio of 3:2.
5. **Medulloblastomas** (see Figure 5.3)
   - found in the infratentorial compartment and are thought to arise from the external granular layer of the cerebellar cortex.
   - represent ~20% of the primary intracranial tumors found in children.

CLINICAL CORRELATES   **Pituitary adenomas** are slow-growing, benign tumors mostly of the anterior pituitary gland. They are common—about 1 in 10 people will develop a pituitary adenoma in their lifetime. Those that secrete hormones are "functional adenomas," the most common of which produce prolactin, a **prolactinoma**.

IV. NERVE CELL DEGENERATION AND REGENERATION (See Figure 5.2)

A. Retrograde degeneration
- occurs toward the proximal end of an axon and the cell body.
- takes place in both the CNS and the PNS.
- reaction begins 2 days (or sooner) after insult and reaches a maximum at ~20 days.
- involves the following changes:
  1. Disappearance of Nissl substance (chromatolysis)
  2. Swelling of the cell body
  3. Flattening and displacement of the nucleus to the periphery

B. Anterograde (Wallerian) degeneration (see Figure 5.2)
- occurs toward the distal end of the axon.
- takes place in both the PNS and the CNS.
- characterized by successive fragmentation and disappearance of axons and myelin sheaths and by secondary proliferation of Schwann cells.

C. Regeneration of the peripheral nerve fiber (see Figure 5.2)

- If the severed distal nerve fiber maintains its integrity and the basement membrane and endoneurium are maintained, an axon sprout may grow into it.
- Schwann cells proliferate along a degenerating axon and myelinate a new axonal sprout, which grows at the rate of ~3 mm/d.
- If the path of regenerating axons is blocked, a neuroma forms at the site of obstruction. A neuroma comprises a proliferative mass of axons and Schwann cells.

D. Regeneration of axons in the CNS

- No Schwann cell basement membranes or endoneurial investments surround axons of the CNS.
- Effective regeneration does not occur in the CNS because of the formation of an astroglial scar after axonal injury, specific proteins in the CNS myelin, lack of growth factors, and slow debris clearance relative to the PNS.

V. AXONAL TRANSPORT

- mediates the intracellular distribution of secretory proteins, organelles, and cytoskeletal elements.
- inhibited by colchicine that depolymerizes microtubules.

A. Fast anterograde transport

- microtubule dependent.
- responsible for transporting newly synthesized membranous organelles (vesicles) and precursors of neurotransmitters.
- rate of 200 to 400 mm/d.
- mediated by microtubules and **kinesin**.

B. Slow anterograde transport

- responsible for transporting cytoskeletal and cytoplasmic elements.
- rate of 1 to 5 mm/d.
- moves unidirectionally away from the cell body.
- transports neurofilaments and microtubules.

C. Fast retrograde transport

- returns used materials from the axon terminal to the cell body for degradation and recycling.
- rate of 100 to 200 mm/d.
- transports nerve growth factor and neurotropic viruses and toxins (herpes simplex, rabies, polioviruses, and tetanus toxin).
- mediated by microtubules and **dynein**.

VI. CAPILLARIES OF THE CENTRAL NERVOUS SYSTEM (Figure 5.4)

- have a higher density in gray matter than in white matter and are of two types:

A. Nonfenestrated capillaries

- ubiquitous in white and gray matter.
- have endothelial cells with tight junctions surrounded by a continuous basement membrane and an outer investment of astrocytic foot processes; the endothelial cells and their tight junctions constitute the **blood-brain barrier**.

B. Fenestrated capillaries

- consist of endothelial cells with fenestrations that permit the passage of blood-borne substances into the extracellular spaces of the CNS.
- located in specialized areas of the brain that lack a blood-brain barrier (eg, circumventricular organs).

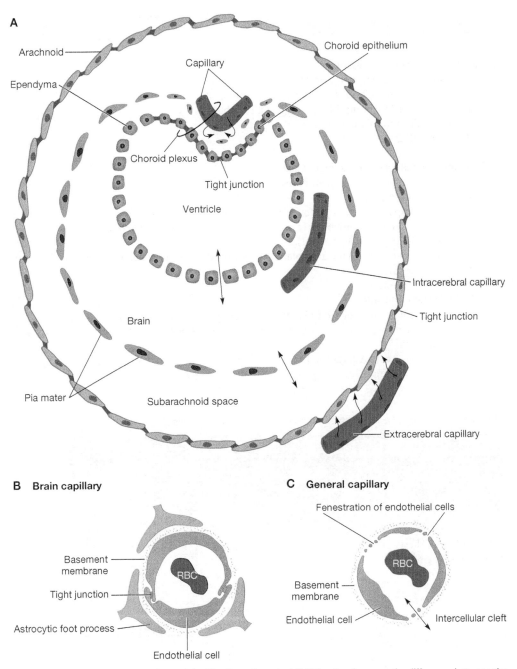

FIGURE 5.4. The blood-brain barrier and the blood-cerebrospinal fluid barrier. Compare the difference between the intracerebral capillaries (**B**), the extracerebral capillaries (**C**), and the capillaries of the choroid plexus (**A**). Barrier function is mediated by tight junctions between the endothelial cells and between choroid plexus epithelial cells. Tumors and cerebrovascular accidents disrupt the endothelial wall and cause cerebral edema (vasculotoxic edema). RBC, red blood cell. (Adapted from Nolte J. *The Human Brain: An Introduction to Its Functional Anatomy.* 2nd ed. Mosby; 1988. Copyright © 1988 Elsevier. With permission.)

VII. SENSORY RECEPTORS

A. Pain and temperature receptors

- free (nonencapsulated) nerve endings.
- found throughout the body (eg, epidermis, cornea).
- associated with A-δ (group III) and C (group IV) fibers.
- project via the anterolateral system.
- slowly adapting.

B. Cutaneous mechanoreceptors (Figure 5.5)

- endings that respond to touch and pressure.

1. Merkel tactile disks

- nonencapsulated endings found in the basal layer of the epidermis.
- mediate light (crude) touch (eg, stroking the skin with a wisp of cotton).
- associated with A-β (group II).
- project centrally via the anterolateral system and the posterior column-medial lemniscus pathway.
- slowly adapting.

2. Meissner corpuscles

- encapsulated endings found in the dermal papillae of glabrous skin.
- mediate fine discriminative tactile sensation via the posterior column-medial lemniscus pathway.
- associated with A-β (group II).
- rapidly adapting.

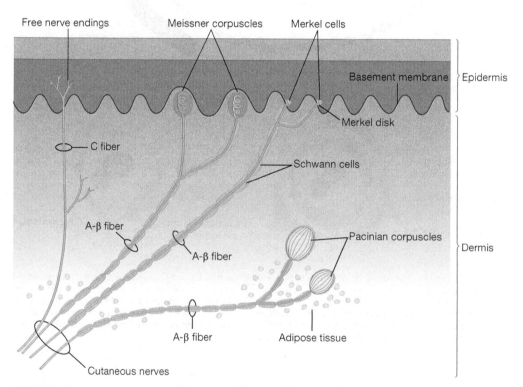

FIGURE 5.5. Four cutaneous receptors: free nerve endings—mediate pain and temperature sensation; Meissner corpuscles of the dermal papillae—mediate tactile two-point discrimination; Pacinian corpuscles of the dermis—mediate touch, pressure, and vibration sensation; and Merkel disks—mediate light touch. (Adapted with permission from Fix JD. *High-Yield Neuroanatomy.* 3rd ed. Lippincott Williams & Wilkins; 2005:53.)

3. **Pacinian corpuscles**
   - found in the dermis, mesenteries, and periosteum.
   - respond to pressure and vibratory sense via the posterior column-medial lemniscus pathway.
   - associated with A-β (group II).
   - rapidly adapting.

C. **Muscle and tendon receptors**
   1. **Muscle spindles**
      - encapsulated mechanoreceptors and proprioceptors.
      - consist of capsules containing intrafusal fibers (ie, nuclear bag and nuclear chain fibers).
      - arranged parallel with the extrafusal fibers of the muscle.
      - mediate via group Ia afferents, the muscle stretch reflex (MSR), and the myotatic reflex (eg, patellar reflex).
      - sense the relative length of the muscle (static function) and the rate of change of length (dynamic function).
      - the activity of the gamma motor neurons regulates the sensitivity of the muscle spindle to stretch.
      a. **Nuclear bag fibers**
         - receive group Ia primary afferent fibers (annulospiral endings) and static and dynamic gamma efferent fibers.
         - respond primarily to the rate of change of muscle length.
      b. **Nuclear chain fibers**
         - receive group Ia primary and group II secondary afferent fibers (flower spray endings) and static gamma efferent fibers.
         - respond primarily to muscle length.
   2. **Gamma motor neurons**
      - consist of static and dynamic motor neurons.
      - found in the anterior horn with alpha motor neurons.
      - receive input from descending motor pathways (eg, corticospinal and reticulospinal tracts).
      - modify the sensitivity of muscle spindles.
      - coactivated along with alpha motor neurons.
   3. **Golgi tendon organs**
      - found at the junction of the muscle and its tendon and are connected with the muscle fibers in series.
      - respond to muscle tension during muscle stretch and contraction and are also sensitive to the velocity of tension development.
      - innervated by group Ib fibers.

Review Test

1. Peripheral nerve fibers regenerate at the rate of _____ mm/d.

(A) 0.1
(B) 3
(C) 100
(D) 200
(E) 400

2. Fast pain has a conduction velocity of _____ m/s.

(A) 1
(B) 5
(C) 15
(D) 50
(E) 100

3. A 10-year-old boy has severed his radial nerve. Which of the following cells plays a major role in axonal regrowth?

(A) Fibrous astrocytes
(B) Fibroblasts
(C) Oligodendrocytes
(D) Protoplasmic astrocytes
(E) Schwann cells

4. Which of the following receptors initiates the MSR?

(A) Free nerve endings
(B) Merkel disks
(C) Muscle spindles
(D) Ruffini end bulbs
(E) Pacinian corpuscles

5. Wallerian degeneration involves:

(A) chromatolysis.
(B) only the CNS.
(C) successive fragmentation of the axon.
(D) swelling of the cell body.
(E) the proximal end of the axon.

6. A 46-year-old woman complains of right-sided hearing loss and vertigo (dizziness). A small tumor was demonstrated within the internal auditory canal. Which structure listed below accounts for the hearing loss and vertigo?

(A) Arachnoid cyst
(B) Ependymoma
(C) Epidermoid cyst
(D) Meningioma
(E) Schwannoma

7. A 9-year-old boy has a stumbling gait, dizziness, diplopia, headache, vomiting, and coarse nystagmus toward the side of the lesion. He scans his speech. Tests for dysdiadochokinesia, papilledema, elevated CSF protein, and intention tremor are positive. Match this symptom complex with the best-fitting choice.

(A) Craniopharyngioma
(B) Medulloblastoma
(C) Meningioma
(D) Oligodendroglia
(E) von Hippel-Lindau disease

8. A 45-year-old man presented to his primary care physician with a complaint about chronic headaches that are now affecting his vision. Upon examination, a right homonymous upper quadrantanopia is demonstrated, which has only recently developed and "is closing in." The patient also presents with a shuffling gait because of an inability to appropriately move his right lower limb. Imaging reveals multiple tumors with an obvious rim around them, all confined to the left side of the patient's frontal and temporal lobes. Based on these characteristics, what is the most likely diagnosis?

(A) Astrocytoma
(B) Germinoma
(C) Glioblastoma
(D) Meningioma
(E) Oligodendroglioma

9. A 76-year-old man with previously diagnosed Parkinson disease passes away peacefully in his sleep. Having had treatment since diagnosis at a large academic medical center, he had agreed to an autopsy while capable of making sound decisions. Brain autopsy, investigation, and imaging focus on the substantia nigra and reveal

a multitude of eosinophilic intracytoplasmic inclusion bodies, known as:

(A) Lewy bodies.
(B) lipofuscin granules.
(C) Nissl substance.
(D) psammoma bodies.
(E) Rosenthal fibers.

Questions 10 to 14

The response options for items 10 to 14 are the same. Select one answer for each item in the set.

(A) Astrocytes
(B) Microglial cells
(C) Oligodendrocytes
(D) Schwann cells
(E) Tanycytes

Match each of the following descriptions with the corresponding type of nerve cell.

10. Are a variety of ependymal cells found in the wall of the third ventricle

11. Arise from monocytes

12. Are neural crest derivatives

13. Contain glial filaments and glycogen granules

14. Are perineuronal satellite cells in the CNS

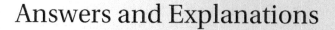

Answers and Explanations

1. **B.** Peripheral nerve fibers regenerate at 3 mm/d.

2. **C.** Fast pain has a nerve fiber (A-δ) conduction velocity of 12 to 30 m/s. Slow pain has a nerve fiber (C) conduction velocity of 0.5 to 2 m/s.

3. **E.** Schwann cells play a major role in axon regeneration (axon regrowth) in the PNS. Fibrous and protoplasmic astrocytes, as well as oligodendrocytes are found in the CNS. Fibroblasts are a component of connective tissue throughout the body and are not involved with nerve regeneration.

4. **C.** The MSR is initiated by muscle spindles. The other peripheral receptors function in somatosensation (eg, pain and temperature, touch, pressure, vibratory sense).

5. **C.** Wallerian, or anterograde degeneration, occurs toward the distal end of the axon in both the CNS and PNS and is characterized by successive fragmentation and disappearance of axons and myelin sheaths and by secondary proliferation of Schwann cells. Retrograde degeneration occurs toward the proximal end of the axon and in the cell body. It takes place in both the CNS and PNS and is characterized by chromatolysis, cell body swelling, and flattening and displacement of the nucleus to the periphery.

6. **E.** A schwannoma is a benign tumor derived from Schwann cells of the vestibular division of CN VIII (acoustic neuroma of CN VIII). Schwannomas occur twice as frequently in females as in males. Symptoms arise from pressure on the vestibular division, resulting in vertigo, and pressure on the cochlear division, resulting in nerve deafness (sensorineural). Acoustic neuromas represent 8% of intracranial neoplasms. When bilateral, they are diagnostic of type II neurofibromatosis. The internal auditory canal contains the facial and vestibulocochlear nerves and the labyrinthine artery. An arachnoid cyst is a congenital disorder; it is a CSF sac that forms in the cranium or spinal cord. An ependymoma is a slow-growing, benign circumscribed neoplasm typically found within the ventricles. An epidermoid cyst is a benign cyst derived from ectodermal tissue. A meningioma is a slow-growing intracranial tumor of mesenchymal origin.

7. **B.** Medulloblastomas are malignant neoplasms comprising one-third of the tumors in the posterior cranial fossa of children. They are radiosensitive. Metastatic spread within the neuraxis is frequent. Meningiomas are benign tumors originating from arachnoid cells; they contain psammoma bodies that are calcified and visible on computed tomography. Oligodendroglia are the myelin-producing cells of the CNS. Craniopharyngiomas, congenital epidermoid tumors, are the commonest supratentorial tumors found in children. Von Hippel-Lindau disease is a rare genetic disorder that results in tumor growth in blood-rich areas of the body.

8. **C.** Glioblastomas are characterized by well-formed rings around their perimeter and multiple tumors, and they are often found in the frontal and temporal lobes. Astrocytomas are most commonly found in children and more commonly in males. Germinomas are found deep within the brain in the pineal region and often lead to hydrocephalus. Meningiomas are associated with the meninges and indent the brain from the outside, pushing it in. Oligodendrogliomas are more common in males, tend to calcify, and have a characteristic "fried egg" appearance.

9. **A.** Lewy bodies are commonly found in the substantia nigra in patients with Parkinson disease. Lipofuscin granules are a common finding during aging; they are not concentrated in the substantia nigra and are not directly related to Parkinson disease. Nissl substance is a normal protein synthesis part of a cell. Psammoma bodies are associated with meningiomas and are not related to Parkinson disease. Rosenthal fibers are also eosinophilic inclusions, but are found more dispersed and often associated with astrocytomas.

10. **E.** Tanycytes are a variety of ependymal cells found in the wall of the third ventricle. The processes of these cells extend from the lumen of the third ventricle to the capillaries of the hypophyseal portal system and also to the neurosecretory neurons of the arcuate nucleus.

11. **B.** Microglial cells, the scavenger cells of the CNS, arise from blood-born monocytes.

12. **D.** Schwann cells are derived from the neural crest; they myelinate the axons of the PNS.

13. **A.** Astrocytes are characterized by the presence of glial filaments and glycogen; glial filaments contain GFAP, a marker for astrocytes.

14. **C.** Oligodendrocytes are perineuronal satellite cells; they myelinate the axons of the CNS.

6 Spinal Cord

Objectives

- Identify external parts of the spinal cord, including attachments and structural characteristics.
- Describe the spinal nerve, including components, derivatives, and locations.
- Describe a nerve plexus—somatic and autonomic.
- Identify the various internal parts of the spinal cord, including the subdivisions of the gray and white matter.
- Identify unique features of various spinal cord levels.
- Describe the myotatic reflex.

I. INTRODUCTION (Figure 6.1)

- derived from the caudal part of the neural tube.
- maintains segmental organization throughout development.
- surrounded by three membranes, the **meninges**.
- weighs approximately 30 g.

II. EXTERNAL MORPHOLOGY

A. Location

- extends, in adults, from the foramen magnum to the inferior border of the first lumbar vertebra; in newborns, it extends to the third lumbar vertebra.
- continuous with the **medulla oblongata** at the spinomedullary junction, a plane defined by three structures: the foramen magnum, the pyramidal decussation, and the emergence of the first cervical nerve anterior rootlets.
- lies within the **subarachnoid space** that extends caudally to the level of the second sacral vertebra (see Figure 2.2).

B. Attachments

- suspend and anchor the spinal cord within the dural sac.
- arise from the **pia mater**, which closely invests the spinal cord.

  #### 1. Denticulate ligaments

  - consist of a lateral flattened band of pial tissue on each side of the spinal cord.
  - adhere to the spinal dura mater with 21 pairs of tooth-like extensions.

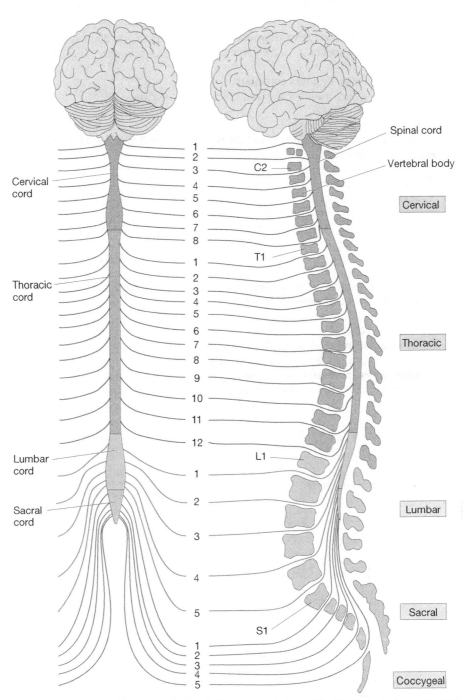

FIGURE 6.1. Diagram of the position of the spinal cord with reference to the vertebral bodies and spinous processes. The conus medullaris lies in the L1-L2 interspace. The dural sac ends at S2. (Adapted with permission from Bear MF, Connors BW, Paradiso MA. *Neuroscience: Exploring the Brain.* 2nd ed. Lippincott Williams & Wilkins; 2001, Figure 12.10.)

2. Filum terminale

▓ an extension of pia mater that extends from the conus medullaris to the dural sac (internus) and from the dural sac to the coccyx (externus).

3. Spinal nerve roots

▓ provide anchorage and fixation of the spinal cord to the vertebral canal.

C. Shape

- an elongated and nearly cylindrical structure, approximately 1 cm in diameter.
- **cervical** (C5-T1) and **lumbar** (L1-S2) **enlargements** for the nerve supply of the upper and lower extremities.
- terminates caudally as the **conus medullaris**.
- length: averages 45 cm in adult males and 42 cm in adult females.

D. Spinal nerves (Figure 6.2)

- consist of 31 pairs of nerves that emerge from the spinal cord: **8 cervical**, **12 thoracic**, **5 lumbar**, **5 sacral**, and **1 coccygeal**.
- contain both motor and sensory fibers.

1. Special considerations

- the first cervical nerve and the coccygeal nerve usually have neither the posterior (sensory) roots nor corresponding dermatomes.
- the first cervical nerve passes between the atlas and the skull.
- the second cervical nerve passes between the atlas and the axis.
- with the exception of C1, spinal nerves exit the vertebral canal via intervertebral or sacral foramina.

2. Functional components of spinal nerve fibers (Figure 6.3; see also Table 4.1)

- **General somatic afferent (GSA) fibers**
  - a. convey sensory input from skin, muscle, bone, and joints to the central nervous system (CNS).
- **General visceral afferent (GVA) fibers**
  - a. convey sensory input from visceral organs to the CNS.
- **General somatic efferent (GSE) fibers**
  - a. convey motor output from anterior horn motor neurons to skeletal muscle.

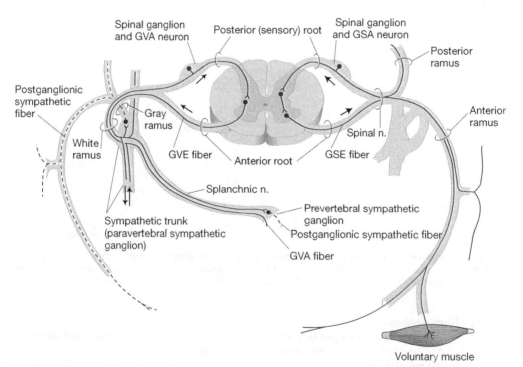

FIGURE 6.2. The typical thoracic spinal nerve and its branches and reflex connections. White communicating rami are found only at thoracolumbar levels T1 to L2. Gray communicating rami are found at all spinal cord levels. GSA, general somatic afferent; GSE, general somatic efferent; GVA, general visceral afferent; GVE, general visceral efferent.

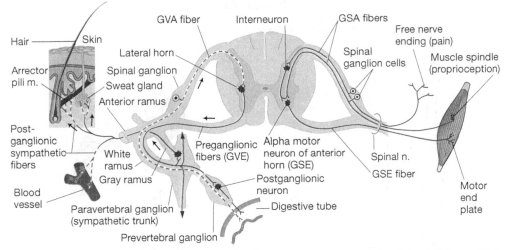

FIGURE 6.3. Diagram of the four functional components of the thoracic spinal nerve: general visceral afferent (GVA), general somatic afferent (GSA), general somatic efferent (GSE), and general visceral efferent (GVE). Proprioceptive, cutaneous, and visceral reflex arcs are shown. The muscle stretch (myotatic) reflex (MSR) includes the muscle spindle, GSA spinal ganglion cell, GSE anterior horn motor neuron, and skeletal muscle.

■ **General visceral efferent (GVE) fibers**
    a. convey motor output from intermediolateral cell column neurons, via paravertebral or prevertebral ganglia, to glands, smooth muscle, and visceral organs (sympathetic divisions of the autonomic nervous system).
    b. convey motor output from the sacral parasympathetic nucleus to the pelvic viscera via intramural ganglia.
    c. contribute to autonomic plexuses of the thorax, abdomen, and pelvis (Figure 6.4).
    d. fibers from the intermediolateral cell column (lateral horn) participate in plexuses and are found in anterior and posterior rami to innervate body wall targets: erector pili, sweat glands, and blood vessels via gray rami communicans.

3. Components and branches of spinal nerves
  ■ the spinal nerve is formed by the union of posterior and anterior roots within the intervertebral foramen, resulting in a mixed nerve.
  a. Posterior root
    ■ enters the posterior lateral sulcus as posterior rootlets and conveys sensory input from the body via the spinal ganglion.
    ■ contains, distally, the spinal ganglion.
    ■ joins the anterior root distal to the spinal ganglion and within the intervertebral foramen to form the spinal nerve.
  b. Spinal ganglion
    ■ located within the posterior root and within the **intervertebral foramen**.
    ■ contains **pseudounipolar neurons** of neural crest origin that transmit sensory input from the periphery (GSA and GVA) to the spinal cord via the posterior roots.
  c. Anterior root
    ■ emerges as anterior rootlets from the anterior lateral sulcus and conveys motor output from visceral and somatic motor neurons.
    ■ joins the posterior roots distal to the spinal ganglion and within the intervertebral foramen to form the spinal nerve.
  d. Cauda equina
    ■ consists of lumbosacral (posterior and anterior) nerve roots (L2-Co) that descend from the spinal cord through the subarachnoid space to exit through their respective intervertebral or sacral foramina.
  e. Spinal nerve rami
    ■ **Posterior ramus**
      (1) innervates the skin and muscles of the back.

Autonomic Plexus

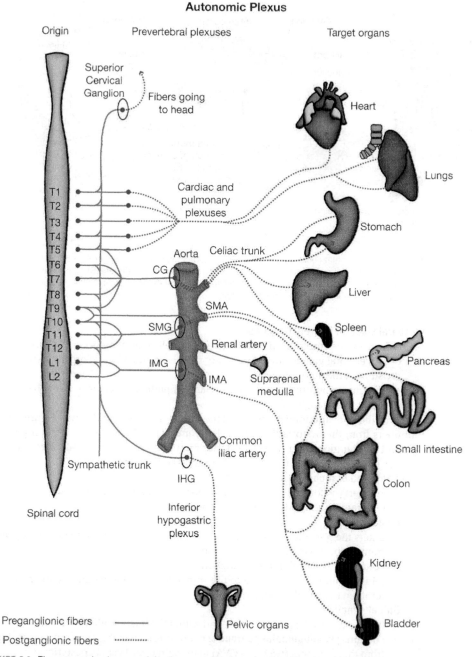

FIGURE 6.4. The autonomic plexuses of the thorax, abdomen, and pelvis. The plexus is composed of preganglionic and postganglionic sympathetic fibers, preganglionic parasympathetic fibers, and visceral afferent fibers. CG, ciliary ganglion and plexus; IHG, inferior hypogastric ganglia and plexus (pelvic plexus or ganglia); IMA, inferior mesenteric artery; IMG, inferior mesenteric ganglion and plexus; SMA, superior mesenteric artery; SMG, superior mesenteric ganglion and plexus.

- **Anterior ramus (Figure 6.5)**
    - **(1)** innervates the anterior and lateral muscles and skin of the trunk, limbs, and visceral organs.
    - **(2)** contribute to the presence of somatic plexuses in regions serving the neck and limbs, which facilitates multiple spinal cord levels in various peripheral nerves.
    - **(3)** stay segmental in thorax/trunk region, that is, do not form or contribute to plexuses.

Somatic Plexuses

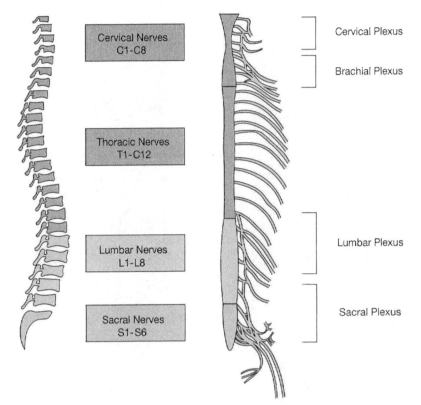

FIGURE 6.5. The somatic plexuses of the body supply cervical and limb musculature.

■ **Meningeal ramus**
  (1) innervates the meninges and vertebral column.
■ **Gray communicating rami**
  (1) contain **unmyelinated** postganglionic sympathetic fibers.
  (2) associated with *all* spinal nerves.
■ **White communicating rami**
  (1) contain **myelinated** preganglionic sympathetic fibers and myelinated GVA fibers (splanchnic nerves).
  (2) found only in thoracolumbar segments of the spinal cord (T1-L2).

E. **Spinal nerve innervation (Figure 6.6)**
  ■ one spinal nerve innervates the derivatives from one **somite** that includes the following:
  1. **Dermatome** (see Figure 6.6)
    ■ consists of a **cutaneous area** innervated by the fibers of one spinal nerve.
  2. **Myotome**
    ■ consists of **muscles** innervated by the fibers of one spinal nerve.
  3. **Sclerotome**
    ■ consists of **bones and ligaments** innervated by the fibers of one spinal nerve.

F. **Surface structures and sulci (Figure 6.7)**
  1. **Anterior median fissure**
    ■ a deep anterior midline groove in which the anterior spinal artery is found superficially.
  2. **Anterior lateral sulcus**
    ■ a shallow groove from which the anterior rootlets emerge.
  3. **Posterior lateral sulcus**
    ■ a shallow groove into which the posterior rootlets enter.

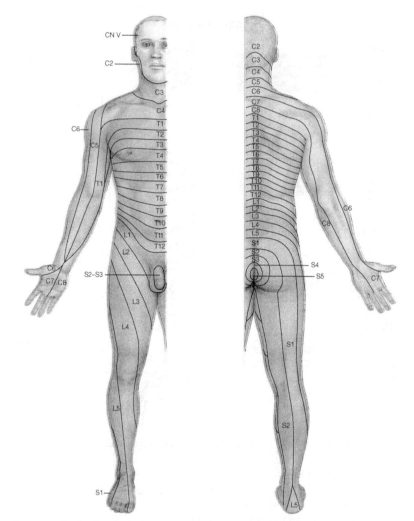

FIGURE 6.6. Cutaneous distribution of spinal nerves, the dermatomes. (Adapted from Haymaker W, Woodhall B. *Peripheral Nerve Injuries.* 2nd ed. WB Saunders; 1952:32. Copyright © 1952 Elsevier. With permission.)

4. **Posterior intermediate sulcus**
   - a shallow groove that is continuous with the posterior intermediate septum.
   - found between the posterior lateral and the posterior median sulci but only rostral to T6.
   - separates the fasciculus gracilis from the fasciculus cuneatus.
5. **Posterior median sulcus**
   - a shallow posterior midline groove that is continuous with the posterior median septum.

III. INTERNAL MORPHOLOGY (See Figure 6.7)

- in transverse sections, the spinal cord consists of central gray matter and peripheral white matter.

A. Gray matter
   - toward the center of the spinal cord.
   - butterfly- or **H-shaped**, the shape of which varies according to spinal cord level.
   - contains a central canal.

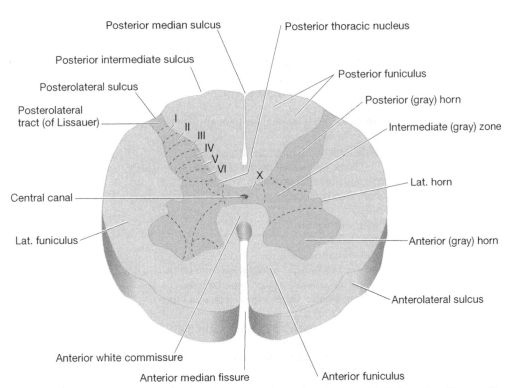

FIGURE 6.7. Topography of the spinal cord in transverse section: horns (columns), sulci, funiculi, and Rexed laminae. The lateral horn is found only at thoracolumbar cord levels (T1-L2). The posterior intermediate sulcus and septum are found only above T6.

- divided into cytoarchitectural areas called **Rexed laminae**, expressed with Roman numerals (see Figure 6.7).
- divided into three horns or cell columns on each side:
  1. Posterior horn (column)
  - receives and processes sensory input.
  - found at all levels.
  - includes the following nuclei:
    a. Posteromarginal nucleus (Rexed lamina I)
    - found at all cord levels.
    - associated with light touch, pain, and temperature sensation.
    - origin of some fibers of anterolateral system.
    b. Substantia gelatinosa (Rexed lamina II)
    - found at all cord levels.
    - homologous to the spinal trigeminal nucleus.
    - associated with light touch, pain, and temperature sensation.
    - origin of some fibers of anterolateral system.
    c. Nucleus proprius (Rexed laminae III and IV)
    - found at all cord levels.
    - associated with light touch, pain, and temperature sensation.
    - origin of some fibers of anterolateral system.
    d. Posterior thoracic nucleus (also known as nucleus dorsalis of Clarke) (Rexed lamina VII)
    - found at the base of the posterior horn.
    - extends from (C8) T1 to L2.
    - homologous to the **accessory cuneate nucleus** of the medulla.

▓ subserves unconscious proprioception from muscle spindles and Golgi tendon organs (GTOs).

▓ the origin of the posterior spinocerebellar tract.

2. Lateral horn (column) (Rexed lamina VII)

▓ receives viscerosensory input.

▓ found between the posterior and anterior horns.

▓ extends from T1 to L2.

▓ contains the **intermediolateral nucleus** (column), a visceromotor nucleus that extends from T1 to L2.

▓ contains preganglionic sympathetic neurons (GVE).

▓ contains, at T1-T2, the **ciliospinal center of Budge** (sympathetic innervation of the eye).

3. Anterior horn (column) (Rexed laminae VII, VIII, and IX)

▓ contains predominantly motor nuclei.

▓ found at all levels.

▓ includes the following nuclei:

a. Spinal border cells

▓ extend from L2 to S3.

▓ subserve unconscious proprioception from GTOs and muscle spindles.

▓ the origin of the anterior spinocerebellar tract.

b. Sacral parasympathetic nucleus (Rexed lamina VII)

▓ extends from S2 to S4.

▓ gives rise to preganglionic parasympathetic fibers that innervate the pelvic viscera via the pelvic splanchnic nerves.

c. Somatic motor nuclei (Rexed lamina IX)

▓ found at all levels.

▓ subdivided into medial and lateral groups that innervate axial and appendicular muscles, respectively.

d. Spinal accessory nucleus (Rexed lamina IX)

▓ extends from C1 to C6.

▓ gives rise to the **spinal accessory nerve** (CN XI).

▓ innervates the sternocleidomastoid and trapezius.

e. Phrenic nucleus (Rexed lamina IX)

▓ extends from C3 to C5.

▓ innervates the diaphragm.

B. White matter (see Figure 6.7)

▓ consists of bundles of myelinated fibers that surround the gray matter.

▓ consists of ascending and descending fiber pathways called tracts.

▓ divided bilaterally by sulci into three major divisions.

1. Posterior funiculus (posterior column)

▓ located between the posterior median sulcus and the posterior lateral sulcus.

▓ is subdivided above T6 into two fasciculi:

a. Fasciculus gracilis

▓ located between the posterior median sulcus and the posterior intermediate sulcus and septum.

▓ found at all cord levels.

b. Fasciculus cuneatus

▓ located between the posterior intermediate sulcus and septum and the posterior lateral sulcus.

▓ found only at the upper thoracic and cervical cord levels (C1-T6).

2. Lateral funiculus

▓ located between the posterior lateral and the anterior lateral sulci.

3. Anterior funiculus

▓ located between the anterior median fissure and the anterior lateral sulcus.

▓ contains the **anterior white commissure**:

a. located between the central canal and the anterior median fissure.

b. contains decussating spinothalamic fibers.

C. Characterization of spinal cord levels

- based on regional variation in the shape of the gray matter and the presence of the posterior intermediate sulci and septa.

    1. Cervical cord
    - posterior intermediate sulci and septa are present.
    - anterior horns are massive from C3 to C8.

    2. Thoracic cord
    - posterior intermediate sulci and septa are present from T1 to T6.
    - the posterior thoracic nucleus is present at all thoracic levels but is most prominent at T11 and T12.
    - lateral horns are present at all thoracic levels.
    - posterior and anterior horns are typically slender and **H**-shaped.

    3. Lumbar cord
    - the posterior thoracic nucleus is very prominent at L1 and L2.
    - contains massive anterior and posterior horns from L2 to L5; the substantia gelatinosa is greatly enlarged.
    - the lumbar section is difficult to distinguish from upper sacral segments.
    - the lateral horn is prominent only at L1.

    4. Sacral cord
    - contains massive anterior and posterior horns; the substantia gelatinosa is greatly enlarged.
    - greatly reduced in overall diameter from S3 to S5.

    5. Coccygeal segment
    - contains posterior horns that are more voluminous than the anterior horns.
    - has a greatly reduced overall diameter.

IV. MYOTATIC REFLEX (See Figure 6.3)

A. Afferent limb
- includes a muscle spindle (receptor) and a spinal ganglion neuron and its Ia fiber.

B. Efferent limb
- includes an anterior horn motor neuron that innervates striated muscle (effector).

Review Test

1. Which of the following reflexes is monosynaptic?

(A) Achilles
(B) Babinski
(C) Corneal
(D) Extensor plantar
(E) Pupillary light

2. The spinal cord of a newborn baby terminates at:

(A) VL1
(B) VL3
(C) VS1
(D) VS3
(E) VS5

3. Which spinal nerve rami contain unmyelinated postganglionic sympathetic nerve fibers?

(A) Anterior primary
(B) Gray communicating
(C) Meningeal
(D) Posterior primary
(E) White communicating

4. The efferent limb of a myotatic reflex includes a(n):

(A) anterior horn motor neuron.
(B) lateral horn visceromotor nucleus.
(C) muscle spindle.
(D) preganglionic sympathetic neuron.
(E) spinal ganglion neuron.

5. A 45-year-old man was thrown from his horse during an equestrian competition. He landed awkwardly on his head, breaking his neck. The injury caused severe spinal cord damage at C2, leaving him paralyzed from the neck down and in need of a ventilator, as he was unable to breathe on his own. The C2 injury damaged descending influence to what spinal cord nucleus to cause the need for breathing assistance?

(A) Nucleus proprius
(B) Phrenic
(C) Posterior thoracic
(D) Spinal accessory
(E) Substantia gelatinosa

6. A 35-year-old woman presents to her primary care physician for a chief complaint of a worsening pain that started in her back and is beginning to extend into her lower limb. She describes the pain as sharp and shooting. The patient reveals that she had started back to regular workouts about a month prior and the pain is worse at the gym; she finds relief when laying down. Imaging reveals an intervertebral disk herniation at L4/L5. Which of the following spinal nerves would be affected by this herniation to produce the patient's symptoms?

(A) C7
(B) T10
(C) L4
(D) L5
(E) S2

Questions 7 to 11

The response options for items 7 to 11 are the same. Select one answer for each item in the set.

(A) Cervical
(B) Coccygeal
(C) Lumbar
(D) Inferior thoracic
(E) Sacral
(F) Superior thoracic

Match each characteristic below with the spinal cord level it best describes.

7. Contains preganglionic parasympathetic neurons

8. Subserves the brachial plexus

9. Has a ciliospinal center (of Budge)

10. Contains the spinal accessory nucleus (CN XI)

11. Contains the phrenic nucleus

Answers and Explanations

1. **A.** The Achilles reflex, or ankle jerk reflex, is a myotatic monosynaptic reflex that is mediated by cord segment S1. The other reflexes listed are polysynaptic.

2. **B.** In the newborn, the spinal cord ends at the level of the third lumbar vertebra (VL3). In the adult, the spinal cord ends at the lower border of the first lumbar vertebra (VL1), and the dural sac ends at the level of the second sacral vertebra (VS2).

3. **B.** Gray communicating rami contain unmyelinated postganglionic sympathetic fibers, and white communicating rami contain myelinated preganglionic sympathetic fibers and myelinated GVA fibers. The meningeal ramus innervates the meninges and vertebral column, the posterior primary ramus innervates the skin and muscles of the back, and the anterior primary ramus innervates the anterolateral muscles and skin of the trunk, extremities, and visceral.

4. **A.** The myotatic reflex is a monosynaptic and ipsilateral muscle stretch reflex (MSR). The efferent limb consists of the axon of an anterior horn alpha motor neuron that innervates striated muscle fibers (effector); the afferent limb consists of a muscle spindle (receptor) and an Ia fiber (axon) of a spinal ganglion neuron. The quadriceps (patellar) and triceps surae (ankle) MSRs are myotatic reflexes.

5. **B.** The phrenic nucleus (C3-C5) contains the lower motor neurons that innervate the diaphragm, an injury at C2 may damage descending influence on this nucleus, leading to diaphragmatic paralysis. None of the other nuclei listed are involved with respiration: nucleus proprius and substantia gelatinosa—touch, pain and temperature, posterior thoracic—unconscious proprioception, and spinal accessory—innervation of sternocleidomastoid and trapezius.

6. **D.** Beyond the cervical region, spinal nerves emerge from the vertebral canal inferior to the vertebra of the same number. The L4 spinal nerve would emerge and exit inferior to the L4 vertebra, just superior to the herniation, while L5 would be nearing its exit inferior to L5 and be compressed. C7 and T10 are well above the herniation and would not be affected. S2 is too far below the herniation to be affected.

7. **E.** The sacral cord contains the sacral parasympathetic nucleus (S2-S4), which gives rise to preganglionic fibers that synapse in the intramural ganglia of the pelvic viscera. Other preganglionic nuclei are found in the brainstem.

8. **A.** The cervical cord contains massive anterior horns, which give rise to the brachial plexus (C5-C8).

9. **F.** The ciliospinal center (of Budge) is found in the lateral horn at T1. This sympathetic nucleus innervates the dilator pupillae and the nonstriated superior and inferior tarsal muscles.

10. **A.** The spinal accessory nucleus extends from C1 to C6 and gives rise to the spinal accessory nerve; it innervates the sternocleidomastoid and trapezius.

11. **A.** The phrenic nucleus extends from C3 to C5 and innervates the diaphragm.

Tracts of the Spinal Cord

Objectives

- List the three major ascending spinal cord pathways and describe the location of their primary, secondary, and tertiary neurons and the sensory modalities each is concerned with.
- List the major descending spinal cord pathways and describe the function of each.
- Describe somatotopic organization and list the spinal cord tracts that possess somatotopic organization and describe how the fibers are organized in each.

I. ASCENDING TRACTS

- represent functional pathways that convey sensory information from the periphery to higher levels.
- consist of a chain of three neurons: first-, second-, and third-order neurons. The first-order neuron is always in a spinal ganglion. Exception: the olfactory system does not follow the three-neuron "rule"; olfactory input has the most direct connection to the brain.
- mostly decussate at some point along their course.
- give rise to collateral branches that serve in local spinal reflex arcs.

A. Posterior column-medial lemniscus pathway (Figure 7.1)

- mediates fine touch, conscious proprioception, and vibratory sense.
- somatotopically organized.
- receives input from Pacinian and Meissner corpuscles, joint receptors, muscle spindles, and Golgi tendon organs (GTOs).

1. First-order neurons

- located in the spinal ganglia at all levels.
- give rise to the **fasciculus gracilis** from the lower extremity.
- give rise to the **fasciculus cuneatus** from the upper extremity.
- give rise to axons that ascend in the posterior columns and terminate in the gracile and cuneate nuclei of the medulla.

2. Second-order neurons

- located in the gracile and cuneate nuclei of the caudal medulla.
- give rise to axons, **internal arcuate fibers** that decussate and form a compact fiber bundle, the **medial lemniscus**. The medial lemniscus ascends through the contralateral brainstem to terminate in the ventral posterolateral (**VPL**) nucleus of the thalamus.

3. Third-order neurons

- located in the VPL nucleus of the thalamus.
- project via the posterior limb of the internal capsule to the postcentral gyrus, the **somatosensory cortex** (areas 3, 1, and 2).

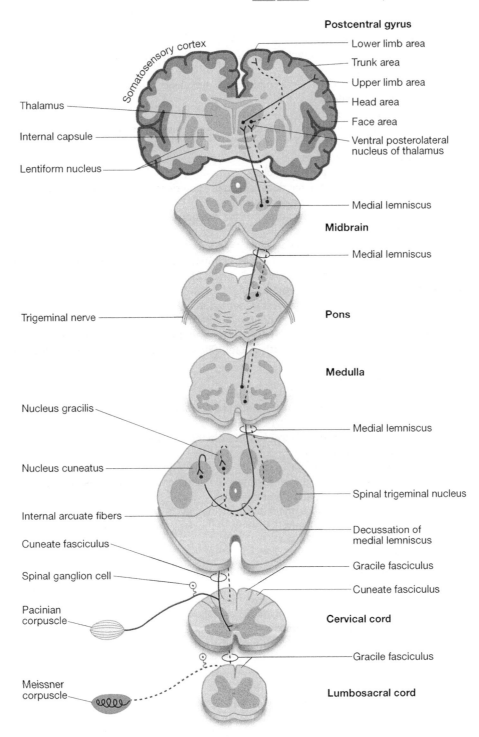

FIGURE 7.1. The posterior column-medial lemniscus pathway. (Adapted with permission from Carpenter MB, Sutin J. *Human Neuroanatomy.* 8th ed. Williams & Wilkins; 1983:266.)

B. **Anterolateral system**[1]
   1. **Anterior spinothalamic tract**
      - concerned with **crude touch**, the sensation produced by stroking glabrous skin with a wisp of cotton.
      - receives input from free nerve endings and Merkel tactile disks.
      a. **First-order neurons**
         - found in spinal ganglia at all levels.
         - project axons into the medial root entry zone to second-order neurons in the posterior horn.
      b. **Second-order neurons**
         - located in the **posterior horn**.
         - give rise to axons that decussate in the anterior white commissure and ascend in the contralateral anterior funiculus.
         - terminate in the VPL nucleus of the thalamus.
      c. **Third-order neurons**
         - found in the **VPL nucleus** of the thalamus.
         - project via the posterior limb of the internal capsule to the somatosensory cortex of the postcentral gyrus (areas 3, 1, and 2).
   2. **Lateral spinothalamic tract** (Figure 7.2)
      - mediates itch, pain, and temperature sensation.
      - receives input from free nerve endings and thermal receptors.
      - receives input from A-δ and C fibers (ie, fast- and slow-conducting pain fibers).
      - somatotopically organized with sacral fibers posterolaterally and cervical fibers anterolaterally.
      a. **First-order neurons**
         - found in spinal ganglia at all levels.
         - project axons via the **posterolateral tract (of Lissauer)** to second-order neurons in the posterior horn.
         - synapse with second-order neurons in the posterior horn.
      b. **Second-order neurons**
         - found in the posterior horn.
         - give rise to axons that decussate in the **anterior white commissure** and ascend in the anterior half of the lateral funiculus.
         - project collaterals to the reticular formation.
         - terminate contralaterally in the VPL nucleus and bilaterally in the intralaminar nuclei of the thalamus.
      c. **Third-order neurons**
         - found in the VPL nucleus and in the intralaminar nuclei.
         (1) **VPL neurons**
            - project via the posterior limb of the internal capsule to the somatosensory cortex of the postcentral gyrus (areas 3, 1, and 2).
         (2) **Intralaminar neurons**
            - project to the striatum and to the frontal and parietal cortex.

C. **Cerebellar**
   1. **Posterior spinocerebellar tract** (Figure 7.3)
      - transmits unconscious proprioceptive information to the cerebellum.
      - receives input from muscle spindles, GTOs, and pressure receptors.
      - involved in fine coordination of posture and the movement of individual muscles of the lower limb.
      - an uncrossed tract.
      a. **First-order neurons**
         - found in the spinal ganglia from C8 to S3.
         - project via the medial root entry zone to synapse in the **posterior thoracic nucleus**.

---

[1]The anterolateral system (tract) not only contains the anterior and lateral spinothalamic tracts but also includes spinomesencephalic, spinoreticular, and spinolimbic fibers.

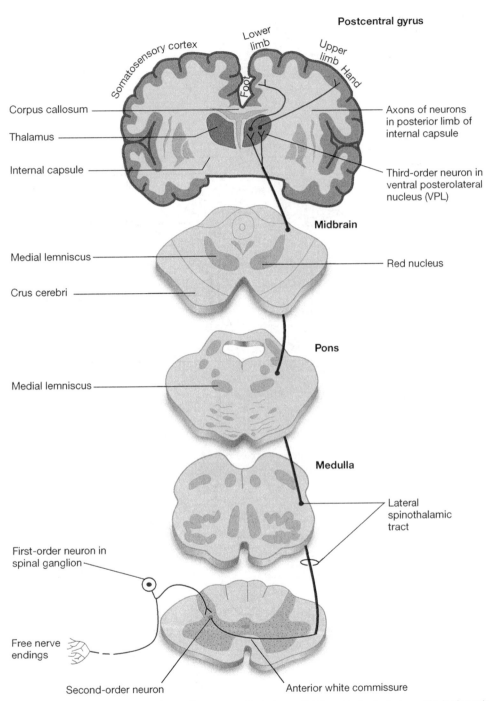

FIGURE 7.2. The lateral spinothalamic tract. Numerous collaterals are distributed to the brainstem reticular formation. (Adapted with permission from Carpenter MB, Sutin J. *Human Neuroanatomy*. 8th ed. Williams & Wilkins; 1983:274.)

b. **Second-order neurons**
  ▪ found in the posterior thoracic nucleus (C8-L3).
  ▪ give rise to axons that ascend in the lateral funiculus and reach the cerebellum via the inferior cerebellar peduncle.
  ▪ contain axons that terminate ipsilaterally as mossy fibers in the cortex of the rostral and caudal cerebellar vermis.

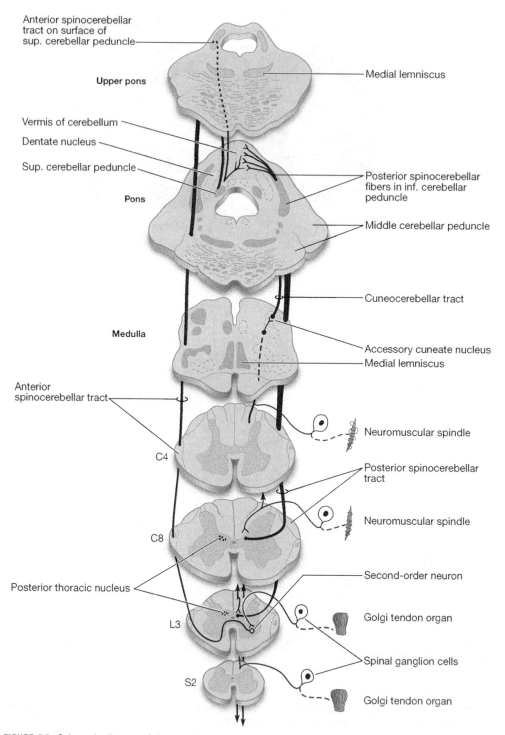

FIGURE 7.3. Schematic diagram of the anterior and posterior spinocerebellar tracts and the cuneocerebellar tract. (Adapted with permission from Carpenter MB, Sutin J. *Human Neuroanatomy.* 8th ed. Williams & Wilkins; 1983:277.)

2. **Anterior spinocerebellar tract** (see Figure 7.3)
   - transmits unconscious proprioceptive information to the cerebellum.
   - concerned with coordinated movement and posture of the lower limb as a whole.
   - receives input from muscle spindles, GTOs, and pressure receptors.
   - a crossed tract.
   a. **First-order neurons**
      - found in the spinal ganglia from L1 to S2.
      - synapse on **spinal border cells**.
   b. **Second-order neurons**
      - spinal border cells found in the anterior horns (L1-S2).
      - give rise to axons that decussate in the anterior white commissure and ascend lateral to the lateral spinothalamic tract in the lateral funiculus.
      - give rise to axons that enter the cerebellum via the **superior cerebellar peduncle** and terminate contralaterally as mossy fibers in the cortex of the rostral cerebellar vermis.
3. **Cuneocerebellar tract** (see Figure 7.3)
   - the upper extremity equivalent of the posterior spinocerebellar tract.
   a. **First-order neurons**
      - found in the spinal ganglia from C2 to T7.
      - project their axons via the fasciculus cuneatus to the caudal medulla, where they synapse in the **accessory cuneate nucleus**—a homolog of the posterior thoracic nucleus.
   b. **Second-order neurons**
      - located in the accessory cuneate nucleus of the medulla.
      - give rise to axons that project ipsilaterally to the cerebellum via the **inferior cerebellar peduncle**.

II. DESCENDING TRACTS (Figures 7.4 and 7.5)

- concerned with somatic and visceral motor activities.
- have their cells of origin (ie, upper motor neurons) in the cerebral cortex or in the brainstem.

A. Lateral corticospinal (pyramidal) tract (see Figure 7.4)
- not fully myelinated until the end of the second year of life.
- concerned with **volitional skilled motor activity**, primarily of the digits of the upper limb.
- receives input from the **paracentral lobule**, a medial continuation of the motor and sensory cortices, and subserves the muscles of the contralateral leg and foot.
- arises from lamina V of the cerebral cortex from three cortical areas: the **premotor cortex** (area 6); the **precentral motor cortex** (area 4); and the **postcentral sensory cortex** (areas 3, 1, and 2).
- terminates via interneurons on anterior horn motor neurons and sensory neurons of the posterior horn.
- the axons of the **giant cells of Betz** contribute large diameter fibers to the tract.
- passes through the posterior limb of the internal capsule.
- passes through the **crus cerebri** (basis pedunculi) of the midbrain and the basilar pons.
- constitutes the pyramid of the medulla.
- 90% of the fibers decussate at the pyramidal decussation in the medulla.
- lies in the posterior aspect of the lateral funiculus of the spinal cord.
- transection results in spastic hemiparesis with positive Babinski sign.

B. Anterior corticospinal tract (see Figure 7.4)
- a small uncrossed tract that decussates at spinal cord levels in the anterior white commissure.
- concerned with the control of axial muscles.

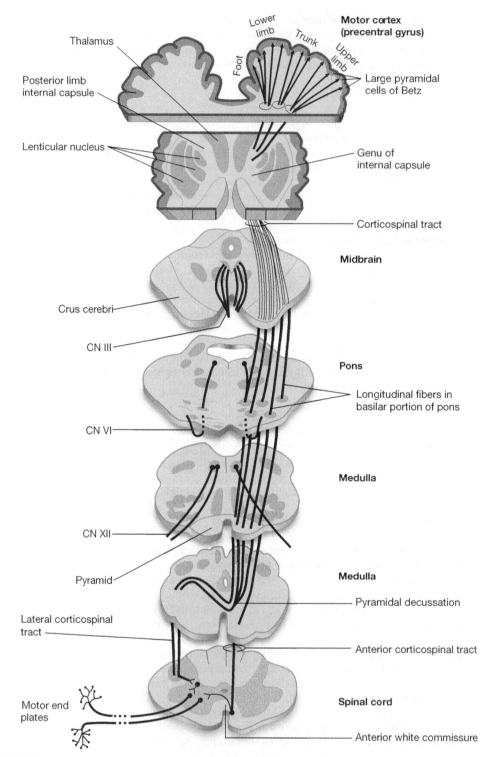

FIGURE 7.4. The lateral and anterior corticospinal tracts (the pyramidal tracts). (Adapted with permission from Carpenter MB, Sutin J. *Human Neuroanatomy*. 8th ed. Williams & Wilkins; 1983:285.)

Ascending tracts   Descending tracts

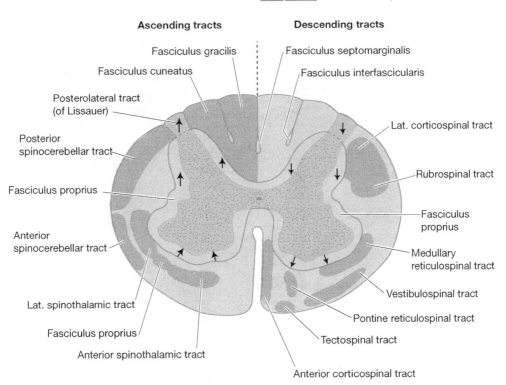

FIGURE 7.5. Schematic diagram of the major ascending and descending pathways of the spinal cord. (Adapted with permission from Carpenter MB. *Core Text of Neuroanatomy.* 3rd ed. Williams & Wilkins; 1985:97.)

C. Rubrospinal tract (see Figure 7.5)

- arises in the contralateral red nucleus of the midbrain.
- plays a role in the control of flexor tone.
- anterior to the lateral corticospinal tract.
- fibers terminate primarily at cervical cord levels.

D. Vestibulospinal tracts (see Figure 7.5)

- arise from the giant cells of Deiters in the ipsilateral lateral vestibular nuclei.
- medial and lateral tracts play a role in the control of extensor tone.
- located in the anterior funiculus.

E. Reticulospinal tracts

- medial (pontine) tract arises from the oral and caudal pontine reticular nuclei; facilitate limb extension.
- lateral (medullary) tract arises from gigantocellular and ventral reticular nuclei; facilitate limb flexion.

F. Descending autonomic tracts (Figure 7.6)

- project to sympathetic (T1-L2) and parasympathetic (S2-S4) centers in the spinal cord.
- innervate the ciliospinal center (T1-T2), a pupillary center; interruption of this hypothalamospinal tract (found in the posterior quadrant of the lateral funiculus) results in **Horner syndrome**.

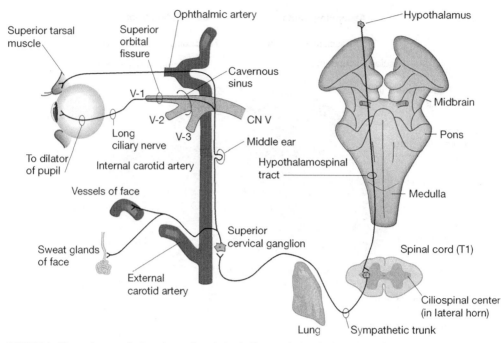

FIGURE 7.6. The oculosympathetic pathway. Hypothalamic fibers project to the ipsilateral ciliospinal center (of Budge) of the inter-mediolateral cell column at T1. The ciliospinal center projects preganglionic sympathetic fibers to the superior cervical ganglion. The superior cervical ganglion projects perivascular postganglionic sympathetic fibers through the tympanic cavity, cavernous sinus, and superior orbital fissure to the dilator pupillae. (Adapted with permission from Fix, JD. *High-Yield Neuroanatomy.* 3rd ed. Lippincott Williams & Wilkins; 2005:67.)

III. INTEGRATIVE PATHWAYS (Figure 7.5)

A. Ascending pain pathways
- pain ascends in all three funiculi.
- tracts that carry pain include the lateral spinothalamic and the following:
  1. Spinoreticular—ascend as part of the anterolateral system, originate in the contralateral posterior horn, and terminate diffusely throughout the reticular formation.
  2. Spinomesencephalic—ascend as part of the anterolateral system, originate in the contralateral posterior horn, and terminate on multiple nuclei of the midbrain.
  3. Spinocervical—travel in the posterior aspect of the lateral funiculus, originate in the nucleus proprius, and terminate in the cervical spinal cord.
  4. Postsynaptic fibers in the posterior columns.

B. Posterolateral tract (of Lissauer)
- (predominantly) white matter tract capping the posterior horn.
- mainly pain and temperature fibers ascending or descending 1-2 spinal cord segments before synapsing.
- serves to provide central overlap of pain and temperature.

C. Fasciculus proprius
- white matter tract surrounding the margins of gray matter at all spinal cord levels.
- contains fibers ascending or descending multiple levels, which then reenter the gray matter.
- serves as an intersegmental connection between adjacent cord levels.

IV. CLINICAL CONSIDERATIONS

A. Upper motor neurons (UMNs)
- cortical neurons that give rise to corticobulbar or corticospinal tracts.
- found in brainstem nuclei that influence lower motor neurons (LMNs).
- terminate directly or via interneurons on LMNs.

B. UMN lesions
- caused by damage to the neurons (or their axons) that innervate LMNs.
  1. **Acute-stage lesions**
     - result in transient spinal shock, including:
       a. **Flaccid paralysis**
       b. **Areflexia**
       c. **Hypotonia**
  2. **Chronic-stage lesions**
     - result in:
       a. **Spastic paresis**
       b. **Hypertonia**
          - occurs with increased tone in antigravity muscles (ie, flexors of upper limbs and extensors of lower limbs).
       c. **Reduction or loss of superficial abdominal and cremasteric reflexes**
       d. **Extensor toe response (Babinski sign)**
       e. **Clonus**
          - a repetitive and sustained muscle stretch reflex (MSR) (eg, ankle clonus).

C. Lower motor neurons
- neurons that directly innervate skeletal muscles.
- found in the anterior horns of the spinal cord.
- found in the motor nuclei of CN III, CN IV to CN VII, and CN IX to CN XII.

D. LMN lesions
- result from damage to motor neurons or their peripheral axons.
- result in:
  1. **Flaccid paralysis**
  2. **Areflexia**
  3. **Muscle atrophy**
  4. **Fasciculations and fibrillations**

Review Test

1. The ability to recognize an unseen familiar object placed in the hand depends on the integrity of which of the following?

(A) Fasciculus proprius
(B) Posterior columns
(C) Posterior spinocerebellar tract
(D) Spino-olivary tract
(E) Spinothalamic tract

2. Which of the following tracts is involved with the control of trunk muscles?

(A) Anterior corticospinal
(B) Anterior spinocerebellar
(C) Cuneocerebellar
(D) Lateral corticospinal
(E) Rubrospinal

3. The sensation produced by a wisp of cotton on one's fingertip is mediated by which of the following tracts?

(A) Anterior corticospinal
(B) Anterior spinocerebellar
(C) Anterior spinothalamic
(D) Cuneocerebellar
(E) Posterior column-medial lemniscus pathway

4. First-order neurons of the anterior spinocerebellar tract:

(A) are found in spinal ganglia at all levels.
(B) give rise to the fasciculus cuneatus.
(C) project axons into the medial root entry zone.
(D) project axons via the posterolateral tract (of Lissauer).
(E) provide the afferent limb for MSRs.

5. Acute-stage UMN lesions result in:

(A) hypertonia.
(B) extensor toe response.
(C) clonus.
(D) flaccid paralysis.
(E) spastic paresis.

6. A 65-year-old man, previously diagnosed with amyotrophic lateral sclerosis, presents to his neurologist for an evaluation of the progression of his disease. In addition to cramping, fasciculations, and weakness, examination reveals bilateral thenar wasting (atrophy). What structure/region is compromised to lead to this constellation of symptoms?

(A) Anterior horn
(B) Lateral corticospinal tract
(C) Lateral spinothalamic tract
(D) Medial lemniscus
(E) Posterior columns

7. A 25-year-old woman is brought to the emergency department following a fall from a high ladder at work. The fall onto a pile of branches caused a deep laceration in her back. Imaging reveals a spinal cord hemisection at T0 on the right side. What symptoms should be expected from such an injury below T10? Loss of:

(A) crude touch, right side of body.
(B) fine touch, conscious proprioception and vibratory sense, left side of body.
(C) motor control, left side of body.
(D) pain and temperature, left side of body.
(E) unconscious (reflex) proprioception, left side of body.

Questions 8 to 12

The response options for items 8 to 12 are the same. Select one answer for each item in the set.

(A) Cuneocerebellar tract
(B) Cuneate fasciculus
(C) Lateral corticospinal tract
(D) Lateral spinothalamic tract
(E) Posterior spinocerebellar tract
(F) Posterolateral tract
(G) Vestibulospinal tract

Match each statement below with the appropriate spinal cord tract.

8. Contains axons from the giant cells of Deiters

9. Is the upper limb equivalent of a tract that arises from the cells of the posterior thoracic nucleus (of Clarke)

10. Conveys nociceptive input from the contra-lateral side of the body

11. Contains axons from the giant cells of Betz

12. Contains ipsilateral pain fibers that have their second-order neurons in the posterior horn

Questions 13 to 20

Match the description of a spinal cord tract in items 13 to 20 with the appropriate lettered structure shown in the figure.

13. Projects to the cerebellum via the inferior cerebellar peduncle

14. Mediates pain and temperature sensation

15. Cells of origin are found in the precentral gyrus

16. Mediates two-point tactile discrimination from the hand

17. Myelination is not fully achieved until the end of the second year

18. Transection results in spasticity

19. Plays a role in regulating extensor tone

20. Transmits vibration sensation from the ankle

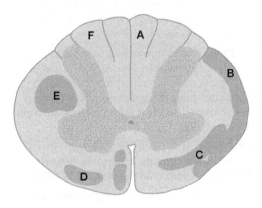

Answers and Explanations

1. **B.** The ability to recognize the form and texture of an unseen familiar object is called stereognosis. This is an important function of the posterior column-medial lemniscus system. Fasciculus proprius connects adjacent cord levels together. The posterior spinocerebellar tract conveys proprioceptive information to the cerebellum. The spino-olivary tract conveys sensory information to the inferior olivary nucleus, which relays movement-related sensory information into the cerebellum. The spinothalamic tract is part of the anterolateral system and conveys pain and temperature information.

2. **A.** The anterior corticospinal tract is concerned with the control of axial muscles, including the muscles of the trunk and head. The anterior spinocerebellar and cuneocerebellar tracts convey proprioceptive information. The lateral corticospinal tract is concerned with control of appendicular muscles, particularly those of the hand. The rubrospinal tract plays a role in flexor tone, primarily the flexors of the upper limb.

3. **C.** The anterior spinothalamic tract is concerned with crude touch, the sensation produced by stroking glabrous skin with a wisp of cotton. The anterior corticospinal tract is a descending tract and not concerned with sensory perception. The anterior spinocerebellar and cuneocerebellar tracts convey proprioceptive information. The posterior column-medial lemniscus pathway conveys fine touch, conscious proprioception, and vibratory sense.

4. **E.** First-order neurons of the anterior spinocerebellar tract provide the afferent limb for MSRs. They are found in the spinal ganglia from L1 to S2 and synapse on spinal border cells. First-order neurons of the anterior spinothalamic and posterior spinocerebellar tracts project axons into the medial root entry zone; first-order neurons of the posterior column-medial lemniscus pathway give rise to the fasciculus gracilis and cuneatus; and first-order neurons of the lateral spinothalamic tract project axons via the posterolateral tract (of Lissauer).

5. **D.** Acute-stage UMN lesions result in transient spinal shock, which includes flaccid paralysis, areflexia, and hypotonia. Chronic-stage lesions result in spastic paresis, hypertonia, reduction or loss of superficial abdominal and cremasteric reflexes and extensor toe response, and clonus.

6. **A.** The anterior horn of the spinal cord contains lower motor neurons, the lesion of which leads to fasciculations, flaccid paralysis, hyporeflexia, and muscular atrophy. The lateral corticospinal tract contains the upper motor neurons that innervate the anterior horn cells—lesion of this tract, composed of upper motor neurons, leads to many of the same symptoms as lesion of the anterior horn cells initially (acute phase), but transitions into spastic paralysis, hyperreflexia and hypertonia over time. The lateral spinothalamic, medial lemniscus, and posterior columns are all ascending/sensory pathways and are unrelated to the motor-related symptoms in this patient.

7. **D.** Spinal cord hemisection on the right side would damage the lateral spinothalamic tract, the tract conveys paint and temperature information, and is formed of fibers that cross the midline upon entering the cord (ie, from the left side). Crude touch also crosses the midline upon entering the spinal cord, so crude touch would also be lost on the side contralateral to the lesion (ie, left side). The posterior column modalities (fine touch, conscious proprioception, and vibratory sense) would also be lost, but they ascend the cord ipsilaterally, so the loss would be on the same side as the lesion (ie, right side). The corticospinal tract crosses the midline in the medulla and so is uncrossed in the spinal cord, lesion would result in loss of descending motor influence ipsilateral to the lesion (ie, right side). Unconscious proprioception is primarily conveyed via the uncrossed posterior spinocerebellar tract and so loss, albeit not as straightforward to detect, would be on the same side as the lesion.

8. **G.** The vestibulospinal tract arises from the giant cells of Deiters found in the ipsilateral lateral vestibular nucleus of the pons. The vestibulospinal tracts facilitate extensor muscle tone.

9. **A.** The cuneocerebellar tract is the upper extremity equivalent of the posterior spinocerebellar tract, which arises from the cells of the posterior thoracic nucleus (of Clarke). The cuneocerebellar tract arises from cells of the accessory cuneate nucleus, a homolog of the posterior thoracic nucleus.

10. **D.** The anterolateral system conveys nociceptive input from the contralateral side of the body; the lateral spinothalamic tract is part of the anterolateral system.

11. **C.** The lateral corticospinal tract contains axons from the giant cells of Betz. The giant pyramidal cells of Betz are found in the precentral gyrus and in the anterior paracentral lobule.

12. **F.** The posterolateral tract (of Lissauer) contains ipsilateral pain fibers that have their second-order neurons in the posterior horn.

13. **B.** The posterior spinocerebellar tract projects unconscious proprioceptive information (muscle spindles and GTOs) to the cerebellum via the inferior cerebellar peduncle.

14. **C.** The anterolateral tract lies between the anterior spinocerebellar tract and the anterior horn. It mediates pain and temperature sensation.

15. **E.** The lateral corticospinal tract has its cells of origin in the premotor, motor, and sensory cortices. The precentral gyrus and the anterior paracentral lobule are motor cortices and contain the motor homunculus. The lateral corticospinal gives rise to one-third of the fibers of the corticospinal (pyramidal) tract.

16. **F.** The fasciculus cuneatus mediates two-point tactile discrimination from the hand.

17. **E.** The corticospinal (pyramidal) tracts are not fully myelinated until the end of the second year. For this reason, the Babinski sign may be elicited in young children.

18. **E.** Transection of the lateral corticospinal tract results in spastic paresis (exaggerated MSRs and clonus).

19. **D.** The vestibulospinal tracts, found in the anterior funiculus, play a role in regulating extensor tone.

20. **A.** The fasciculus gracilis transmits vibratory sensation (pallesthesia) from the lower extremities.

chapter 8

Lesions of the Spinal Cord

Objectives

- Describe the difference between upper and lower motor neuron lesions and include examples of each.
- Give examples of sensory versus motor pathway lesions, peripheral nervous system lesions, and combined lesions.

I. LOWER MOTOR NEURON LESIONS (Figure 8.1A)

- result from damage to somatic motor neurons of the anterior horns of the spinal cord or somatic motor neuron nuclei of the brainstem, including oculomotor, trochlear, trigeminal, abducens, facial, ambiguus, and hypoglossal.
- result from interruption of the final common pathway connecting the neuron via its axon with the muscle fibers it innervates (the motor unit).

A. Neurologic deficits resulting from lower motor neuron (LMN) lesions
1. **Flaccid paralysis**
2. **Muscle atrophy (amyotrophy)**
3. **Hypotonia**
4. **Areflexia**
   - consists of loss of muscle stretch reflexes (MSRs) (eg, knee and ankle jerk) and loss of superficial reflexes (eg, abdominal and cremasteric).
5. **Fasciculations** (spontaneous muscle contraction and relaxation, or muscle twitches)
6. **Fibrillations** (rapid, unsynchronized contraction of muscle fibers)

B. Diseases of LMNs (see Figure 8.1A)
1. **Poliomyelitis**
   - an acute inflammatory viral infection affecting LMNs caused by the polio virus (an enterovirus).
   - cases have decreased 99% since mid-1980s.
   - results in a flaccid paralysis, mostly in children younger than 5 years of age.
2. **Progressive infantile muscular atrophy (Werdnig-Hoffmann disease)**
   - a hereditary degenerative disease of infants that affects LMNs of the anterior horn of the spinal cord and the brainstem.
   - characterized by hypotonia and hyporeflexia with preservation of intellect and higher order functions.
   - 50% mortality rate before birth, mostly fatal before 2 years of age.

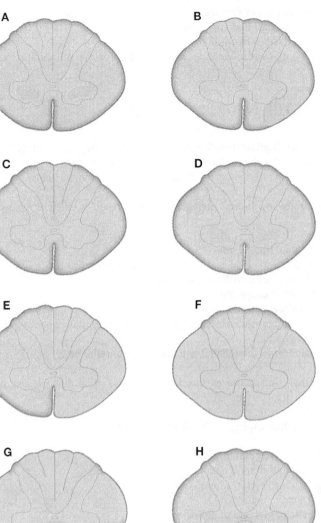

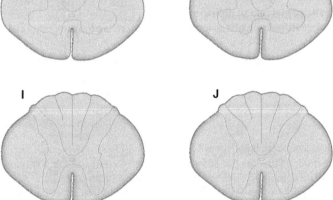

FIGURE 8.1. Lesions of the spinal cord. **(A)** Poliomyelitis and progressive infantile muscular atrophy (Werdnig-Hoffmann disease). **(B)** Multiple sclerosis. **(C)** Posterior column disease (tabes dorsalis). **(D)** Amyotrophic lateral sclerosis. **(E)** Hemisection of the spinal cord (Brown-Séquard syndrome). **(F)** Complete anterior spinal artery occlusion of the spinal cord. **(G)** Subacute combined degeneration (vitamin B_{12} neuropathy). **(H)** Syringomyelia. **(I)** Charcot-Marie-Tooth disease (hereditary motor-sensory neuropathy type 1). **(J)** Complete posterior spinal artery occlusion. (Modified with permission from Fix JD. *High-Yield Neuroanatomy*. 3rd ed. Lippincott Williams & Wilkins; 2005:70.)

3. **Kugelberg-Welander disease** (juvenile hereditary LMN disease)
   - genetic disorder that appears at 3 to 20 years of age.
   - characterized by hypotonia.
   - affects upper and lower limbs starting with proximal musculature and moves distally.

II. UPPER MOTOR NEURON LESIONS

- known as **pyramidal tract lesions**: lesions of the corticospinal and corticobulbar tracts.
- may occur at all levels of the neuraxis from the cerebral cortex to the spinal cord.
- when rostral to the pyramidal decussation, they result in deficits below the lesion, on the contralateral side.
- when caudal to the pyramidal decussation, they result in deficits below the lesion, on the ipsilateral side.

A. **Lateral corticospinal tract lesion**
   - results in the following ipsilateral motor deficits found below the lesion:
   1. **Spastic hemiparesis with muscle weakness**
   2. **Hyperreflexia (exaggerated MSRs)**
   3. **Clasp-knife spasticity**
      - when a joint is moved briskly, resistance occurs initially and then fades (like the opening of a pocketknife).
   4. **Loss of superficial (abdominal and cremasteric) reflexes**
   5. **Clonus**
      - rhythmic contractions of muscles in response to sudden, passive movements (eg, wrist, patellar, or ankle clonus).
   6. **Babinski sign**
      - plantar reflex response—dorsiflexion of big toe.

B. **Anterior corticospinal tract lesion**
   - results in **mild contralateral motor deficit**. Anterior corticospinal tract fibers decussate at spinal levels via the anterior white commissure.

C. **Hereditary spastic paraplegia or diplegia**
   - caused by defective function of transport proteins, therefore long tracts affected first, for example, corticospinal tracts.
   - gradual development of spastic weakness of the lower limbs with increased difficulty in walking.

III. SENSORY PATHWAY LESIONS

A. **Posterior column syndrome (see Figure 8.1C)**
   - includes the fasciculi gracilis (T6-S5) and cuneatus (C2-T6) and the posterior roots.
   - seen in subacute combined degeneration (vitamin B_{12} neuropathy).
   - seen in neurosyphilis as **tabes dorsalis** and in nonsyphilitic sensory neuropathies.
   - results in the following **ipsilateral sensory deficits** found below the level of the lesion:
   1. **Loss of tactile discrimination**
   2. **Loss of position (joint) and vibratory sensation**
   3. **Stereoanesthesia** (asterognosis)
   4. **Sensory (posterior column) dystaxia**
   5. **Paresthesias and pain** (posterior root irritation)
   6. **Hyporeflexia or areflexia** (posterior root deafferentation)
   7. **Urinary incontinence, constipation, and impotence** (posterior root deafferentation)
   8. **Romberg sign** (sensory dystaxia) (standing patient is more unsteady with eyes closed)

B. Lateral spinothalamic tract lesion
- contralateral loss of pain and temperature sensation beginning one segment below the level of the lesion.

C. Anterior spinothalamic tract lesion
- contralateral loss of crude touch sensation three or four segments below the level of the lesion.
- does not appreciably reduce touch sensation if the posterior columns are intact.

D. Posterior spinocerebellar tract lesion
- ipsilateral lower limb dystaxia; patient has difficulty performing the heel-to-shin test.

E. Anterior spinocerebellar tract lesion
- contralateral lower limb dystaxia; patient has difficulty performing the heel-to-shin test.

IV. PERIPHERAL NERVOUS SYSTEM LESIONS

- may be sensory, motor, or combined.
- affect spinal roots, spinal ganglia, and peripheral nerves.

CLINICAL CORRELATES Herpes zoster (shingles) is a common (4:1,000) **viral infection** of the nervous system. It involves an acute inflammatory reaction in the spinal or cranial nerve ganglia and is usually limited to the territory of one dermatome; the most common sites are from **T5 to T10**. The irritation of the ganglion cells, results in pain, itching, burning sensation, and vesicular eruption over the affected dermatome(s).

CLINICAL CORRELATES Acute idiopathic polyneuritis (Guillain-Barré syndrome), also known as postinfectious polyneuritis, produces lower motor neuron symptoms (muscle weakness, flaccid paralysis, and areflexia). Symptoms are symmetric and begin in the lower limbs and ascend to the trunk and upper limbs; the facial nerve is frequently (bilaterally) involved. It affects 1 to 2:100,000 individuals, and those older than 50 years of age are at greatest risk.

V. COMBINED UPPER MOTOR NEURON AND LOWER MOTOR NEURON LESIONS

A. Characteristics
- muscle weakness and wasting without sensory deficits.

B. Prototypic disease—amyotrophic lateral sclerosis (ALS) (see Figure 8.1D)
- also called **Lou Gehrig disease**, motor neuron disease, or motor system disease.
- usually occurs in persons of 50 to 70 years.
- affects nearly twice as many men as women.
- involves both LMNs and lower motor neurons (UMNs).
- progressive (spinal) muscular atrophy or progressive bulbar palsy refers to an LMN component.
- pseudobulbar palsy or primary lateral sclerosis refers to a UMN component.

VI. COMBINED MOTOR AND SENSORY LESIONS

A. Spinal cord hemisection (Brown-Séquard syndrome) (Figures 8.2 and 8.3; see Figure 8.1E)

1. **Posterior column transection**
   - results in ipsilateral loss of tactile discrimination, form perception, and position and vibration sensation below the level of the lesion.
2. **Lateral spinothalamic tract transection**
   - results in contralateral loss of pain and temperature sensation, starting one segment below the level of the lesion.
3. **Anterior spinothalamic tract transection**
   - results in contralateral loss of crude touch sensation starting three or four segments below the level of the lesion.
4. **Posterior spinocerebellar tract transection**
   - loss of unconscious/reflex proprioception.
   - results in ipsilateral lower limb dystaxia.
5. **Anterior spinocerebellar tract transection**
   - loss of unconscious/reflex proprioception.
   - results in contralateral lower limb dystaxia.
6. **Hypothalamospinal tract transection rostral to T2**
   - results in Horner syndrome.
7. **Lateral corticospinal tract transection**
   - results in ipsilateral spastic paresis below the UMN lesion with Babinski sign.
8. **Anterior corticospinal tract transection**
   - results in minor contralateral muscle weakness below the level of the lesion.

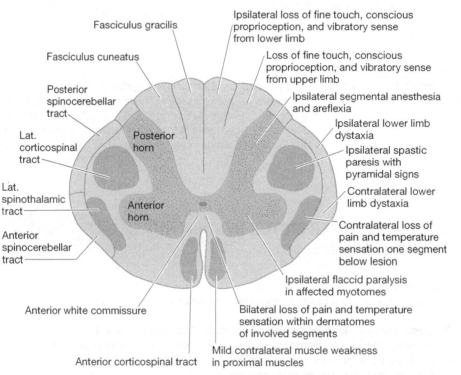

FIGURE 8.2. Transverse section of the cervical spinal cord. Clinically important pathways are shown on the left side; clinical deficits resulting from the interruption of these pathways are shown on the right side. Destructive lesions of the posterior horns result in anesthesia and areflexia, and destructive lesions of the anterior horns result in lower motor neuron lesions and areflexia. Destruction of the anterior white commissure interrupts the central transmission of pain and temperature impulses bilaterally via the anterolateral system.

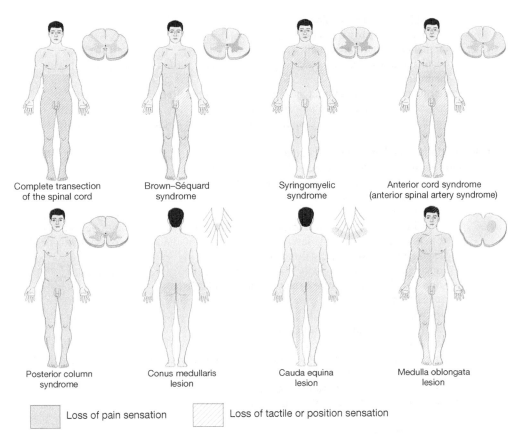

Complete transection
of the spinal cord

Brown–Séquard
syndrome

Syringomyelic
syndrome

Anterior cord syndrome
(anterior spinal artery syndrome)

Posterior column
syndrome

Conus medullaris
lesion

Cauda equina
lesion

Medulla oblongata
lesion

☐ Loss of pain sensation   ▨ Loss of tactile or position sensation

FIGURE 8.3. Localization of sensory disorders.

9. Anterior horn destruction
- results in ipsilateral flaccid paralysis of somatic muscles (LMN lesion).

10. Posterior horn destruction
- results in ipsilateral dermatomic anesthesia and areflexia.

B. Complete transection of the spinal cord
- results in the following conditions:
  1. Exitus letalis if between C1 and C3
  2. Quadriplegia if between C4 and C5
  3. Paraplegia if below T1
  4. Spastic paralysis of all voluntary movements below the level of the lesion
  5. Complete anesthesia below the level of the lesion
  6. Urinary and fecal incontinence (although reflex emptying may occur)
  7. Anhidrosis and loss of vasomotor tone
  8. Paralysis of volitional and automatic breathing, if the transection is above C5 (the phrenic nucleus is found at C3-C5)

C. Anterior spinal artery occlusion (see Figure 8.1F)
- causes infarction of the anterior two-thirds of the spinal cord.
- typically spares the posterior columns and posterior horns.
- paralysis of voluntary and automatic respiration in cervical segments; it also results in bilateral Horner syndrome.
- loss of voluntary bladder and bowel control, with preservation of reflex emptying.
- anhidrosis and loss of vasomotor tone.
  1. Anterior horn destruction
  - complete flaccid paralysis and areflexia at the level of the lesion.

2. Corticospinal tract transection
- results in a spastic paresis below the level of the lesion.

3. Spinothalamic tract transection
- results in loss of pain and temperature sensation, starting one segment below the level of the lesion.

4. Posterior spinocerebellar tract and anterior spinocerebellar tract transection
- loss of unconscious/reflex proprioception
- results in cerebellar incoordination, which is masked by LMN and UMN paralysis.

D. Conus medullaris and epiconus syndromes
- include neurologic deficits and signs that are mostly bilateral.
- often presents as a mixture of UMN and LMN deficits.

1. Conus medullaris syndrome
- involves segments S3-Co.
- typically caused by small intramedullary tumor metastases or hemorrhagic infarcts.
- results in destruction of the sacral parasympathetic nucleus, which causes paralytic bladder, fecal incontinence, and impotence.
- causes perianogenital sensory loss in dermatomes S3-Co (saddle anesthesia).
- shows an absence of motor deficits in the lower limbs.

2. Epiconus syndrome
- involves segments L4-S2.
- caused by ossification of the ligamentum flavum.
- results in reflex functioning of the bladder and rectum but loss of voluntary control.
- characterized by considerable motor disability (external rotation and extension of the thigh are most affected).
- affects the anterior horns and longitudinal spinal cord tracts.
- associated with absent Achilles tendon reflex.

E. Cauda equina syndrome
- classically involves spinal roots L3-Co.
- typically caused by large disk herniation.
- preferentially affects women, 30 to 50 years of age.
- produces neurologic deficits similar to those seen in conus or epiconus lesions.
- results in signs that frequently predominate on one side.
- may result from intervertebral disk herniation.
- commonly results in severe spontaneous radicular pain (pain that radiates along a dermatome).

F. Filum terminale (tethered cord) syndrome
- results from a thickened, shortened filum terminale that adheres to the sacrum and causes traction on the conus medullaris.
- characterized by sphincter dysfunction, gait disorders, and deformities of the feet.

G. Subacute combined degeneration (vitamin B$_{12}$ neuropathy) (see Figure 8.1G)
- a spinal cord disease associated with pernicious anemia.
- consists of demyelination of posterior columns, resulting in loss of vibration and position sensation.
- consists of demyelination of spinocerebellar tracts, resulting in arm and leg dystaxia.
- consists of demyelination of corticospinal tracts, resulting in spastic paresis (UMN signs).

H. Friedreich hereditary ataxia (see Figure 8.1G)
- the commonest hereditary ataxia with autosomal recessive inheritance.
- results in spinal cord pathology and spinal cord symptoms that are similar to subacute combined degeneration with posterior column, spinocerebellar, and corticospinal tract involvement.
- cerebellar involvement (Purkinje cells and dentate nucleus) is frequent with progressive ataxia.
- commonly leads to cardiomyopathy, pes cavus (high plantar arch), and kyphoscoliosis.

I. Syringomyelia (see Figures 8.1H and 8.3)

- a central cavitation of the spinal cord of unknown etiology, typically found in upper spinal cord regions.
- results in destruction of the anterior white commissure and interruption of decussating spinothalamic fibers, causing bilateral loss of pain and temperature sensation.
- may result in extension of the syrinx into the anterior horn, causing an LMN lesion with muscle wasting and hyporeflexia. Atrophy of lumbricals and interosseous muscles of the hand is a common finding.
- may result in extension of the syrinx into the lateral funiculus, affecting the lateral corticospinal tract and resulting in spastic paresis (UMN lesion).
- may result in caudal extension of the syrinx into the lateral horn at T1 or lateral extension into the lateral funiculus (interruption of descending autonomic pathways), resulting in Horner syndrome.
- may be associated with Chiari malformation.

J. Charcot-Marie-Tooth disease (hereditary motor-sensory neuropathy type I) (see Figure 8.1I)

- also called fibular (peroneal) muscular atrophy.
- the commonest inherited neuropathy, manifest between 5 and 15 years of age.
- more common in women than men.
- affects the posterior columns, resulting in a loss of conscious proprioception.
- affects the anterior horn motor neurons, resulting in muscle weakness (atrophy) below the knee.

CLINICAL CORRELATES   **Multiple sclerosis** (Figure 8.1B) is the commonest form of demyelinating disease (3.5:1,000). The autoimmune disorder is more common in women than men and affects individuals who are 15 to 50 years of age. It is characterized by asymmetric sclerotic lesions in the brain and spinal cord, formed when the myelin is destroyed. In the spinal cord, lesions occur most frequently at cervical levels.

VII. INTERVERTEBRAL DISK HERNIATION

A. Overview

- consists of prolapse or herniation of the **nucleus pulposus** through a defective **annulus fibrosus** into the vertebral canal. The nucleus pulposus impinges on spinal roots, resulting in root pain (radiculopathy) or muscle weakness.
- may compress the spinal cord.
- recognized as the major cause of severe and chronic low back and lower limb pain.
- appears in 90% of cases at the L4-L5 or L5-S1 interspaces; usually a single nerve root is compressed, but several may be involved at the L5-S1 interspace (cauda equina).
- appears in 10% of cases in the cervical region, usually at the C5-C6 or C6-C7 interspaces.
- characterized by **spinal root symptoms** that include paresthesias, pain, sensory loss, hyporeflexia, and muscle weakness.

B. Cervical spondylosis with myelopathy

- the most commonly observed myelopathy.
- consists of spinal cord or spinal cord root compression by calcified disk material extruded into the vertebral canal.
- presents as painful stiff neck, upper limb pain and weakness, and spastic lower limb weakness with dystaxia; sensory disorders are frequent.

Review Test

Questions 1 to 3

Questions 1 to 3 relate to the figure.

Neuropathologic examination of the spinal cord reveals two lesions labeled A and B. Lesion A is restricted to five segments.

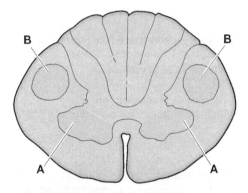

1. The result of lesion A is best described as

(A) bilateral upper limb dystaxia with dysdiadochokinesia.

(B) flaccid paralysis of the upper limbs.

(C) loss of pain and temperature sensation below the level of the lesion.

(D) urinary and fecal incontinence.

(E) spastic paresis of the lower limbs.

2. The result of lesion B is best described as

(A) bilateral apallesthesia.

(B) dyssynergia of movements affecting both upper and lower limbs.

(C) flaccid paralysis of the upper limbs.

(D) impaired two-point tactile discrimination in both upper limbs.

(E) spastic paresis affecting primarily the muscles distal to the knee joint.

3. Lesions A and B may result from

(A) ALS.

(B) an extramedullary tumor.

(C) an intramedullary tumor.

(D) multiple sclerosis.

(E) thrombosis of a spinal artery.

4. Neurologic examination reveals an extensor plantar reflex and hyperreflexia on the left side, a loss of pain and temperature sensation on the right side, and ptosis and miosis on the left side. A lesion that causes this constellation of deficits would most likely be found in the

(A) cervical spinal cord.

(B) crus cerebri, right side.

(C) lumbar spinal cord.

(D) paracentral lobule, left side.

(E) posterolateral medulla, left side.

5. A 50-year-old woman complains of clumsiness in her hands while working in the kitchen. She recently burned her hands on the stove without experiencing any pain. Neurologic examination reveals bilateral weakness of the shoulder girdles, arms, and hands as well as a loss of pain and temperature sensation covering the shoulder and upper limb in a cape-like distribution of sensory loss. Severe atrophy is present in the intrinsic muscles of the hands. The most likely diagnosis is

(A) ALS.

(B) subacute combined degeneration.

(C) syringomyelia.

(D) tabes dorsalis.

(E) Werdnig-Hoffmann disease.

6. A 50-year-old man has a 2-year history of progressive muscle weakness in all limbs, with severe muscle atrophy and reduced MSRs in both lower limbs. In his upper limbs, the muscle atrophy is less pronounced and the MSRs are exaggerated. Which of the following types of neuronal degeneration would postmortem examination most likely reveal?

(A) Demyelination of axons in the posterior and lateral columns

(B) Demyelination of axons in the posterior limb of the internal capsule

(C) Loss of neurons from the globus pallidus

(D) Loss of neurons from the paracentral lobule and from the anterior horns of the spinal cord

(E) Loss of Purkinje cells

7. Transection of the anterolateral tract may result in

(A) areflexia.
(B) cerebellar incoordination.
(C) complete flaccid paralysis.
(D) loss of pain and temperature sensation.
(E) spastic paresis.

8. Which of the following is a characteristic of Lou Gehrig disease?

(A) Loss of tactile discrimination
(B) Loss of vibratory sensation
(C) Posterior root irritation
(D) Progressive bulbar palsy
(E) Stereoanesthesia

9. Clasp-knife spasticity results from a lesion in the

(A) anterior corticospinal tract.
(B) anterior spinothalamic tract.
(C) lateral corticospinal tract.
(D) lateral spinothalamic tract.
(E) posterior spinocerebellar tract.

10. Which of the following syndromes is associated with an absent Achilles tendon reflex?

(A) Cauda equina
(B) Conus medullaris
(C) Epiconus
(D) Filum terminale
(E) Syringomyelia

11. An example of a peripheral nervous system lesion is

(A) Brown-Séquard syndrome.
(B) Charcot-Marie-Tooth disease.
(C) Friedreich ataxia.
(D) Guillain-Barré syndrome.
(E) Lou Gehrig disease.

12. A patient has the ability to stand with open eyes but falls with closed eyes. A lesion of which pathway is likely responsible for this symptom?

(A) Anterior spinocerebellar tract
(B) Anterior spinothalamic tract
(C) Lateral spinothalamic tract
(D) Posterior column syndrome
(E) Posterior spinocerebellar tract

13. A 20-year-old woman, previously diagnosed with multiple sclerosis, presents to her neurologist for evaluation of her condition. She reports that during her last "episode," in addition to well-described visual symptoms that

she experienced significant bilateral muscle weakness in all limbs. Examination revealed a high degree of spasticity, particularly in the lower limbs. Lesion of which of the following spinal cord tracts would lead to the patient's symptoms?

(A) Anterior corticospinal
(B) Anterior spinocerebellar
(C) Lateral corticospinal
(D) Posterior column
(E) Spinothalamic

14. A 10-year-old boy is brought to his pediatrician by his mother who is concerned about repeated sprained ankles during physical activity and what she observes as poorly developed, weak calf musculature. She is concerned that her son may have some type of neuropathy, as she reports it runs in her family. The pediatrician orders electromyography (EMG) testing, which reveals axonal loss and demyelination. Genetic testing confirms which of the following?

(A) Brown-Séquard syndrome
(B) Cauda equina syndrome
(C) Charcot-Marie-Tooth disease
(D) Friedreich hereditary ataxia
(E) Multiple sclerosis

Questions 15 to 20

The response options for items 15 to 20 are the same. Select one answer for each item in the set.

(A) ALS
(B) Cauda equina syndrome
(C) Cervical spondylosis
(D) Friedreich ataxia
(E) Guillain-Barré syndrome
(F) Multiple sclerosis
(G) Subacute combined degeneration
(H) Tabes dorsalis
(I) Werdnig-Hoffmann disease

Match each statement below with the syndrome that corresponds best to it.

15. A pure LMN disease

16. Elevated cerebrospinal fluid (CSF) protein with a normal CSF cell count

17. Characterized by asymmetric lesions found in the white matter of cervical segments

18. May result from intervertebral disk herniation

19. Symptoms include a painful stiff neck, arm pain and weakness, spastic leg weakness with dystaxia; sensory disorders are frequent.

20. Associated with a loss of Purkinje cells

Questions 21 to 28

Match the statement in items 21 to 28 with the lesion shown in the figure that corresponds best to it.

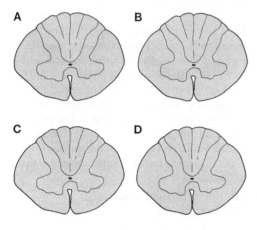

21. Neurologic manifestation of vitamin B_{12} deficiency

22. Lesion owing to vascular occlusion

23. Loss of vibration sensation on the right side; loss of pain and temperature sensation on the left side

24. Bilateral loss of pain and temperature sensation in the lower limbs

25. Bilateral loss of pain and temperature sensation in the hands; muscle atrophy in both hands; spastic paresis on the right side only

26. Urinary incontinence and quadriplegia

27. No muscle atrophy or fasciculations

28. Demyelinating disease

Answers and Explanations

1. **B.** Lesion A involves degeneration of the anterior horns bilaterally at midcervical levels and results in flaccid paralysis in the upper limbs.

2. **E.** Lesion B involves degeneration of the lateral corticospinal tracts bilaterally, resulting in spastic paresis of the lower limbs, primarily affecting the muscles distal to the knee. Spastic paresis of the upper limbs is masked by flaccid paralysis resulting from lesion A. Apallesthesia is the inability to perceive a vibrating tuning fork.

3. **A.** Lesions A and B are the result of ALS, a motor disease.

4. **A.** A lesion of the cervical spinal cord could result in ipsilateral Horner syndrome, ipsilateral spastic paresis, and contralateral loss of pain and temperature sensation. Horner syndrome manifests on the ipsilateral side. This lesion produces a classic Brown-Séquard syndrome.

5. **C.** Syringomyelia is a cavitation of the spinal cord most commonly seen in the cervicothoracic segments. This condition results in bilateral loss of pain and temperature sensation in a cape-like distribution as well as wasting of the intrinsic muscles of the hands. ALS is a purely motor syndrome. Subacute combined degeneration includes both sensory and motor deficits. Werdnig-Hoffmann disease is a purely motor disease. Tabes dorsalis is a purely sensory syndrome (neurosyphilis).

6. **D.** ALS affects both UMN and LMNs. It is also referred to as motor systems disease. A loss of Purkinje cells, as seen in cerebellar cortical atrophy (cerebello-olivary atrophy) results in cerebellar signs. Cell loss in the globus pallidus and putamen is seen in Wilson disease (hepatolenticular degeneration). Demyelination of axons in the posterior and lateral columns is seen in subacute combined degeneration. Demyelination of axons in the posterior limb of the internal capsule results in contralateral spastic hemiparesis.

7. **D.** Transection of the anterolateral tract results in loss of pain and temperature sensations, starting one segment below the level of the lesion. Anterior horn destruction results in flaccid paralysis and areflexia at the level of the lesion. Corticospinal tract transection results in spastic paresis below the level of the lesion. Posterior spinocerebellar tract and ventral spinocerebellar tract transection results in cerebellar incoordination.

8. **D.** Progressive bulbar palsy is an LMN component of ALS, or Lou Gehrig disease. Disease characteristics are muscle weakness and wasting without sensory deficits. Loss of tactile discrimination, loss of vibratory sensation, stereoanesthesia, and dorsal root irritation are all sensory deficits found in posterior column syndrome.

9. **C.** Clasp-knife spasticity is an ipsilateral motor deficit found below a lesion of the lateral corticospinal tract. It is characterized by initial but fading resistance of a briskly moved joint.

10. **C.** Epiconus syndrome involves spinal cord segments L4-S2 and results in loss of voluntary control of the bladder and rectum, motor disability, and an absent Achilles tendon reflex.

11. **D.** Acute idiopathic polyneuritis, or Guillain-Barré syndrome, is a peripheral nervous system disorder. It typically follows an infectious illness and results from a cell-mediated immunologic reaction.

12. **D.** Posterior column syndrome results in a sensory deficit known as sensory dystaxia or Romberg sign. Patients are Romberg positive when they are able to stand with the eyes open but fall with the eyes closed.

13. **C.** Lesion of the lateral corticospinal tract, which is often seen in multiple sclerosis, commonly presents as paraplegia or paraparesis and spastic paralysis, particularly in the lower limbs. Lesion of the anterior corticospinal tract would have a milder effect and would not be as evident in the limbs. The anterior spinocerebellar (reflex proprioception), posterior columns (fine touch, conscious proprioception, and vibratory sense), and spinothalamic (pain and temperature) tracts are all ascending/sensory tracts and lesion would not produce spastic paralysis.

14. C. Charcot-Marie-Tooth disease is a genetic disorder that affects the lower motor neurons of the anterior horn, particularly below the knee, resulting in an increase in sprained ankles, muscle atrophy, and difficulty walking and running. It typically manifests in the first decade of life. Brown-Séquard syndrome is caused by spinal cord hemisection and produces a much larger and more widespread constellation of symptoms than seen in this patient. Cauda equina syndrome typically produces pain on one side of the body, not the symptoms of the current patient. Friedreich hereditary ataxia is also a genetic disease that causes progressive ataxia, which is often accompanied by posterior column sign. Multiple sclerosis is also a demyelinating disease, but it produces widespread asymmetric lesions, most commonly seen in the cervical region.

15. I. Werdnig-Hoffmann disease is a hereditary degenerative disease of infants that affects only LMNs.

16. E. Guillain-Barré syndrome is characterized by elevated CSF protein with normal CSF cell count (albuminocytologic dissociation).

17. F. Multiple sclerosis is characterized by asymmetric lesions frequently found in the white matter of cervical spinal cord segments.

18. B. Cauda equina syndrome frequently results from intervertebral disk herniation; severe spontaneous radicular pain is common.

19. C. Cervical spondylosis is the most commonly observed myelopathy. Its symptoms include a painful stiff neck, arm pain and weakness, and spastic leg weakness with dystaxia; sensory disorders are frequent.

20. D. Friedreich ataxia is the most common hereditary ataxia with autosomal recessive inheritance. Posterior columns, spinocerebellar tracts, and the corticospinal tracts show demyelination. Friedreich ataxia results in a loss of Purkinje cells in the cerebellar cortex and a loss of neurons in the dentate nucleus.

21. C. A neurologic manifestation of vitamin B_{12} deficiency is subacute combined degeneration. There is no involvement of LMNs.

22. A. Lesion A shows the territory of infarction resulting from occlusion of the anterior spinal artery.

23. D. A spinal cord hemisection (Brown-Séquard syndrome) results in a loss of vibratory sense on the right side and a loss of pain and temperature sensation on the left side (dissociated sensory loss).

24. A. Total occlusion of the anterior spinal artery that involves five cervical segments and results in infarction of the anterior two-thirds of the spinal cord and interrupts the anterolateral system. The patient will have a loss of pain and temperature sensation caudal to the lesion.

25. B. Lesion B shows a cervical syringomyelic lesion involving the anterior white commissure, both anterior horns, and the right corticospinal tract. The patient will have a bilateral loss of pain and temperature sensation in the hands, muscle wasting in both hands, and a spastic paresis on the right side.

26. A. In lesion A, both lateral and anterior funiculi have been infarcted by arterial occlusion. Bilateral destruction of the lateral corticospinal tracts at upper cervical levels results in quadriplegia (spastic paresis in upper and lower limbs). Bilateral destruction of the anterolateral quadrants results in urinary and fecal incontinence.

27. C. In lesion C, subacute combined degeneration, there is no involvement of LMNs, hence no flaccid paralysis, muscle atrophy, or fasciculations.

28. C. In lesion C, subacute combined degeneration, there is symmetric degeneration of the white matter, both in the posterior columns and in the lateral funiculi. In this degenerative disease, both the myelin sheaths and the axon are involved. Subacute combined degeneration is classified under nutritional diseases (in this case, a vitamin B_{12} neuropathy). In true demyelinative diseases (eg, multiple sclerosis), the myelin sheaths are involved, but the axons and nerve cells are relatively spared.

chapter

Objectives

■ List the parts of the brainstem and external characteristics of each part.
■ List the major pathways (ascending and descending) and nuclei found in the medulla, pons, and midbrain and include a general description of the significance of each.
■ Identify the components of representative brainstem sections based on the diagrams provided in the text.

I. OVERVIEW (Figure 9.1)

▨ includes the **medulla**, **pons**, and **mesencephalon** (midbrain).
▨ extends from the pyramidal decussation to the posterior commissure.
▨ gives rise to cranial nerves III to XII.
▨ receives blood supply from the vertebrobasilar system.
▨ contains the **reticular formation** as its central core: phylogenetically old—functions as the core integrating structure of the central nervous system (CNS) as it receives collaterals from most afferent and efferent systems.

II. MEDULLA OBLONGATA (MYELENCEPHALON)

A. Overview: the medulla

▨ contains autonomic centers that regulate respiration, circulation, and gastrointestinal motility.
▨ extends from the pyramidal decussation to the inferior pontine sulcus.
▨ gives rise to cranial nerves IX to XII. The nuclei of CN V and CN VIII extend caudally into the medulla.
▨ connected to the cerebellum by the inferior cerebellar peduncle.

B. Internal structures of the medulla (Figures 9.2 through 9.5)

1. Ascending pathways and relay nuclei

▨ **Fasciculus gracilis and fasciculus cuneatus**
  a. convey posterior column modalities.
  b. terminate in the nucleus gracilis and nucleus cuneatus.
▨ **Nucleus gracilis and nucleus cuneatus**
  a. contain second-order neurons of the posterior column-medial lemniscus pathway.
  b. give rise to internal arcuate fibers, which cross the midline.
  c. project via the medial lemniscus to the ventral posterolateral nucleus of the thalamus.

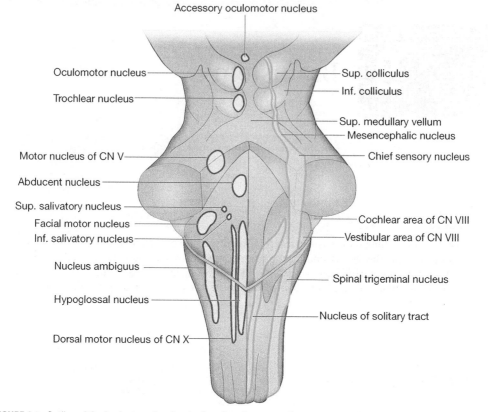

FIGURE 9.1. Outline of the brainstem showing the location of motor and sensory cranial nerve nuclei. Motor nuclei are shown on the left side of the figure and sensory nuclei are shown on the right side.

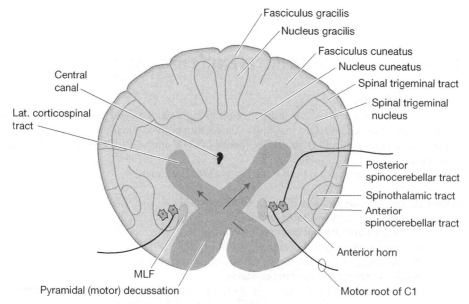

FIGURE 9.2. Transverse section of the caudal medulla at the level of the pyramidal (motor) decussation. MLF, medial longitudinal fasciculus.

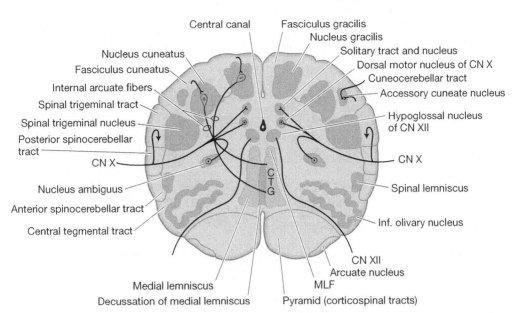

FIGURE 9.3. Transverse section of the caudal medulla at the level of the decussation of the medial lemniscus. The internal arcuate fibers decussate and form the medial lemniscus. General somatic afferent fibers of the vagal nerve (CN X) enter the spinal trigeminal tract of CN V (arrow). CTG, cuneate (arm), trunk, and gracile (leg) components of the medial lemniscus; MLF, medial longitudinal fasciculus.

- **Internal arcuate fibers**
    - **a.** arise from the nucleus gracilis and nucleus cuneatus and form the contralateral medial lemniscus.
- **Decussation of the medial lemniscus** (see Figure 9.3)
    - **a.** formed by decussating internal arcuate fibers.
    - **b.** also known as the sensory decussation.
- **Medial lemniscus**
    - **a.** conveys posterior column modalities to the ventral posterolateral nucleus of the ipsilateral thalamus.

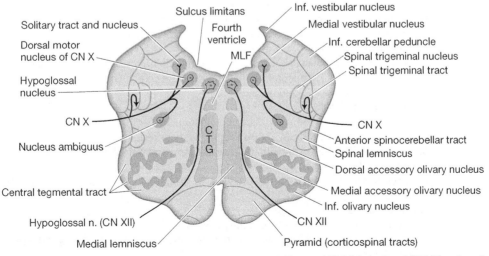

FIGURE 9.4. Transverse section of the medulla at the midolivary level. The vagal (CN X), hypoglossal (CN XII), and vestibular (CN VIII) nerves are prominent in this section. The nucleus ambiguus gives rise to special visceral efferent fibers in CN IX and CN X. The posterior spinocerebellar tract is in the inferior cerebellar peduncle. CTG, cuneate (arm), trunk, and gracile (leg) components of the medial lemniscus; MLF, medial longitudinal fasciculus.

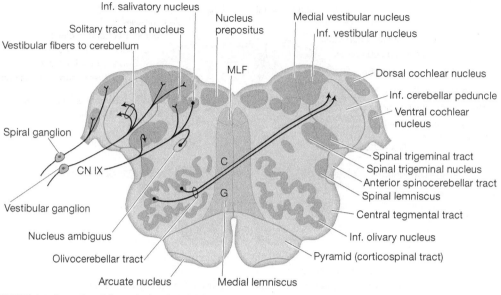

FIGURE 9.5. Rostral medulla at the level of the dorsal and ventral cochlear nuclei (of CN VIII). The glossopharyngeal nerve (CN IX) is also found at this level. The hypoglossal nucleus (of CN XII) has been replaced by the nucleus prepositus. General somatic afferent fibers of the glossopharyngeal nerve (CN IX) enter the spinal trigeminal tract of CN V (*arrow*). C, cuneate (arm); G, gracile (leg); MLF, medial longitudinal fasciculus.

  ■ **Spinal lemniscus**
   a. contains the lateral and anterior spinothalamic tracts and the spinotectal tract.
 2. Descending pathways
  ■ **Pyramidal decussation** (see Figure 9.2)
   a. located at the spinomedullary junction.
   b. consists of crossing corticospinal fibers.
  ■ **Pyramids** (see Figures 9.4 and 9.5)
   a. constitute the base of the medulla.
   b. contain uncrossed corticospinal fibers.
 3. Cerebellar pathways and relay nuclei
  ■ **Accessory (lateral) cuneate nucleus**
   a. contains second-order neurons of the cuneocerebellar tract.
   b. projects to the cerebellum via the inferior cerebellar peduncle.
  ■ **Inferior olivary nucleus**
   a. cerebellar relay nucleus that projects olivocerebellar fibers via the inferior cerebellar peduncle to the contralateral cerebellar cortex and cerebellar nuclei.
   b. receives input from the red nucleus.
  ■ **Central tegmental tract**
   a. well-defined tract within the reticular formation.
   b. extends from the midbrain to the inferior olivary nucleus.
   c. contains rubro-olivary, hypothalamospinal, taste and reticulothalamic fibers.
  ■ **Lateral reticular nucleus**
   a. a cerebellar relay nucleus that projects via the inferior cerebellar peduncle to the cerebellum.
  ■ **Arcuate nucleus**
   a. located on the anterior surface of the pyramids.
   b. gives rise to arcuatocerebellar fibers that become the striae medullares of the rhomboid fossa.

■ **Posterior spinocerebellar tract**
   a. mediates unconscious proprioception from the lower limbs to the cerebellum via the inferior cerebellar peduncle.
■ **Anterior spinocerebellar tract**
   a. mediates unconscious proprioception from the lower limbs to the cerebellum via the superior cerebellar peduncle.
■ **Inferior cerebellar peduncle**
   a. connects the medulla to the cerebellum.
   b. largely contains fibers entering the cerebellum from the spinal cord.

4. **Cranial nerve nuclei and associated tracts**
   ■ **Medial longitudinal fasciculus (MLF)**
      a. yokes together cranial nerve nuclei, particularly important for coordination of eye movement.
      b. contains vestibular fibers of CN VIII that coordinate eye movements via CN III, CN IV, and CN VI.
      c. mediates nystagmus and lateral conjugate gaze.
   ■ **Solitary tract**
      a. receives general visceral afferent (GVA) input from CN IX and CN X.
      b. receives special visceral afferent (SVA) (taste) input from CN VII, CN IX, and CN X.
   ■ **Solitary nucleus**
      a. projects GVA and SVA input ipsilaterally via the central tegmental tract to the parabrachial nucleus of the pons and to the ventral posteromedial nucleus of the thalamus.
   ■ **Dorsal motor nucleus of CN X** (see Figures 9.1, 9.3, and 9.4)
      a. gives rise to vagal preganglionic parasympathetic general visceral efferent (GVE) fibers that synapse in the terminal (intramural) ganglia of the thoracic and abdominal viscera.
   ■ **Inferior salivatory nucleus of CN IX**
      a. gives rise to preganglionic parasympathetic (GVE) fibers that synapse in the otic ganglion.
   ■ **Hypoglossal nucleus of CN XII** (see Figures 9.1, 9.3, and 9.4)
      a. gives rise to general somatic efferent (GSE) fibers that innervate the ipsilateral intrinsic and extrinsic muscles of the tongue.
   ■ **Nucleus ambiguus of CN IX and CN X** (see Figures 9.1 and 9.3 through 9.5)
      a. represents a special visceral efferent (SVE) cell column whose axons innervate pharyngeal arch muscles of the larynx and pharynx. These fibers contribute to parts of CN IX and CN X; they exit the medulla via the postolivary sulcus.
   ■ **Spinal trigeminal tract** (Figure 9.6; see Figures 9.2 through 9.4)
      a. replaces the posterolateral tract (of Lissauer) of the spinal cord.
      b. contains first-order neuron general somatic afferent (GSA) fibers that mediate pain, temperature, and light touch sensations from the face via CNs V, VII, IX, and X.
      c. projects to the spinal trigeminal nucleus.
   ■ **Spinal trigeminal nucleus** (see Figures 9.1 through 9.6)
      a. replaces the substantia gelatinosa of the spinal cord.
      b. gives rise to decussating axons that form the anterior trigeminothalamic tract. This tract terminates in the ventral posteromedial nucleus of the thalamus.
   ■ **Inferior and medial vestibular nuclei of CN VIII**
      a. receive proprioceptive (special somatic afferent [SSA]) input from the semicircular ducts, utricle, saccule, and cerebellum.
      b. project to the cerebellum and MLF.

5. **Area postrema**
   ■ lies rostral to the obex in the floor of the fourth ventricle.
   ■ a circumventricular organ with no blood-brain barrier.

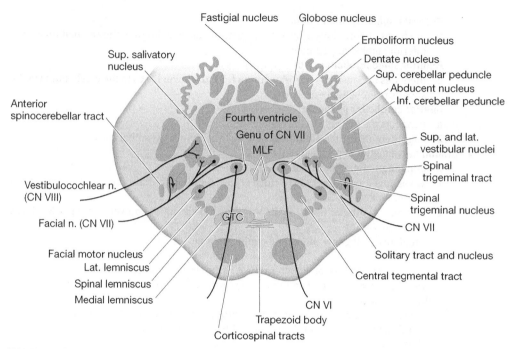

FIGURE 9.6. Caudal pons at the level of the abducens (CN VI) and facial (CN VII) nuclei. The intra-axial abducens fibers pass through the medial lemniscus and the descending corticospinal fibers. Note the looping course of the intra-axial facial nerve fibers that exit the brainstem in the cerebellopontine angle. The four cerebellar nuclei overlie the fourth ventricle. Note also the looping course of the facial nerve fibers. GTC, gracile (leg), trunk, and cuneate (arm) components of the medial lemniscus; MLF, medial longitudinal fasciculus.

III. PONS

A. Overview
- extends from the inferior pontine sulcus to the superior pontine sulcus.
- consists of a **base** that contains corticobulbar, corticospinal, and corticopontine tracts and pontine nuclei and the **tegmentum** that contain cranial nerve nuclei, reticular nuclei, and the major ascending pathways.
- connected to the cerebellum by the middle cerebellar peduncle.
- contains auditory relay nuclei and vestibular nuclei; the latter regulate postural mechanisms and vestibulo-ocular reflexes.
- contains, in its caudal portion, the facial motor nucleus of CN VII, which innervates the muscles of facial expression.
- contains, in the mid pons, the trigeminal motor nucleus of CN V; its axons innervate the muscles of mastication (masseter, temporalis, medial, and lateral pterygoid), tensor palati, tensor tympani, anterior belly of digastric, and mylohyoid.
- contains a center for lateral gaze.
- gives rise to cranial nerves V to VIII.

B. Internal structures of the pons (Figure 9.7; see Figure 9.6)
1. **Ascending pathways and relay nuclei**
   - **Dorsal and ventral cochlear nuclei** (see Figure 9.5)
     a. receive auditory input from the cochlea through SSA fibers via the cochlear branch of CN VIII.
     b. are auditory relay nuclei that give rise to the lateral lemnisci.

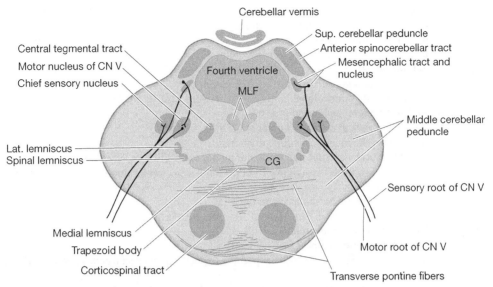

FIGURE 9.7. Mid pons at the level of the motor and chief sensory nuclei of the trigeminal nerve (CN V). The mesencephalic tract and nucleus provide the afferent limb of the myotatic jaw jerk reflex; the trigeminal motor nucleus is the efferent limb. CG, cuneate (arm) and gracile (leg); MLF, medial longitudinal fasciculus.

- **Trapezoid body**
  - **a.** formed by decussating fibers of the ventral cochlear nuclei.
  - **b.** contains the acoustic striae, medial lemnisci, exiting abducens (CN VI) fibers, and aberrant corticobulbar fibers.
- **Superior olivary nucleus**
  - **a.** an auditory relay nucleus at the level of the trapezoid body.
  - **b.** receives input from the cochlear nuclei.
  - **c.** contributes bilaterally to the lateral lemniscus.
  - **d.** functions in sound localization.
- **Lateral lemniscus**
  - **a.** a pontine auditory pathway extending from the trapezoid body to the nucleus of the inferior colliculus.
  - **b.** conducts a preponderance of contralateral cochlear input.
- **Medial lemniscus**
- **Spinal lemniscus**
2. **Descending pathways (base of the pons)**
- **Corticobulbar tract**
  - **a.** synapses in the somatic motor nuclei of cranial nerves.
- **Corticospinal tract (pyramidal tract)**
  - **a.** synapses in the anterior horn of the spinal cord.
- **Corticopontine tract**
  - **a.** synapses in the pontine nuclei.
3. **Cerebellar pathways and relay nuclei**
- **Central tegmental tract**
- **Juxtarestiform body**
  - **a.** forms part of the inferior cerebellar peduncle.
  - **b.** contains vestibulocerebellar, cerebellovestibular, and cerebelloreticular fibers.
- **Middle cerebellar peduncle**
  - **a.** contains pontocerebellar fibers.
  - **b.** connects the pons to the cerebellum.
  - **c.** largest cerebellar peduncle.

- **Superior cerebellar peduncle**
  - **a.** connects the cerebellum to the pons and midbrain.
  - **b.** contains the dentatorubrothalamic fibers and the anterior spinocerebellar tract.
  - **c.** contains the majority of cerebellar outflow.
- **Pontine nuclei**
  - **a.** cerebellar relay nuclei in the base of the pons.
  - **b.** give rise to pontocerebellar fibers that constitute the middle cerebellar peduncle.

4. **Cranial nerve nuclei and associated tracts**
  - **Dorsal and ventral cochlear nuclei of CN VIII**
    - **a.** found at the medullopontine junction.
  - **Medial, lateral, and superior vestibular nuclei of CN VIII** (see Figure 9.6)
    - **a.** receive proprioceptive (SSA) input from the semicircular ducts, utricle, saccule, and cerebellum.
    - **b.** project into the cerebellum and the MLF.
    - **c.** give rise to the medial and lateral vestibulospinal tracts.
  - **Medial longitudinal fasciculus**
  - **Abducens nucleus of CN VI** (see Figure 9.6)
    - **a.** underlies, in the caudal medial pontine tegmentum, the facial colliculus of the rhomboid fossa.
    - **b.** projects exiting fibers through the trapezoid body and through the corticospinal tract of the base of the pons.
    - **c.** gives rise to GSE fibers that innervate the lateral rectus.
    - **d.** gives rise to fibers that project via the MLF to the contralateral oculomotor nucleus.
    - **e.** near the **pontine center for lateral conjugate gaze**, which receives commands from the contralateral frontal eye field (area 8). It innervates (via the MLF) the contralateral medial rectus and (via abducens fibers) the ipsilateral lateral rectus to execute conjugate lateral gaze.
  - **Facial nucleus of CN VII** (see Figure 9.6)
    - **a.** gives rise to SVE fibers that innervate the muscles of facial expression.
    - **b.** receives bilateral corticobulbar input for upper facial muscles and contralateral input for lower facial muscles.
    - **c.** contains neurons that project axons dorsomedially, encircle the abducens nucleus as a genu (forming the facial colliculus), and pass anterolaterally between the facial nucleus and spinal trigeminal nucleus to exit the brainstem in the cerebellopontine angle.
  - **Superior salivatory nucleus of CN VII**
    - **a.** gives rise to GVE preganglionic parasympathetic fibers that synapse in the pterygopalatine and submandibular ganglia.
  - **Spinal trigeminal tract and nucleus of CN V**
  - **Trigeminal motor nucleus**
    - **a.** lies in the lateral midpontine tegmentum at the level of the trigeminal nerve.
    - **b.** lies medial to the principal sensory nucleus.
    - **c.** receives bilateral corticobulbar input.
    - **d.** gives rise to SVE fibers that innervate muscles of mastication, anterior belly of digastric, mylohyoid, tensor palati, and tensor tympani.
  - **Chief sensory nucleus of CN V**
    - **a.** lies lateral to the trigeminal motor nucleus.
    - **b.** receives discriminative tactile and pressure input from the face.
    - **c.** gives rise to trigeminothalamic fibers that join the contralateral anterior trigeminothalamic tract.
    - **d.** gives rise to the uncrossed posterior trigeminothalamic tract, which terminates in the ventral posteromedial nucleus of the thalamus.
  - **Mesencephalic nucleus and tract of CN V** (Figures 9.8 and 9.9; see Figure 9.7)
    - **a.** extend from the upper pons to the upper midbrain.

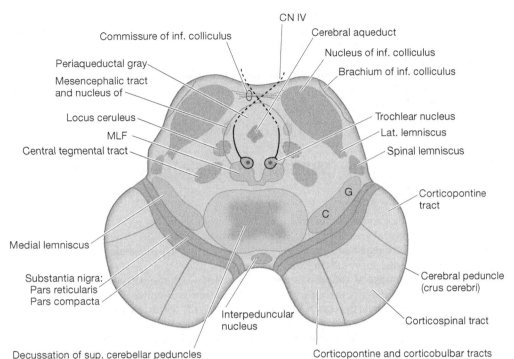

FIGURE 9.8. Midbrain at the level of the inferior colliculus, the decussation of the superior cerebellar peduncles, and the trochlear nucleus (of CN IV). C, cuneate (arm); G, gracile (leg); MLF, medial longitudinal fasciculus.

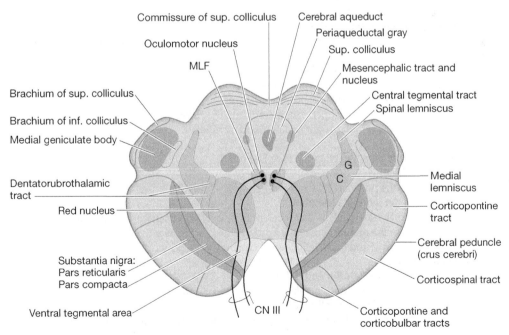

FIGURE 9.9. Midbrain at the level of the superior colliculus, the oculomotor nucleus, and the red nucleus. Oculomotor fibers pass laterally through the red nucleus and basis pedunculi and exit in the interpeduncular fossa. C, cuneate (arm); G, gracile (leg); MLF, medial longitudinal fasciculus.

   b. contain the only population of pseudounipolar neurons in the CNS.
   c. receive input from muscle spindles and pressure receptors (muscles of mastication and extraocular muscles).

   5. Locus ceruleus
   - a melanin-containing nucleus in the pons and midbrain.
   - an important nucleus of the monoamine system that projects noradrenergic axons to all parts of the CNS.

IV. MESENCEPHALON (MIDBRAIN) (See Figures 9.8 and 9.9)

A. Overview
- mediates auditory and visual reflexes.
- contains a center for vertical conjugate gaze in its rostral extent.
- contains the **substantia nigra**, the largest nucleus of the midbrain; degeneration of this extrapyramidal motor nucleus results in Parkinson disease.
- contains the **paramedian reticular formation**; lesions of which result in coma.
- extends from the superior medullary velum to the posterior commissure.
- gives rise to two cranial nerves **CN III** (oculomotor) and **CN IV** (trochlear), which innervate the extraocular muscles of the eye.
- consists of three parts: the **tectum**, the **tegmentum**, and the **base** (**basis pedunculi**).

B. Structures of the midbrain
   ### 1. Tectum
   - located posterior to the cerebral aqueduct.
   - forms the roof of the midbrain, includes the superior and inferior colliculi.
   ### 2. Tegmentum
   - located between the tectum and the base.
   - contains cranial nerve nuclei and sensory pathways.
   ### 3. Basis pedunculi (crus cerebri)
   - forms the base of the midbrain and contains corticospinal, corticobulbar, and corticopontine tracts.
   ### 4. Pedunculus cerebri (cerebral peduncle)
   - includes the tegmentum and basis pedunculi.
   ### 5. Pretectum (pretectal area)
   - located between the superior colliculus and the habenular trigone.
   - mediates the pupillary light and optokinetic reflexes.

C. Inferior collicular level of the midbrain (see Figure 9.8)
   ### 1. Inferior colliculus
   - contains the nucleus of the inferior colliculus.
   ### 2. Nucleus of the inferior colliculus
   - an auditory relay nucleus that receives binaural input from the lateral lemniscus.
   - projects to the medial geniculate body via the brachium of the inferior colliculus.
   - functions in sound localization and frequency perception.
   ### 3. Lateral lemniscus
   ### 4. Commissure of the inferior colliculus
   - interconnects the inferior collicular nuclei of both sides.
   ### 5. Brachium of the inferior colliculus
   - conducts auditory information from the inferior collicular nucleus to the medial geniculate body.

6. **Cerebral aqueduct**
   - located between the tectum and tegmentum.
   - surrounded by the periaqueductal gray matter.
   - interconnects the third and fourth ventricles.
   - blockage (aqueductal stenosis) results in **hydrocephalus**.
7. **Periaqueductal gray matter**
   - the central gray matter that surrounds the cerebral aqueduct.
   - contains several nuclear groups.
     a. **Locus ceruleus**
     b. **Mesencephalic nucleus and tract**
     c. **Dorsal tegmental nucleus**
        - contains enkephalinergic neurons that play a role in endogenous pain control.
     d. **Raphe nuclei**
        - contains serotonergic neurons.
8. **Trochlear nucleus of CN IV** (see Figure 9.8)
   - gives rise to GSE fibers that encircle the periaqueductal gray matter, decussate in the superior medullary velum, and exit the midbrain from its posterior aspect to innervate the superior oblique.
9. **Medial longitudinal fasciculus**
10. **Decussation of the superior cerebellar peduncles** (see Figure 9.8)
    - most conspicuous structure of this level.
11. **Interpeduncular nucleus**
    - receives input from the habenular nuclei via the habenulointerpeduncular tract (fasciculus retroflexus of Meynert).
12. **Substantia nigra** (see Figures 9.8 and 9.9)
    - divided into the posterior pars compacta containing large pigmented (melanin) cells and the anterior pars reticularis.
    - receives gamma-aminobutyric acid-ergic (GABA-ergic) input from the caudatoputamen (striatonigral fibers).
    - projects dopaminergic fibers to the caudatoputamen (nigrostriatal fibers).
    - projects nondopaminergic fibers to the ventral anterior nucleus, ventral lateral nucleus, and mediodorsal nucleus of the thalamus (nigrothalamic fibers).
13. **Medial lemniscus**
14. **Spinal lemniscus**
15. **Central tegmental tract**
16. **Basis pedunculi (crus cerebri)** (see Figures 9.8 and 9.9)

D. **Superior collicular level of the midbrain (see Figure 9.9)**
   1. **Superior colliculus**
      - receives visual input from the retina and from frontal (area 8) and occipital (area 19) eye fields.
      - receives auditory input from the inferior colliculus to mediate audiovisual reflexes.
      - concerned with detection of movement in visual fields, thus facilitating visual orientation, searching, and tracking.
   2. **Commissure of the superior colliculus**
      - interconnects the two superior colliculi.
   3. **Brachium of the superior colliculus**
      - conducts retinal and corticotectal fibers to the superior colliculus and to the pretectum, thus mediating optic and pupillary reflexes.
   4. **Cerebral aqueduct and periaqueductal gray matter**
   5. **Oculomotor nucleus of CN III** (see Figure 9.9)
      - gives rise to GSE fibers that innervate four extraocular muscles (medial, inferior, superior recti, and inferior oblique) and the levator palpebrae superioris.

- projects crossed fibers to the superior rectus.
- innervates the levator palpebrae superioris bilaterally.
6. **Accessory oculomotor (Edinger-Westphal) nucleus of CN III**
    - gives rise to GVE preganglionic parasympathetic fibers that terminate in the ciliary ganglion.
    - postganglionic fibers from the ciliary ganglion innervate the ciliary body (accommodation) and sphincter pupillae.
7. **Medial longitudinal fasciculus**
8. **Central tegmental tract**
9. **Red nucleus** (see Figure 9.9)
    - located in the tegmentum at the level of the oculomotor nucleus (the level of the superior colliculus).
    - receives bilateral input from the cerebral cortex.
    - receives contralateral input from the cerebellar nuclei.
    - gives rise to the crossed rubrospinal tract.
    - gives rise to the uncrossed rubro-olivary tract.
    - exerts facilitatory influence on flexor muscles.
10. **Medial lemniscus**
11. **Spinal lemniscus**
12. **Substantia nigra**

E. **Posterior commissural level (pretectal region)**
- a transition area between the mesencephalon and the diencephalon.
    1. **Posterior commissure**
        - marks the caudal extent of the third ventricle.
        - marks the rostral extent of the cerebral aqueduct.
        - interconnects pretectal nuclei, thus mediating consensual pupillary light reflexes.
    2. **Pretectal nucleus**
        - receives retinal input via the brachium of the superior colliculus.
        - projects to the ipsilateral and contralateral accessory oculomotor nuclei, thus mediating the pupillary light reflexes.

V. CORTICOBULBAR (CORTICONUCLEAR) FIBERS (Figure 9.10)

- arise from precentral and postcentral gyri.
- may synapse directly on motor neurons or indirectly via interneurons (corticoreticular fibers).
- innervate sensory nuclei (gracile, cuneate, solitary, and trigeminal).
- innervate cranial nerve motor nuclei bilaterally, with the exception of part of the facial nucleus (CN VII). The upper face division of the facial nucleus receives bilateral input; the lower face division of the facial nucleus receives only contralateral input (Figure 9.11).
- innervate the ipsilateral spinal nucleus of CN XI that supplies the sternocleidomastoid and the contralateral spinal nucleus of CN XI that innervates the trapezius.
- the orbicularis oculi receives a variable number of crossed and uncrossed fibers; the paresis therefore varies from patient to patient.

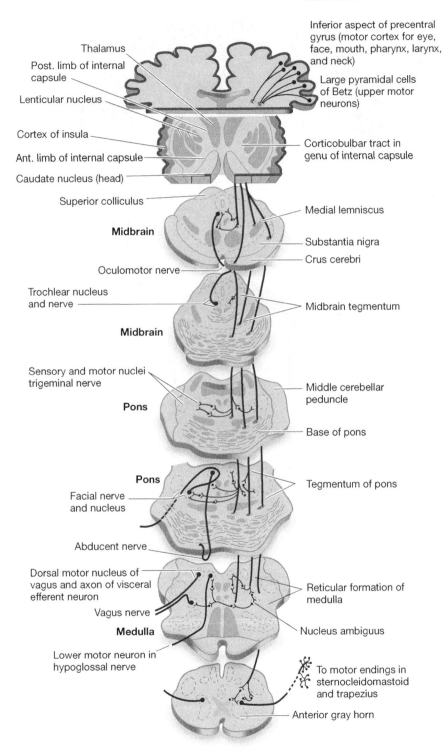

FIGURE 9.10. Corticobulbar pathways of the brainstem. Corticobulbar fibers arise from the facial area of the motor cortex and innervate motor (general somatic efferent [GSE]) and (special visceral efferent [SVE]) cranial nerve nuclei of CN V, CN VII, CN IX, CN X, CN XI, and CN XII. Direct corticobulbar fibers to the ocular motor nerves, CN III, CN IV, and CN VI, have not been demonstrated. Interruption of the corticobulbar fibers results in an upper motor neuron lesion. (Adapted with permission from Carpenter MC. *Core Text of Neuroanatomy.* 3rd ed. Williams & Wilkins; 1985:129.)

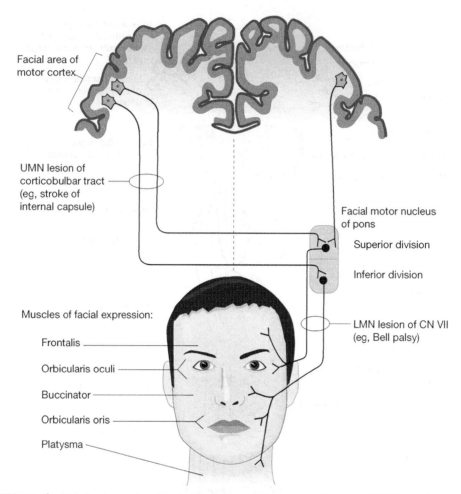

Facial area of motor cortex

UMN lesion of corticobulbar tract (eg, stroke of internal capsule)

Facial motor nucleus of pons

Superior division

Inferior division

Muscles of facial expression:

Frontalis

Orbicularis oculi

Buccinator

Orbicularis oris

Platysma

LMN lesion of CN VII (eg, Bell palsy)

FIGURE 9.11. Corticobulbar innervation of the facial motor nucleus. An upper motor neuron (UMN) lesion (eg, a stroke involving the internal capsule) results in contralateral weakness of the inferior face and spares the superior face. A lower motor neuron (LMN) lesion (eg, Bell palsy) results in paralysis of the ipsilateral facial muscles in both the superior and the inferior face.

Review Test

1. A 40-year-old woman is brought to the emergency department by her neighbor. Neurologic examination reveals the following: blood pressure 160/90 mm Hg, numbness on the right side of the inferior aspect of her face, no weakness in the upper or lower limbs, tongue deviates to the right side upon protrusion, and her uvula deviates to the left side when she says "ah." In which of the following loci is the lesion causing these symptoms found?

(A) Anterior limb of internal capsule
(B) Claustrum
(C) Genu of internal capsule, left side
(D) Paracentral lobule, right side
(E) Posterior limb internal capsule

2. A 30-year-old man is brought to the imaging suite for an x-ray subsequent to a diagnosis of noncommunicating hydrocephalus. Given that the causative lesion was located in the cerebral aqueduct, what part of the brainstem should be imaged?

(A) Diencephalon
(B) Mesencephalon
(C) Metencephalon
(D) Myelencephalon
(E) Telencephalon

3. A 25-year-old woman with a past medical history of a vascular lesion that affected her lateral lemniscus would most likely have issues with what function?

(A) Hearing
(B) Olfaction
(C) Proprioception
(D) Taste
(E) Vision

4. A 40-year-old man presents to the emergency department after waking with a constellation of issues, including difficulty breathing and a loss of sensation over the left side of his face and the right side of his body. The physician suspects a lesion in which part of the nervous system to produce the patient's symptoms?

(A) Cerebral cortex
(B) Diencephalon
(C) Midbrain
(D) Medulla
(E) Spinal cord

5. A 35-year-old woman presents to her neurologist as part of her routine visit to manage her multiple sclerosis. She reveals that, in addition to previously described weakness, tingling, and vision problems, she has developed a problem swallowing. Based on this new symptom, the physician suspects a sclerotic plaque is now affecting which nucleus?

(A) Ambiguus
(B) Chief sensory
(C) Hypoglossal
(D) Solitarius
(E) Spinal trigeminal

Questions 6 to 13

The response options for items 6 to 13 are the same. Select one answer for each item in the set.

(A) Base of pons
(B) Midbrain, at level of superior colliculus
(C) Midbrain, at level of inferior colliculus
(D) Medial medulla
(E) Lateral medulla
(F) Tegmentum of pons

Match the following structures with the appropriate brainstem division.

6. Decussation of the superior cerebellar peduncle

7. Inferior olivary nucleus

8. Nucleus ambiguus

9. Abducens nucleus

10. Facial motor nucleus

11. Oculomotor nucleus

12. Red nucleus

13. Trochlear nucleus

Answers and Explanations

1. **C.** A lesion of the genu of the internal capsule destroys corticobulbar fibers. The facial nucleus receives bilateral corticobulbar input, the upper face division receives bilateral input, and the lower face division receives only contralateral input. The hypoglossal nucleus receives only contralateral corticobulbar input. When the tongue is protruded, it deviates to the weak side owing to the unopposed activity of the intact genioglossus. The uvula deviates to the intact side when the patient says "ah." The muscles of the uvula and palatal arches are innervated by the vagus nerve (CN X).

2. **B.** The cerebral aqueduct is found in the mesencephalon; it connects the third ventricle to the fourth ventricle.

3. **A.** The lateral lemniscus carries ascending fibers mediating hearing from the cochlear nuclei on both sides.

4. **D.** A lesion that causes sensory loss on one side of the face and the contralateral side of the body must be located in the brainstem, as this is the only place in the body where sensory fibers ascending from the body have crossed, whereas those from the face have not. By the time the ascending fibers from the body and face reach the midbrain, all crossing has been accomplished, so lesions in the midbrain and "up" would produce ipsilateral sensory loss from the face and body—ruling out cerebral cortex, diencephalon, and midbrain. The fibers from the body cross in the very caudal-most part of the medulla, whereas sensory fibers from the face enter more cranially. Lesions of the spinal cord would not produce sensory deficits of the face.

5. **A.** Nucleus ambiguus is the somatic motor nucleus that controls the skeletal muscle associated with cranial nerves IX and X. It is the nucleus that controls the muscles of the pharynx and larynx. The chief sensory, solitarius and spinal trigeminal are all sensory nuclei and so would not be involved with the motor problem of swallowing. The hypoglossal nucleus is a lower motor neuron nucleus, but it is involved with tongue movement, not swallowing per se, but more the initiation of swallowing—a reflexive act that begins when a bolus of food is moved into the oropharynx by the tongue.

6. **C.** The decussation of the superior cerebellar peduncle is found in the midbrain at the level of the inferior colliculus.

7. **E.** The inferior olivary nucleus, a cerebellar relay nucleus, is the most prominent nucleus in the lateral medulla.

8. **E.** The nucleus ambiguus is found in the lateral medulla; it gives rise to the SVE components of cranial nerves IX and X.

9. **F.** The abducens nucleus (CN VI) is located in the dorsomedial tegmentum of the pons. All brainstem cranial nerve nuclei are found in the tegmentum.

10. **F.** The facial nucleus (CN VII) is located in the lateral tegmentum of the pons.

11. **B.** The oculomotor nucleus (CN III) lies in the dorsomedial tegmentum of the midbrain at the level of the superior colliculus; it lies medial to the medial longitudinal fasciculus.

12. **B.** The red nucleus is found in the midbrain at the level of the superior colliculus; it lies between the oculomotor nucleus (CN III) and the substantia nigra.

13. **C.** The trochlear nerve (CN IV) is located in the dorsomedial tegmentum of the midbrain at the level of the inferior colliculus.

Objectives

■ List the cranial nerves.
■ Describe the general characteristics, components, and functions of each cranial nerve.
■ Describe the effects of a lesion of each cranial nerve.
■ Refer to Appendix for a table of cranial nerve components.

I. OVERVIEW

▓ the pairs of nerves that arise from the brain (Figures 10.1 through 10.3; see Figures 1.1 and 1.7).

II. NERVUS TERMINALIS (CN 0)

▓ first identified in humans approximately 100 years ago, often not included in texts because of difficulty in identifying the nerve, its function, and its origin.
▓ located anteromedial to the filia olfactoria, pierces the cribriform plate with CN I.
▓ most likely a special visceral afferent (SVA) nerve that mediates the perception of pheromones and functions in reproductive systems.
▓ consists of unmyelinated nerve fibers associated with gyrus rectus.
▓ projects posteriorly to the medial and lateral septal nuclei and the preoptic area of the diencephalon.

III. OLFACTORY NERVE (CN I) (See Chapter 17 I and Appendix)

A. General characteristics of CN I
▓ an **SVA** nerve that mediates the **sense of smell** (olfaction).
▓ consists of a collection of unmyelinated axons—the filia olfactoria—of bipolar neurons located in the nasal mucosa, the olfactory epithelium.
▓ enters the skull via the foramina of the cribriform plate of the ethmoid bone.
▓ synapses with mitral and tufted cells found in the olfactory bulb, an outgrowth of the telencephalon.
▓ the only cranial nerve that projects directly to the forebrain.

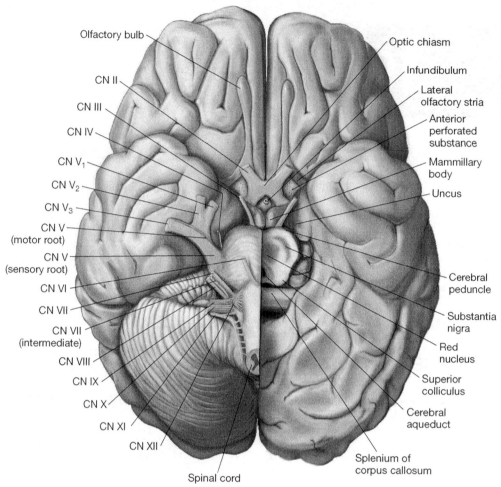

Olfactory bulb

CN II

CN III

CN IV

CN V$_1$

CN V$_2$

CN V$_3$

CN V
(motor root)

CN V
(sensory root)

CN VI

CN VII

CN VII
(intermediate)

CN VIII

CN IX

CN X

CN XI

CN XII

Spinal cord

Optic chiasm

Infundibulum

Lateral
olfactory stria

Anterior
perforated
substance

Mammillary
body

Uncus

Cerebral
peduncle

Substantia
nigra

Red
nucleus

Superior
colliculus

Cerebral
aqueduct

Splenium of
corpus callosum

FIGURE 10.1. The base of the brain with attached cranial nerves. (Modified from Truex RC, Kellner CE. *Detailed Atlas of the Head and Neck.* Oxford University Press; 1958:34. Reproduced with permission of Oxford University Press (Books) through PLSclear.)

B. Clinical consideration: CN I damage
- results in **anosmia**, loss of olfactory sensation (eg, ethmoid bone fracture).
- the olfactory epithelium is capable of regeneration after injury.

IV. OPTIC NERVE (CN II) (See Figures 1.2, 16.2, and 16.4; See Chapter 16 III B)

A. General characteristics of CN II
- a special somatic afferent (**SSA**) nerve that subserves **vision** and the **pupillary light reflex**.
- consists of axons of neurons located in the ganglion cell layer of the retina.
- enters the skull via the optic canal of the sphenoid bone.
- has axons that continue via the optic chiasm and optic tracts to the lateral geniculate body, a thalamic relay nucleus that projects to the visual cortex (area 17) of the occipital lobe.
- **not a true peripheral nerve** but a tract of the diencephalon.
- contains fibers from the nasal retina that decussate in the optic chiasm.
- contains fibers from the temporal retina that continue ipsilaterally through the optic chiasm.
- invested by the dura and pia-arachnoid membranes and lies within the subarachnoid space.

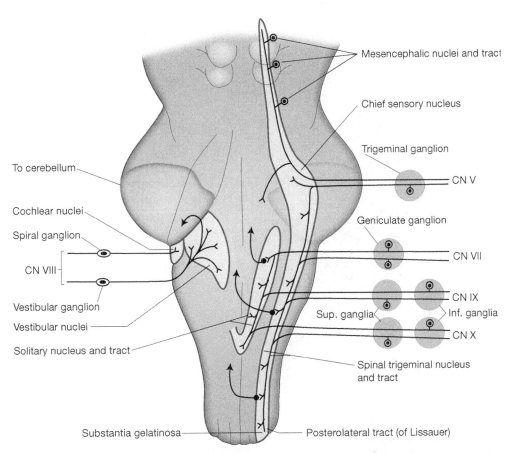

FIGURE 10.2. Location of the sensory cranial nerve nuclei within the brainstem. The spinal trigeminal tract and nucleus extend into the cervical cord (C3). Three sensory areas are prominent: the special somatic afferent area, including the cochlear and vestibular nuclei of CN VIII; the combined general visceral afferent and special visceral afferent column, the solitary nucleus of CN VII, CN IX, and CN X; and the general somatic afferent column, including the spinal trigeminal, chief sensory, and mesencephalic nuclei of CN V, CN VII, CN IX, and CN X. (Modified with permission from Noback CR, Demarest RJ. *The Human Nervous System.* 4th ed. Williams & Wilkins; 1991:222.)

B. **Clinical considerations: CN II**
- when it is transected, **ipsilateral blindness** and **loss of direct pupillary light reflex** result; regeneration of the optic nerve does not occur.
- when subjected to increased intracranial pressure (eg, tumor), **papilledema**, a choked optic disk results.
- when it is constricted, **optic atrophy** (ie, axonal degeneration) results.

V. OCULOMOTOR NERVE (CN III) (See Figures 1.1, 1.7, and 10.3; Chapter 16)

A. **General characteristics of CN III**
- contains general somatic efferent (**GSE**) and general visceral efferent (**GVE**) fibers.
- a purely motor nerve that **moves the eye, constricts the pupil**, and **accommodates**.
- exits the brainstem from the interpeduncular fossa of the midbrain, passes through the lateral wall of the cavernous sinus, and enters the orbit via the superior orbital fissure.

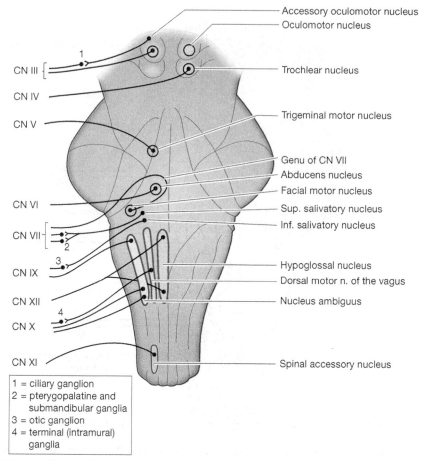

FIGURE 10.3. Location of motor cranial nerve nuclei within the brainstem. Three functional cell columns are visible from medial to lateral; the general somatic efferent column of CN III, CN IV, CN VI, and CN XII; the general visceral efferent column of CN III, CN VII, CN IX, and CN X; and the special visceral efferent column of CN V, CN VII, CN IX, CN X, and CN XI. (Modified with permission from Noback CR, Demarest RJ. *The Human Nervous System*. 4th ed. Williams & Wilkins; 1991:223.)

1. **GSE component**
   - arises from the oculomotor nucleus of the midbrain.
   - innervates four extraocular muscles and the levator palpebrae superioris.
   a. **Medial rectus**
      - adducts the eye.
      - with its opposite partner, converges the eyes.
      - innervated ipsilaterally.
   b. **Superior rectus**
      - elevates, intorts, and adducts the eye.
      - innervated contralaterally.
   c. **Inferior rectus**
      - depresses, extorts, and adducts the eye.
      - innervated ipsilaterally.
   d. **Inferior oblique**
      - elevates, extorts, and abducts the eye.
      - innervated ipsilaterally.
   e. **Levator palpebrae superioris**
      - elevates the upper eyelid.
      - innervated bilaterally.

2. **GVE component**
   ▨ **Composition**
     a. consists of preganglionic parasympathetic fibers.
   ▨ **Pathway**
     a. arises from the accessory oculomotor nucleus (Edinger-Westphal nucleus) of the midbrain.
       ▨ **Accessory oculomotor nucleus**
         (1) projects to the ciliary ganglion of the orbit via CN III.
       ▨ **Ciliary ganglion**
         (1) projects postganglionic parasympathetic fibers via branches of CN V$_1$ to the sphincter pupillae (miosis) and to the ciliaris (accommodation).

B. **Clinical considerations: CN III**
   1. **Transtentorial (uncal) herniation**
      ▨ increased supratentorial pressure, caused by a space-occupying lesion, forces the uncus through the tentorial notch, which compresses the oculomotor nerve.
      ▨ pupilloconstrictor fibers are affected first, as they are found on the outer part of the nerve, resulting in a dilated and fixed pupil; somatic efferent fibers are affected later, resulting in external strabismus (exotropia).
   2. **Aneurysms (eg, of the carotid or posterior communicating arteries)**
      ▨ may compress the oculomotor nerve within the cavernous sinus or the interpeduncular cistern.
      ▨ usually affect the peripheral pupilloconstrictor fibers first, as in uncal herniation.
   3. **Diabetes mellitus (diabetic oculomotor palsy)**
      ▨ frequently affects the oculomotor nerve, damaging the central fibers and sparing the pupilloconstrictor fibers.

CLINICAL CORRELATES   **Oculomotor paralysis** is seen frequently with **transtentorial herniation**. Results include **diplopia** (double vision) when the patient looks in the direction of the paretic muscle. Denervation of the levator palpebrae superioris results in **ptosis** (drooping of the upper eyelid). Denervation of the extraocular muscles causes the affected eye to look **down and out** because the unopposed action of the lateral rectus (CN VI) and superior oblique (CN IV). Interruption of the parasympathetic fibers in CN III results in a **dilated and fixed pupil** and **lack of accommodation (cycloplegia)**.

VI. TROCHLEAR NERVE (CN IV) (See Figures 1.7 and 10.3)

A. **General characteristics of CN IV**
   ▨ a pure **GSE** nerve that **innervates the superior oblique**, which **depresses**, **intorts**, and **abducts** the eye.
   ▨ arises from the contralateral trochlear nucleus of the midbrain.
   ▨ decussates within the midbrain and exits the brainstem on its posterior surface, caudal to the inferior colliculus.
   ▨ encircles the midbrain in the subarachnoid space, passes through the lateral wall of the cavernous sinus, and enters the orbit via the superior orbital fissure.

B. **Clinical considerations: CN IV paralysis (Figure 10.4)**
   ▨ results in the following conditions:
   1. **Extorsion of the eye and weakness of downward gaze**
   2. **Vertical diplopia**, which increases when looking down
   3. **Head tilting**, to compensate for extorsion

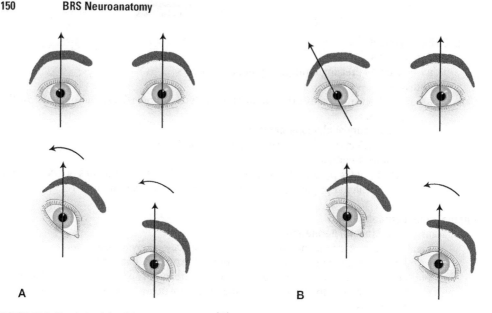

A   **B**

FIGURE 10.4. Paralysis of the right superior oblique. **(A)** A pair of eyes with normal extorsion and intorsion movements. Tilting the chin to the right side results in compensatory intorsion of the left eye and extorsion of the right eye. **(B)** Paralysis of the right superior oblique results in extorsion of the right eye, causing diplopia. Tilting the chin to the right side results in compensatory intorsion of the left eye, thus permitting binocular alignment.

VII. TRIGEMINAL NERVE (CN V) (See Figures 1.1, 1.7, 10.1, and 10.2; See Chapter 11)

A. General characteristics of CN V
- contains general somatic afferent (**GSA**) and special visceral efferent (**SVE**) fibers.
- innervates the **muscles of mastication** and mediates **general sensation** from the face, eye, and nasal and oral cavities.
- the nerve of the first pharyngeal arch (mandibular).
- exits the brainstem from the pons.
- contains first-order sensory neurons in the trigeminal ganglion and in the mesencephalic nucleus.
- contains motor neurons in the trigeminal motor nucleus of the rostral pons.
- three divisions: **ophthalmic** (CN V$_1$), **maxillary** (CN V$_2$), and **mandibular** (CN V$_3$) (see Figures 11.1 and 11.2; see Chapter 11 I A 1–3).
  1. **GSA component** (see Figure 11.1)
     - provides **sensory innervation** to the face; mucous membranes of the nasal and oral cavities; and frontal sinus, teeth, hard palate, soft palate, and deep structures of the head (proprioception from muscles, periodontal ligaments, and the temporomandibular joint).
     - innervates the dura mater of the anterior and middle cranial fossae.
     - innervates the external ear with CN VII, CN IX, and CN X.
  2. **SVE component**
     - innervates the **muscles of mastication** (temporalis, masseter, lateral, and medial pterygoids), the **tensor tympani** and **tensor palati**, the **mylohyoid**, and the **anterior belly of the digastric**.

B. Clinical considerations: lesions of CN V
- result in the following conditions:
  1. **Loss of general sensation** from the face and mucous membranes of the oral and nasal cavities

2. **Loss of the corneal reflex** (afferent limb, CN V_1)
3. **Flaccid paralysis of the muscles of mastication**
4. **Deviation of the jaw to the weak side** because of the unopposed action of the opposite lateral pterygoid
5. **Paralysis of the tensor tympani**, leading to hypacusis (partial deafness to low-pitched sounds)

VIII. ABDUCENS NERVE (CN VI) (See Figures 1.1, 1.7, and 10.3)

A. General characteristics of CN VI

- a pure **GSE** nerve that innervates the lateral rectus, which **abducts the eye**.
- arises from the abducens nucleus of the caudal pons.
- exits the brainstem from the inferior pontine sulcus.
- passes through Dorello canal and the cavernous sinus to enter the orbit via the superior orbital fissure.

B. Clinical considerations: CN VI paralysis

- results in the following conditions:
  1. **Convergent strabismus (esotropia)**, with inability to abduct the eye because of the unopposed action of the medial rectus
  2. **Horizontal diplopia**, with maximum separation of the double images when looking toward the paretic lateral rectus

IX. FACIAL NERVE (CN VII) (See Figures 1.1, 1.7, 10.2, 10.3, and 10.5)

A. General characteristics of CN VII

- contains **GSA**, **SVA**, **SVE**, and **GVE** fibers.
- mediates **facial movements, taste, salivation,** and **lacrimation**.

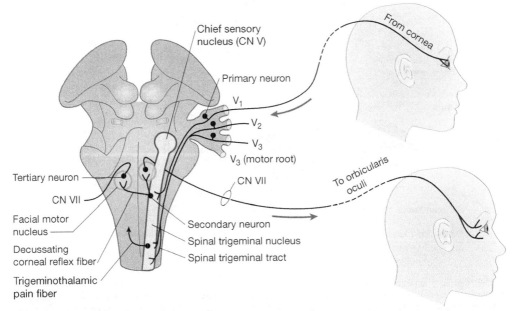

FIGURE 10.5. The corneal reflex pathway showing the three neurons and decussation. This reflex is consensual, like the pupillary light reflex. Second-order pain neurons are found in the caudal region of the spinal trigeminal nucleus. Second-order corneal reflex neurons are found at more rostral levels. (Modified with permission from Fix JD. *High-Yield Neuroanatomy*. 3rd ed. Lippincott Williams & Wilkins; 2005:93.)

- the nerve of the second pharyngeal arch.
- includes the **facial nerve proper** (motor division), which contains the SVE fibers that innervate the muscles of facial expression.
- includes the **intermediate nerve** (sensory division), which contains GSA, SVA, and GVE fibers. All first-order sensory neurons are found in the geniculate ganglion within the temporal bone.
- exits the brainstem at the cerebellopontine (CP) angle.
- enters the internal auditory meatus and the facial canal.
- exits the facial canal and skull via the **stylomastoid foramen**.

1. **GSA component**
   - has cell bodies in the geniculate ganglion.
   - innervates the **posterior surface of the external ear** via the posterior auricular branch of the facial nerve.
   - projects centrally to the spinal trigeminal tract and nucleus.

2. **SVA component**
   - has cell bodies in the geniculate ganglion.
   - projects centrally to the solitary tract and nucleus.
   - innervates the **taste buds** from the anterior two-thirds of the tongue via:

3. **Chorda tympani** (Figure 10.6)
   - located in the tympanic cavity medial to the tympanic membrane and lateral to the malleus.
   - contains **SVA** and **general visceral afferent (GVA)** fibers.
   - joins the lingual nerve (a branch of CN V_3).

4. **GVE component**
   - a parasympathetic component that innervates the **lacrimal, submandibular, and sublingual glands**.
   - contains preganglionic neurons in the superior salivatory nucleus of the caudal pons.

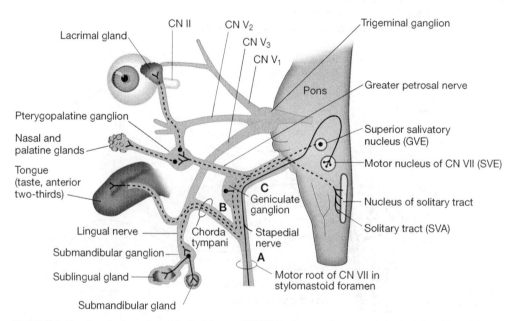

FIGURE 10.6. Functional components of the facial nerve (CN VII). The intermediate nerve is the sensory and visceromotor division of the seventh nerve. **A**, **B**, and **C** indicate three lesions of the nerve. Lesion **A** is at the stylomastoid foramen and spares lacrimation, nasal and palatine secretion, taste to the anterior two-thirds of the tongue, salivation, and the stapedial reflex; the patient has a lower motor neuron lesion involving the ipsilateral muscles of facial expression. Lesion **B** is between the geniculate ganglion and the chorda tympani and spares lacrimation and secretion from the nasal palatine glands. Lesion **C** is proximal to the geniculate ganglion and is total. GVE, general visceral efferent; SVA, special visceral afferent; SVE, special visceral efferent.

a. **Lacrimal pathway** (see Figure 10.6)
- begins in the superior salivatory nucleus, which projects via the intermediate nerve, the greater petrosal nerve, and the nerve of the pterygoid canal to the pterygopalatine ganglion.
- continues as the postganglionic neurons of the pterygopalatine ganglion project through the inferior orbital fissure and via the zygomatic nerve (a branch of CN V_2) and the lacrimal nerve (a branch of CN V_1) to innervate the lacrimal gland.

b. **Submandibular pathway** (see Figure 10.6)
- begins in the superior salivatory nucleus, which projects via the intermediate nerve and chorda tympani to the submandibular ganglion.
- continues as the postganglionic neurons of the submandibular ganglion, which project to and innervate the submandibular and sublingual glands via the lingual nerve (a branch of CN V_3).

5. **SVE component**
- arises from the facial motor nucleus of the caudal pons and exits the brainstem in the CP angle.
- enters the internal auditory meatus, traverses the facial canal, sends a branch to the stapedius, and exits the skull via the stylomastoid foramen.
- innervates the **muscles of facial expression**, the **stylohyoid**, the **posterior belly of the digastric**, and **stapedius**.

B. **Clinical considerations: lesions of CN VII (see Figure 10.6)**
- result in the following conditions:
  1. **Flaccid paralysis** of the ipsilateral muscles of facial expression (upper and lower face)
  2. **Loss of the corneal (blink) reflex** (efferent limb), which may lead to corneal ulceration (keratitis paralytica)
  3. **Loss of taste** (ageusia) from the anterior two-thirds of the tongue
  4. **Hyperacusis** (increased acuity to sounds) because of stapedius paralysis
  5. Central **facial palsy** (supranuclear palsy)
     - results from transection of corticobulbar fibers in the internal capsule.
     - results in contralateral facial weakness below the orbit.
     - an upper motor neuron lesion affecting the muscles of the contralateral lower face.
  6. **Crocodile tears syndrome** (lacrimation during eating)
     - caused by a facial nerve lesion proximal to the geniculate ganglion. Regenerating preganglionic salivatory fibers are misdirected to the pterygopalatine ganglion, which projects to the lacrimal gland.

CLINICAL CORRELATES **Bell palsy** (Figure 9.11) is caused by trauma to the facial nerve within the facial canal, causing paresis or paralysis of the ipsilateral muscles of facial expression, that is, hemiparesis/hemiparalysis of the ipsilateral face. Bell palsy is seen most commonly in people 15 to 45 years old. Risk factors include pregnancy, preeclampsia, obesity, hypertension, diabetes, and upper respiratory ailments.

X. VESTIBULOCOCHLEAR NERVE (CN VIII) (See Figures 1.1, 1.7, and 10.2)

- maintains balance and mediates hearing.
- consists of two functional divisions: the vestibular nerve and the cochlear nerve.
- a purely SSA nerve.
- exits the brainstem at the cerebellopontine (CP) angle.
- enters the internal auditory meatus and is confined to the temporal bone.

A. Vestibular nerve (see Chapters 14 II C 6 and 15)
1. **General characteristics of the vestibular nerve**
   - plays a role in **equilibrium** and **balance**.
   - associated functionally with the cerebellum (flocculonodular lobe).
   - regulates **compensatory eye movements**.
   - has first-order sensory bipolar neurons in the vestibular (Scarpa) ganglion of the internal auditory meatus.
   - projects peripheral processes to the hair cells of the cristae ampullares of the semicircular ducts and into hair cells of the utricular and saccular maculae.
   - projects central processes to the four vestibular nuclei of the brainstem and to the flocculonodular lobe of the cerebellum.
   - conducts efferent fibers to hair cells from the brainstem to decrease the sensation of movement; failure results in motion sickness.
2. **Clinical consideration: lesions of the vestibular nerve**
   - result in disequilibrium, vertigo, and nystagmus.

B. Cochlear nerve (see Chapter 14 III C)
1. **General characteristics of the cochlear nerve**
   - serves **audition** (hearing).
   - has first-order sensory bipolar neurons in the cochlear (spiral) ganglion of the modiolus of the cochlea, within the temporal bone.
   - projects peripheral processes to the hair cells of the organ of Corti.
   - projects central processes to the dorsal and ventral cochlear nuclei of the brainstem.
   - conducts efferent fibers to the hair cells from the brainstem.
2. **Clinical considerations: lesions of the cochlear nerve** (see Chapter 14 V B)
   - results in **hearing loss** (sensorineural deafness) (destructive lesions).
   - causes **tinnitus** (irritative lesions).

XI. GLOSSOPHARYNGEAL NERVE (CN IX) (See Figures 1.1, 1.7, 10.2, and 10.3)

A. General characteristics of CN IX
- contains **GSA, GVA, SVA, SVE,** and **GVE** components.
- mediates **taste** (gustation), **salivation**, and (with CN X and CN XII) **swallowing**.
- mediates **input from the carotid sinus**, which contains baroreceptors that monitor arterial blood pressure.
- mediates **input from the carotid body**, which contains chemoreceptors that monitor the carbon dioxide and oxygen concentration of the blood.
- the nerve of the third pharyngeal arch.
- contains predominantly sensory fibers.
- exits the brainstem (medulla) from the postolivary sulcus with CN X.
- exits the skull via the jugular foramen with CN X and CN XI.
1. **GSA component**
   - innervates the middle ear cavity and part of the external auditory meatus.
   - has cell bodies in the superior glossopharyngeal ganglion.
   - projects its central processes to the spinal trigeminal tract and nucleus.
2. **GVA component**
   - innervates structures derived from endoderm (eg, foregut).
   - innervates the mucous membranes of the posterior third of the tongue, tonsil, upper pharynx (soft palate), tympanic cavity, and auditory tube.
   - innervates the carotid sinus (baroreceptors) and the carotid body (chemoreceptors).
   - has cell bodies in the inferior (petrosal) ganglion.
   - the afferent limb of the gag reflex and the carotid sinus reflex.
3. **SVA component**
   - innervates the **taste buds** of the posterior third of the tongue.

▪ has cell bodies in the inferior (petrosal) ganglion.

▪ projects its central processes to the solitary tract and nucleus.

4. SVE component

▪ innervates the stylopharyngeus.

▪ arises from the nucleus ambiguus of the lateral medulla.

5. GVE component

▪ a parasympathetic component that innervates the **parotid gland**.

▪ consists of preganglionic neurons in the inferior salivatory nucleus of the medulla that project, via the tympanic nerve and the lesser petrosal nerve, to the otic ganglion; postganglionic fibers from the otic ganglion project to the parotid gland via the auriculotemporal nerve (CN V₃).

B. Clinical considerations: lesions of CN IX

▪ Loss of the carotid sinus reflex (interruption of afferent limb)

▪ Loss of taste from the posterior third of the tongue

▪ Glossopharyngeal neuralgia

CLINICAL CORRELATES   Lesion of CN IX causes loss of the **gag (pharyngeal) reflex**, as it serves as the afferent limb of the reflex (CN X serves as the efferent limb of the gag reflex). The gag reflex is evoked through stimulation of the soft palate, oropharynx, or base of the tongue. Testing of the gag reflex is a component of the neurological exam (Figure 10.9).

XII. VAGAL NERVE (CN X) (See Figures 1.1, 1.7, 10.2, and 10.3)

A. General characteristics of CN X

▪ contains **GSA**, **GVA**, **SVA**, **SVE**, and **GVE** components.

▪ mediates **phonation**, **swallowing** (with CN IX and CN XII), **elevation of the palate**, and **taste**.

▪ innervates **viscera of the neck, thorax**, and **abdomen**.

▪ the nerve of the fourth (superior laryngeal) and sixth (recurrent laryngeal) pharyngeal arches.

▪ exits the brainstem (medulla) from the postolivary sulcus.

▪ exits the skull via the jugular foramen with CN IX and CN XI.

1. GSA component

▪ innervates the infratentorial dura (with C2 and C3), posterior surface of the external ear, external auditory meatus, and tympanic membrane.

▪ has cell bodies in the superior (jugular) ganglion.

▪ projects its central processes to the spinal trigeminal tract and nucleus.

2. GVA component

▪ innervates the mucous membranes of the pharynx, larynx, esophagus, trachea, and thoracic and abdominal viscera (to the mid-transverse colon).

▪ has cell bodies in the inferior (nodose) ganglion.

▪ projects its central processes to the solitary tract and nucleus.

3. SVA component

▪ innervates the **taste buds** over the **epiglottis** and soft palate.

▪ has cell bodies in the inferior (nodose) ganglion.

▪ projects its central processes to the solitary tract and nucleus.

4. SVE component

▪ innervates the pharyngeal arch muscles of the larynx and pharynx, striated muscle of the upper esophagus, musculus uvulae, and levator palati and palatoglossus.

▪ arises from the nucleus ambiguus in the lateral medulla.

▪ provides the efferent limb of the gag reflex.

5. GVE component (see Figure 20.2)

▪ innervates the **viscera of the neck** and the **thoracic and abdominal cavities** as far as the mid-transverse colon.

▪ consists of preganglionic parasympathetic neurons in the dorsal motor nucleus of the vagus, which project to the intramural ganglia of the viscera.

B. Clinical considerations: lesions of CN X (Figure 10.7)

■ result in the following conditions:

1. **Ipsilateral paralysis** of the soft palate, pharynx, and larynx leading to **dysphonia** (hoarseness), **dyspnea, dysarthria,** and **dysphagia**
2. Loss of the gag (palatal) reflex (efferent limb)
3. Anesthesia of the pharynx and larynx, leading to unilateral loss of the cough reflex
4. Aortic aneurysms and tumors of the neck and thorax
   ■ frequently compress the vagal nerve.

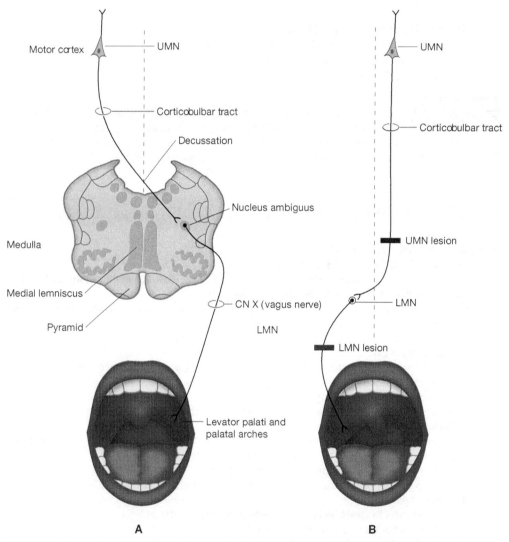

FIGURE 10.7. Innervation of the palatal arches and uvula. Sensory innervation is mediated by the glossopharyngeal nerve (CN IX). Motor innervation of the palatal arches and uvula is mediated by the vagus nerve (CN X). **(A)** A normal palate and uvula in a person saying "ah." **(B)** A patient with an upper motor neuron (UMN) lesion (left) and a lower motor neuron (LMN) lesion (right). When this patient says "ah," the palatal arches sag. The uvula deviates toward the intact (left) side. (Modified with permission of McGraw-Hill Education from DeMyer WE. *Technique of the Neurological Examination: A Programmed Text.* 4th ed. McGraw-Hill; 1994:191. Figure 6–9; permission conveyed through Copyright Clearance Center, Inc.)

XIII. ACCESSORY NERVE (CN XI) (See Figures 1.1, 1.7, and 10.3)

A. General characteristics of CN XI
- not actually a cranial nerve, as it originates in the spinal cord.
- contains **SVE** fibers.
- mediates **head and shoulder movement**.
- arises from the anterior horn of cervical segments C1 to C6.
- spinal roots exit the spinal cord laterally between the anterior and posterior roots, ascend through the foramen magnum, and exit the skull via the jugular foramen.
- innervates the **sternocleidomastoid** (with C2) and **trapezius** (with C3 and C4).

B. Clinical considerations: lesions of CN XI
1. Paralysis of the sternocleidomastoid
- results in difficulty in turning the head to the side opposite the lesion.
2. Paralysis of the trapezius
- results in a shoulder droop.
- results in the inability to shrug the ipsilateral shoulder.

XIV. HYPOGLOSSAL NERVE (CN XII) (See Figures 1.1, 1.7, and 10.3)

A. General characteristics of CN XII
- mediates **tongue movement**.
- a pure **GSE** nerve.
- arises from the hypoglossal motor nucleus of the medulla.
- exits the medulla in the preolivary sulcus.
- exits the skull via the hypoglossal canal.
- innervates **intrinsic and extrinsic muscles of the tongue**.

B. Clinical considerations: CN XII (Figure 10.8)
- when it is transected, hemiparalysis of the tongue results.
- the tongue points toward the weak side because of the unopposed action of the opposite genioglossus upon protrusion.

XV. CRANIAL NERVE TESTING

- testing cranial nerve function is a key part of the neurologic examination.
- able to reveal pathologies in the head and neck.

A. CN I
- not commonly tested.

B. CN II (Figure 10.9)
- visual integrity tested using standard eye chart.
- pupillary light reflex is tested (Chapter 16, Sections IV, V, VI and Figure 16.7).
- visual field test, physician moves object/fingers in the periphery (Figure 10.9).

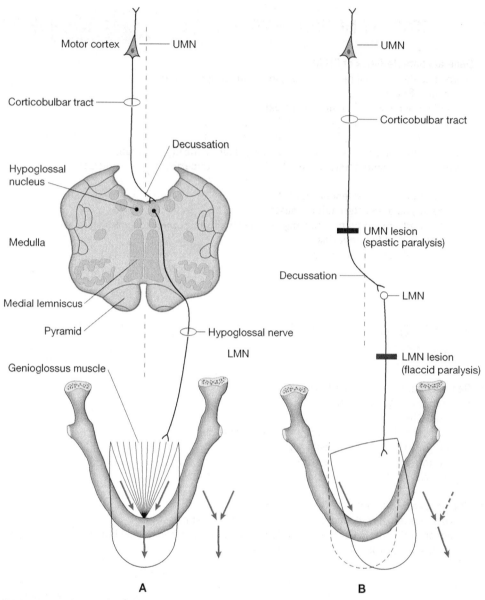

FIGURE 10.8. Motor innervation of the tongue. Corticobulbar fibers project predominantly to the contralateral hypoglossal nucleus. An upper motor neuron (UMN) lesion causes deviation of the protruded tongue to the weak (contralateral) side. A lower motor neuron (LMN) lesion causes deviation of the protruded tongue to the weak (ipsilateral) side. **(A)** Normal tongue. **(B)** Tongue with UMN and LMN lesions. The blue arrows indicate direction of tongue movement. (Modified with permission of McGraw-Hill Education from DeMyer WE. *Technique of the Neurological Examination: A Programmed Text.* 4th ed. McGraw-Hill; 1994:195. Figure 6–11; permission conveyed through Copyright Clearance Center, Inc.)

C. CN III, IV, and VI
- control the extraocular muscles and movement of the eye.
- commonly tested together (Figure 10.10 and Figure 10.4) using the H-test.
- convergence test (Chapter 16, Section VI and Figures 16.6 and 16.7).

D. CN V
- tested with patient's eyes closed.
- swab lightly brushed on forehead, cheek, and mandibular area to test CN V subdivisions: V_1 ophthalmic, V_2 maxillary, and V_3 mandibular nerves (Figure 10.9).

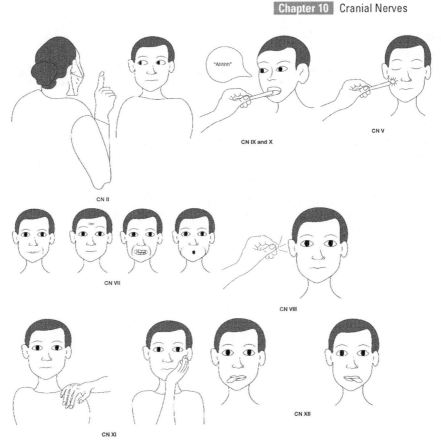

FIGURE 10.9. Cranial nerve testing.

E. CN VII
- test for asymmetrical facial movement.
- ask patient to smile, raise eyebrows, clinch teeth, and puff cheeks (Figure 10.9 and Figure 9.11).

F. CN VIII
- physician rubs fingers near the ear to see if sound is detected (Figure 10.9).
- if negative, more sophisticated tests to examine conduction or nerve deafness may be needed (Chapter 14, Section VI).

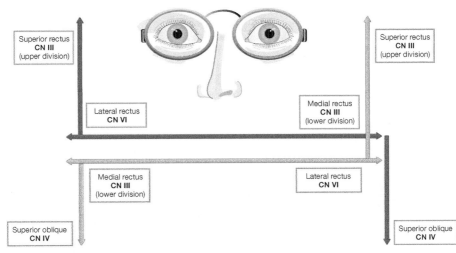

FIGURE 10.10. Normal eye movements and the H-test.

G. **CN IX and X**
   ▩ often tested together.
   ▩ a tongue blade is used to initiate gag reflex—afferent limb CN IX, efferent limb CN X (Figure 10.9).
   ▩ note asymmetrical elevation of the palate, the uvula deviates toward the functional side in CN X testing (Figure 10.7).

H. **CN XI**
   ▩ tested by asking patient to turn head and shrug shoulder against resistance (Figure 10.9).
   ▩ note asymmetry.

I. **CN XII**
   ▩ patient should protrude tongue, note deviation.
   ▩ patient should be tasked with moving tongue to right/left (Figure 10.9).

Review Test

1. A 50-year-old man presents to his primary care physician with a previous diagnosis of vertical diplopia. The patient feels unsure when descending stairs. He can eliminate the double vision by tilting his chin toward the paretic side. Which of the following extraocular muscles is responsible for the ocular malalignment?

(A) Inferior rectus
(B) Inferior oblique
(C) Lateral rectus
(D) Superior oblique
(E) Superior rectus

2. Damage to which cranial nerve will result in anosmia?

(A) I
(B) II
(C) III
(D) IV
(E) V

3. A 50-year-old man presents to his primary care physician with a chief complaint of severe pain in his ear and throat. He describes the pain as episodic and triggered by swallowing, chewing, coughing, and laughing. Examination reveals the loss of the gag (pharyngeal) reflex, analgesia and anesthesia in the region of the tonsils, and dysphagia. Which cranial nerve's lesion most likely produced the neurologic deficits?

(A) Facial
(B) Glossopharyngeal
(C) Hypoglossal
(D) Trigeminal
(E) Vagal

4. A 10-year-old boy is brought to his pediatrician by his mother for a follow-up visit after having a bony growth removed near his stylomastoid foramen that damaged his facial nerve. Given the functions of the facial nerve and the location of the tumor, what function/structure(s) would most likely be affected in this patient?

(A) Ipsilateral facial musculature
(B) Lacrimation
(C) Nasal mucosa
(D) Submandibular gland
(E) Taste from the anterior two-thirds of the tongue

5. A 25-year-old woman's neck was injured in an automobile accident. Upon examination in the emergency department, she reports difficulty in turning her head away from the side of her neck that was injured. She also has a visible shoulder droop. Which nerve was likely damaged?

(A) VIII
(B) IX
(C) X
(D) XI
(E) XII

6. A 40-year-old woman presents to her primary care physician after waking with an inability to move her lips on the left side of her face. Her lips on the left side are angled down and she is drooling on that side. Attempts to smile are asymmetrical, with the right-side elevating and the left side remaining depressed. Physical and neurologic examination reveals nothing else notable in this patient. Prior to any further testing, where should the physician suspect to find a lesion?

(A) Left corticobulbar tract
(B) Left facial motor nucleus
(C) Left facial nerve
(D) Right corticobulbar tract
(E) Right facial motor nucleus
(F) Right facial nerve

7. A 25-year-old woman presents to her primary care physician with a primary complaint of the loss of her blink reflex, which has caused significant irritation. Upon examination—using a cotton swab to stroke the cornea—it is revealed that her blink reflex is working when the left cornea is touched, but not the right cornea. Which nerve(s) is/are most likely lesioned in this patient?

(A) Bilateral ophthalmic
(B) Left facial
(C) Left optic
(D) Right facial
(E) Right ophthalmic

Questions 8 to 12

The response options for items 8 to 12 are the same. Select one nerve for each item in the set.

(A) Accessory
(B) Facial
(C) Glossopharyngeal
(D) Trigeminal
(E) Vagal

Match each description with the appropriate nerve.

8. Innervates the parotid gland

9. Is the efferent limb of corneal blink reflex

10. Is the efferent limb of gag reflex

11. Innervates the infratentorial dura

12. Is a purely motor nerve

Questions 13 to 17

The response options for items 13 to 17 are the same. Select one answer for each item in the set.

(A) Foramen magnum
(B) Foramen ovale
(C) Foramen rotundum
(D) Foramen spinosum
(E) Jugular foramen
(F) Stylomastoid foramen
(G) Superior orbital fissure

Match the anatomic structure(s) below with the foramen or fissure through which it passes.

13. A branch of the maxillary artery

14. The nerve that innervates the buccinator

15. The nerve that innervates the skin of the upper lip

16. CN IX, CN X, and CN XI

17. Four cranial nerves traverse this orifice

Answers and Explanations

1. **D.** The superior oblique depresses, abducts, and intorts the eye when acting independently. When the eyes are adducted (primarily by the actions of medial rectus), the superior oblique depresses the eye, as in reading and walking down stairs. Paralysis of this muscle results in extorsion and weakness of downward gaze. Head tilting compensates for the extorsion. The inferior rectus depresses the abducted eye and causes extorsion and adduction. The inferior oblique and superior rectus both elevate the eye. The lateral rectus is not involved in depression of the eye.

2. **A.** Anosmia, a loss of olfactory sensation, results from damage to the olfactory nerve, CN I.

3. **B.** Glossopharyngeal neuralgia has the following neurologic deficits: paroxysmal pain that comes from the tonsillar area and radiates to the ear; loss of taste sensation from the posterior third of the tongue; and loss of palatal and gag reflexes. Potential causes of glossopharyngeal impairment include fractures of the skull base, thrombosis of the sigmoid sinus, tumors, and aneurysms of the posterior fossa. Pain may be triggered by a blood vessel pressing on the root of the glosso-pharyngeal nerve, and relocation of the vessel may alleviate symptoms. Treatment is with carba-mazepine and other antiepileptic drugs. The facial, hypoglossal, and trigeminal are not involved with the gag reflex, whereas the vagus provides the efferent limb of the gag reflex, but is not in-volved in sensation from the region.

4. **A.** The facial nerve emerges from the stylomastoid foramen; at that point, only the fibers that provide somatic motor innervation to the muscles of the ipsilateral hemiface are still present in the nerve. The facial nerve does convey the preganglionic parasympathetic fibers that eventually innervate the lacrimal gland, nasal mucosa, and submandibular gland; but all of those fibers leave the nerve in the facial canal, before it exits the stylomastoid foramen. Likewise, taste from the anterior two-thirds of the tongue joins the nerve well before it exits the foramen and so are also spared.

5. **D.** The accessory nerve (CN XI) mediates head and shoulder movement. Lesions result in paraly-sis of the sternocleidomastoid, making it difficult to turn the head to the side opposite the lesion, and paralysis of the trapezius, resulting in a shoulder droop and inability to shrug the shoulder on the side of the lesion. The other cranial nerves listed are not involved in shoulder movement.

6. **D.** The corticobulbar tracts provide robust contralateral innervation to the facial motor nuclei, while ipsilaterally, they only innervate the part of the nuclei associated with the top part of the face. Therefore, a lesion of the right corticobulbar tract would leave the contralateral lower face paralyzed, as the upper half of the contralateral face would receive ipsilateral innervation from the corticobulbar fibers on that side. Therefore, a left corticobulbar tract lesion would cause the inferior aspect of the face on the right side to be affected. Lesion of either the left or right facial motor nucleus and lesion of the left or right facial nerve would cause ipsilateral hemiparesis of the face.

7. **E.** The right ophthalmic nerve carries the afferent limb of the corneal blink reflex into the brain-stem; this signal is not arriving there in this patient, as neither the ipsi- or contralateral eye is blinking. As the blink reflex works upon touching the left cornea, we can assume that the left ophthalmic nerve is conveying the signal and that both facial nerves are functioning appropri-ately, that is, ruling out bilateral ophthalmic, left and right facial nerves. The left optic nerve would have an effect on vision and pupillary dilation, but not the blink reflex.

8. **C.** The glossopharyngeal nerve (CN IX) innervates the parotid gland via the tympanic and lesser petrosal nerves, the otic ganglion, and the auriculotemporal nerve.

9. **B.** The facial nerve (CN VII) provides the efferent limb of the corneal reflex (orbicularis oculi).

10. E. The vagus nerve (CN X) provides the efferent limb of the gag reflex (muscles of the soft palate). The glossopharyngeal nerve provides the afferent limb of the gag reflex.

11. E. The vagus nerve (CN X) innervates, via the recurrent meningeal ramus, the infratentorial dura (the dura of the posterior cranial fossa).

12. A. The accessory nerve (CN XI) is a pure SVE motor nerve. It innervates the sternocleidomastoid and the trapezius.

13. D. The middle meningeal artery, a branch of the maxillary artery, traverses the foramen spinosum.

14. F. The facial nerve (CN VII) exits the base of the skull via the stylomastoid foramen; CN VII innervates the muscles of facial expression, including buccinator.

15. C. The maxillary nerve (CN V_2) exits the skull via the foramen rotundum and provides sensory innervation of the cheek and upper lip.

16. E. CN IX, CN X, and CN XI exit the posterior cranial fossa via the jugular foramen.

17. G. CN III, CN IV, CN VI, and CN V_1 pass through the superior orbital fissure.

Objectives

- List the components of the trigeminal sensory system.
- List the divisions of the trigeminal nerve and the fiber types in each.
- Describe the ascending trigeminothalamic pathways, and include a description of the location of their primary, secondary, and tertiary neurons and the modalities each is concerned with.
- List the nuclei associated with the trigeminal system, and include a description of the location and function of each.
- Recognize the function and unique characteristics of the mesencephalic nucleus.
- Recognize the spinal cord homologs for each component of the trigeminal system.

I. TRIGEMINAL NERVE (CN V) (Figure 11.1; See Figures 1.1, 9.1, and 9.7)

- the largest cranial nerve.
- connects to the brainstem at the pons.
- the nerve of the first pharyngeal arch (mandibular nerve).
- contains sensory (general somatic afferent [GSA]) and motor (special visceral efferent [SVE]) fibers.
- provides sensory innervation to the face and oral and nasal cavity.
- innervates the dura mater of the anterior and middle cranial fossae.
- innervates the muscles of mastication.
- consists of a large ganglion that gives rise to three major divisions: the **ophthalmic**, **maxillary**, and **mandibular** nerves.

A. Trigeminal (or semilunar or Gasserian) ganglion

- located in the trigeminal fossa of the temporal bone in the middle cranial fossa.
- covered by dura mater—forms the trigeminal cave.
- contains pseudounipolar neurons, which are the first-order neurons of the trigeminothalamic tracts.

1. Ophthalmic nerve (CN V₁)

- lies in the lateral wall of the cavernous sinus.
- enters the orbit via the superior orbital fissure.
- innervates the forehead, dorsum of the nose, upper eyelid, orbit (cornea and conjunctiva), mucous membranes of the nasal vestibule and frontal sinus, and the cranial dura.
- mediates the afferent limb of the corneal blink reflex.

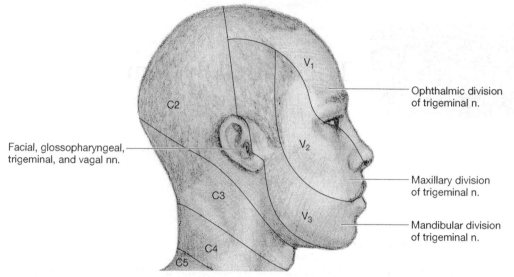

FIGURE 11.1. The cutaneous innervation of the head and neck.

2. Maxillary nerve (CN V₂)
- lies in the lateral wall of the **cavernous sinus**.
- exits the cranial vault via the **foramen rotundum**.
- innervates the upper lip and cheek, lower eyelid, anterior portion of the temple, paranasal sinuses, oral mucosa of the superior aspect of the mouth, nose, pharynx, gums, teeth, hard palate, soft palate, and cranial dura mater.

3. Mandibular nerve (CN V₃)
- exits the cranial vault via the **foramen ovale**.
- consists of a motor component that innervates the **muscles of mastication** (temporalis, masseter, and lateral and medial pterygoids); two suprahyoid muscles: the **mylohyoid** and the **anterior belly of the digastric**; and the **tensor tympani** and **tensor palati**.
- consists of a sensory component that innervates the lower lip and chin, posterior aspect of the temple, external auditory meatus and tympanic membrane, external ear, teeth of the lower jaw, oral mucosa of the cheeks and the floor of the mouth, anterior two-thirds of the tongue, temporomandibular joint, and cranial dura mater.

B. Cranial nerves V, VII, IX, and X
- contribute GSA fibers from various parts of the ear to the trigeminal system.
- send fibers into the trigeminal sensory system.

C. Spinal trigeminal tract
- extends from C3 to the level of the trigeminal nerve in the mid pons.
- a homolog of the posterolateral tract (of Lissauer).
- receives pain, temperature, and fine touch inputs from CN V, CN VII, CN IX, and CN X.
- transection (**tractotomy**) results in ipsilateral facial anesthesia.
- projects to the spinal trigeminal nucleus as follows:
  1. **Pain fibers** terminate in the caudal third of the spinal trigeminal nucleus.
  2. **Corneal blink reflex fibers** terminate in the rostral two-thirds of the spinal trigeminal nucleus.

II. ASCENDING TRIGEMINOTHALAMIC TRACTS

- convey GSA information from the face, oral cavity, and dura mater to the thalamus.

A. Anterior trigeminothalamic tract (Figure 11.2)

- serves as a pain, temperature, and fine touch pathway from the face and oral cavity.
- contains GSA fibers predominantly from CN V and also contributions from CN VII, CN IX, and CN X.
- receives input from free nerve endings and Merkel tactile disks.
- receives discriminative tactile and pressure input from the contralateral chief sensory nucleus, which terminates in the ventral posteromedial (**VPM**) nucleus of the thalamus.
- ascends to the contralateral sensory cortex via three neurons.

1. First-order neurons

- located in peripheral ganglia associated with CNs V (predominant), VII, IX, and X.
- give rise to axons that descend in the spinal trigeminal tract to mediate pain and temperature sensation and axons that enter the chief sensory nucleus to mediate fine touch.

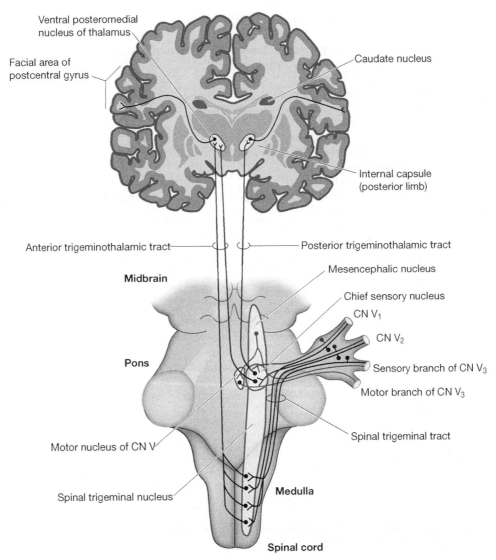

FIGURE 11.2. The anterior and posterior trigeminothalamic pathways. CN, cranial nerve. (Modified with permission from Fix JD. *High-Yield Neuroanatomy*. 3rd ed. Lippincott Williams & Wilkins; 2005:79.)

■ synapse with second-order neurons in the spinal trigeminal nucleus (pain and temperature) and the chief sensory nucleus (fine touch).

2. Second-order neurons

■ located in the spinal trigeminal and chief sensory nuclei.

■ give rise to decussating axons that terminate in the contralateral VPM nucleus of the thalamus.

■ project axons to the reticular formation and to cranial nerve motor nuclei to mediate reflexes (eg, tearing and corneal blink reflexes).

3. Third-order neurons

■ located in the VPM nucleus.

■ project via the posterior limb of the internal capsule to the face area of the postcentral gyrus (areas 3, 1, and 2).

B. Posterior trigeminothalamic tract (see Figure 11.2)

■ subserves discriminative tactile and pressure sensation primarily from the oral cavity via the GSA fibers of CN V.

■ receives input from Meissner and Pacinian corpuscles.

■ an uncrossed tract.

■ the rostral equivalent of the posterior column-medial lemniscus system.

■ ascends to the sensory cortex via three neurons:

1. First-order neurons

■ located in the trigeminal ganglion.

■ synapse in the principal sensory nucleus of CN V.

2. Second-order neurons

■ located in the principal sensory nucleus of CN V.

■ project to the ipsilateral VPM nucleus of the thalamus.

3. Third-order neurons

■ located in the VPM nucleus.

■ project via the posterior limb of the internal capsule to the face area of the postcentral gyrus (areas 3, 1, and 2).

III. TRIGEMINAL SENSORY NUCLEI (See Figures 9.1, 9.7 through 9.9, and 11.2)

A. Chief (principal, main) sensory nucleus

■ located in the rostral pontine tegmentum at the level of the trigeminal motor nucleus.

■ receives fine touch from the face.

■ projects via the uncrossed posterior trigeminothalamic tract to the VPM nucleus of the thalamus.

■ projects via the crossed anterior trigeminothalamic tract to the contralateral VPM nucleus of the thalamus.

■ a homolog of the posterior column nuclei of the medulla.

B. Spinal trigeminal nucleus

■ located in the spinal cord (C1-C3), medulla, and pons.

■ receives pain and temperature inputs from the face and oral cavity.

■ projects via the crossed anterior trigeminothalamic tract to the VPM nucleus of the thalamus.

C. Mesencephalic nucleus (see Figures 9.1, 9.7 through 9.9, and 11.2)

■ subserves **GSA proprioception** from the head.

- contains pseudounipolar neurons.
- receives inputs from muscle spindles and pressure and joint receptors.
- receives inputs from the muscles of mastication, the periodontal ligaments of the teeth, and the temporomandibular joint.
- projects to the trigeminal motor nucleus to mediate the muscle stretch (jaw jerk) reflex and regulate bite force.

D. Trigeminal motor nucleus (SVE) (Figure 11.3; see Figures 9.1, 9.7, and 11.2)
- located in the rostral pontine tegmentum at the level of the chief sensory nucleus.
- innervates the muscles of mastication (temporalis, masseter, medial, and lateral pterygoids), tensor tympani, tensor palati, anterior belly of digastric, and mylohyoid.
- receives bilateral corticobulbar input.
- receives input from the mesencephalic nucleus.

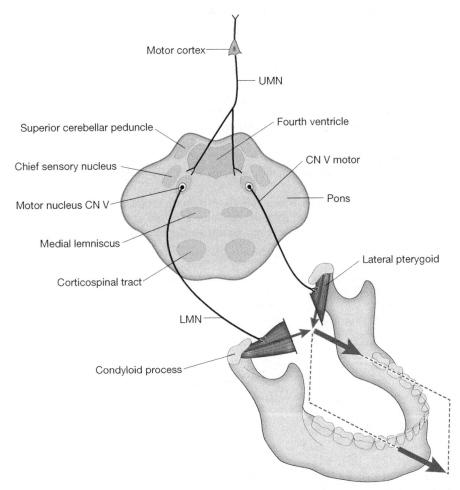

FIGURE 11.3. Function and innervation of the lateral pterygoid muscles (LPMs). The LPM receives its innervation from the motor nucleus of the trigeminal nerve found in the rostral pons. Bilateral innervation of the LPMs results in protrusion of the mandible. The LPMs also open the jaw. Denervation of an LPM results in deviation of the mandible to the ipsilateral, or weak, side. The trigeminal motor nucleus receives bilateral corticobulbar input. CN, cranial nerve; LMN, lower motor neuron; UMN, upper motor neuron. (Adapted with permission of McGraw-Hill Education from DeMyer WE. *Technique of the Neurological Examination: A Programmed Text.* 4th ed. McGraw-Hill; 1994:174. Figure 6–1; permission conveyed through Copyright Clearance Center, Inc.)

IV. TRIGEMINOCEREBELLAR FIBERS

- project from the mesencephalic nucleus via the superior cerebellar peduncle to the cerebellum.
- project from the chief sensory and spinal trigeminal nuclei via the inferior cerebellar peduncle to the cerebellar vermis.

V. TRIGEMINAL REFLEXES

A. Jaw jerk (masseter) reflex (Figure 11.4)

- a monosynaptic myotatic reflex.
  1. The **afferent limb** is the mandibular nerve (**CN V$_3$**).
  2. The **efferent limb** is the mandibular nerve (**CN V$_3$**).

B. Corneal blink reflex

- a consensual and disynaptic reflex.
- has its first-order neuron (afferent limb) in the trigeminal ganglion.
- has its second-order neuron in the rostral two-thirds of the spinal trigeminal nucleus.
- has its third-order neuron (efferent limb) in the facial motor nucleus.
  1. The **afferent limb** is the ophthalmic nerve (**CN V$_1$ motor**).
  2. The **efferent limb** is the facial nerve (**CN VII**).

C. Lacrimal (tearing) reflex

  1. The **afferent limb** is the ophthalmic nerve (**CN V$_1$**); it receives impulses from the cornea and conjunctiva.
  2. The **efferent limb** is the facial nerve (**CN VII**). It transmits impulses via the superior salivatory nucleus, greater petrosal nerve, pterygopalatine ganglion, and the zygomatic (CN V$_2$) and lacrimal (CN V$_1$) nerves to the lacrimal gland (see Figure 10.6).

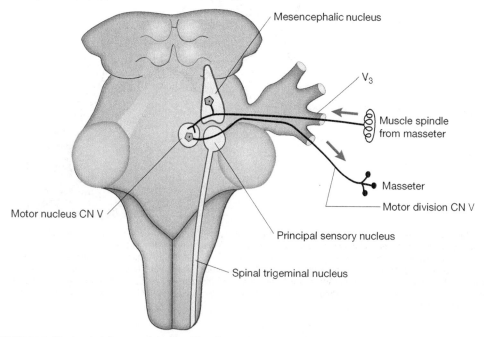

FIGURE 11.4. The jaw jerk (masseteric) reflex. The afferent limb is V$_3$, and the efferent limb is the motor root that accompanies V$_3$. First-order sensory neurons are located in the mesencephalic nucleus. The jaw jerk reflex, like all muscle stretch reflexes, is a monosynaptic myotactic reflex. CN, cranial nerve. (Modified with permission from Fix JD. *High-Yield Neuroanatomy*. 3rd ed. Lippincott Williams & Wilkins; 2005:80.)

VI. CLINICAL CONSIDERATIONS

A. Herpes zoster ophthalmicus
- a viral infection affecting the ophthalmic nerve (CN V$_1$).
- corneal ulceration with infection may result in blindness.

B. Paratrigeminal (Raeder) syndrome
- occurs as a result of lesions of the trigeminal ganglion and sympathetic fibers; the lesion is usually in the parasellar region.
- results in miosis, ptosis, facial pain (similar to trigeminal neuralgia), and trigeminal palsy.
- may involve CN III, CN IV, and CN VI.

C. Central lesions of the spinal trigeminal tract and nucleus
- can result in a **loss of sensation,** occurring in an **onion-skin distribution.**
- the face is represented somatotopically in the spinal trigeminal nucleus as a number of semi-circular territories that extend from the perioral region to the ear.
- fibers innervating the mouth area terminate near the obex; fibers innervating the back of the head terminate in upper cervical levels.

D. Acoustic neuroma (schwannoma)
- an extramedullary tumor of the vestibulocochlear nerve (CN VIII) that is found in the cerebellopontine angle or in the internal acoustic meatus.
- results in initial symptoms that include unilateral **tinnitus** and unilateral **hearing loss** as a result of a CN VIII lesion.
- results in symptoms that include **facial weakness** and **loss of corneal blink reflex** (efferent limb) owing to facial nerve (CN VII) involvement.
- affects the spinal trigeminal tract as the tumor expands and leads to ipsilateral **loss of pain and temperature sensation** and **loss of the corneal blink reflex**.

E. Cavernous sinus syndrome (Figure 11.5)
- most commonly caused by cavernous sinus tumors.

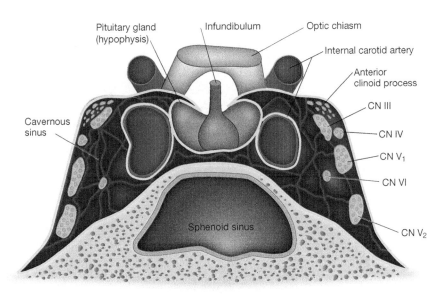

FIGURE 11.5. Coronal diagram of the contents of the cavernous sinus. The wall of the cavernous sinus contains the ophthalmic (CN V$_1$) and maxillary (CN V$_2$) divisions of the trigeminal nerve (CN V) and the trochlear (CN IV) and oculomotor (CN III) nerves. The siphon of the internal carotid artery and the abducens nerve (CN VI) along with postganglionic sympathetic fibers lie within the cavernous sinus. (Modified with permission from Fix JD. *High-Yield Neuroanatomy.* 3rd ed. Lippincott Williams & Wilkins; 2005:81.)

▦ may involve any one or all of the following cranial nerves:
1. **Ocular motor nerves CNs III, IV, and VI**
   ▦ destruction of CN III results in complete **internal ophthalmoplegia** (parasympathetic paresis).
2. **Trigeminal nerve branches of CN V₁ and CN V₂**
3. **Postganglionic sympathetic fibers to the orbit**
   ▦ interruption results in **Horner syndrome**.

CLINICAL CORRELATES　　**Trigeminal neuralgia (tic douloureux)** is characterized by recurrent paroxysms of sharp, severe, stabbing pain in one or more branches of the trigeminal nerve on one side of the face. It usually occurs after 50 years of age and is more common in women than in men. Trigeminal neuralgia may result from a loop of the superior cerebellar artery that impinges on the trigeminal nerve root. Possible treatments include pharmacologic intervention (eg, carbamazepine), rhizotomy, and, as a last result, surgical intervention.

Review Test

1. A 55-year-old woman presents to her primary care physician with a previous diagnosis of idiopathic trigeminal neuralgia. She reports sharp, stabbing pain in her upper lip and nose. Which division of the trigeminal nerve is affected?

(A) Corneal
(B) Mandibular
(C) Maxillary
(D) Lacrimal
(E) Ophthalmic

2. What is the treatment drug of choice for the patient in question 1?

(A) Carbamazepine
(B) Clobazam
(C) Clonazepam
(D) Gabapentin
(E) Lamotrigine

3. For which type of sensation does the posterior trigeminothalamic tract act as a pathway?

(A) Temperature
(B) Fine touch
(C) Pain
(D) Proprioception
(E) Crude touch

4. A 20-year-old woman presents to her primary care physician with a problem opening her jaw. The physician explains that the muscle primarily responsible for jaw opening is:

(A) buccinator.
(B) lateral pterygoid.
(C) masseter.
(D) medial pterygoid.
(E) temporalis.

5. Which one of the following nerves innervates the auricle (pinna) of the external ear?

(A) V_1
(B) V_2
(C) V_3
(D) III
(E) VIII

6. A 30-year-old man presents to his primary care physician with a chief complaint of a dry and irritated right eye. Examination reveals normally moist nasal mucosa, and examination of his facial musculature is unremarkable. Lesion of which of the following cranial nerves or its branches is most likely causing the man's symptoms?

(A) II
(B) III
(C) V_1
(D) V_2
(E) V_3

7. A 55-year-old woman presents to her primary care physician with complaints of an inability to focus that seems worse when reading. On examination, it is observed that the right pupil is constricted; there are no other symptoms of note in the neurologic examination. The physician makes the diagnosis of complete internal ophthalmoplegia. Which cranial nerve is likely involved in this diagnosis?

(A) I
(B) II
(C) III
(D) IV
(E) V

8. A 30-year-old woman presents to a neurosurgeon following several years of failed treatment for temporomandibular disorder, including pharmacologic interventions, corticosteroid injections, and arthroscopic surgery. As a last resort to relieve pain in this patient, the surgeon suggests that a central nervous system tractotomy is performed to relieve pain from the region of the temporomandibular joint (TMJ). Where along the ipsilateral spinal trigeminal tract would a tractotomy occur to eliminate TMJ pain and have minimal effects on other areas?

(A) Basilar pons
(B) Caudal medulla
(C) Cerebral peduncle
(D) Diencephalon
(E) Rostral midbrain

9. An 80-year-old man presents to the emergency department with a chief complaint of numbness over one side of his face. Examination confirms hypesthesia that appeared 1 day prior. Cerebral angiography reveals blockage of the posterior communicating artery, which supplies the thalamus.

Which nucleus is most likely affected in this patient?

(A) Anterior
(B) Mediodorsal
(C) Pulvinar
(D) Ventral posterior lateral
(E) Ventral posterior medial

Answers and Explanations

1. **C.** The affected part is the maxillary branch of the trigeminal nerve (CN V_2) that innervates the upper lip and cheek, inferior eyelid, anterior portion of the temple, paranasal sinuses, oral mucosa, nose, pharynx, gums, teeth hard palate, soft palate, and cranial dura. None of the other branches or divisions listed provide sensory innervation to the upper lip and nose: corneal branches innervate the cornea; the mandibular division innervates the lower lip and skin over the mandible; the lacrimal branches of V_1 innervate the area around the superior lateral aspect of the orbit; and the ophthalmic division innervates the forehead.

2. **A.** Carbamazepine is the drug of choice for treatment of idiopathic trigeminal neuralgia. Carbamazepine, along with lamotrigine, clonazepam, gabapentin, and clobazam, is also used to treat seizure disorders.

3. **B.** The posterior trigeminothalamic tract subserves fine touch and pressure sensation from the face and oral cavity via the GSA fibers of the trigeminal nerve (CN V). Pain, temperature, and crude touch sensations are conveyed via the anterior trigeminothalamic tract.

4. **B.** The lateral pterygoid is one of four muscles of mastication. Unlike the other muscles, it opens the mouth by depressing the jaw. It also helps the medial pterygoids in moving the jaw from side to side. The temporalis, medial pterygoid, and masseter work to close the jaw. The muscles of mastication are innervated by the trigeminal motor nucleus (SVE).

5. **C.** The mandibular nerve, CN V_3, is a division of the trigeminal nerve (CN V) and innervates the external ear, external auditory meatus and tympanic membrane, lower lip and chin, posterior aspect of the temple, teeth of the lower jaw, oral mucosa of the cheeks, floor of the mouth, anterior two-thirds of the tongue, temporomandibular joint, and cranial dura.

6. **C.** The afferent limb of the lacrimal reflex is CN V_1, which receives impulses from the cornea and conjunctiva. The efferent limb CN VII transmits impulses via the superior salivatory nucleus, greater petrosal nerve, pterygopalatine ganglion, and the zygomatic and lacrimal nerves to the lacrimal gland. The lack of other sensory symptoms indicates it is likely a branch of V_1, not the entire nerve that is compromised.

7. **C.** Destruction of CN III results in complete internal ophthalmoplegia—paralysis of the sphincter pupillae and ciliaris.

8. **B.** The somatotopic organization of the spinal trigeminal tract is such that the fibers from the area nearest the ear are the most caudal in the tract. As a side note, the tractotomy would be most effective on the posterior aspect of the tract, sparing the anteriorly disposed fibers, as the mandibular division of the trigeminal, which carries fibers from the region of the TMJ, are most posterior in the tract. The trigeminal sensory system is not found in the basilar pons, cerebral peduncle, or diencephalon. The cranial-most end of the mesencephalic nucleus extends superiorly into the rostral midbrain, but that nucleus is involved with proprioception, not pain.

9. **E.** The ventral posterior medial nucleus of the thalamus receives the trigeminothalamic fibers that convey ascending somatosensory information. The ventral posterior medial receives information from the face, whereas the ventral posterior lateral nucleus receives somatosensory information from the body. The anterior, mediodorsal, and pulvinar do not receive projections from the trigeminal sensory system.

chapter 12

Lesions of the Brainstem

Objectives

■ Describe common vascular lesions of the medulla, pons, and midbrain.
■ List structures affected in the various vascular lesions of parts of the brainstem and predict the functional/clinical manifestation of each.
■ Describe the characteristics of an acoustic neuroma and jugular foramen syndrome.
■ Differentiate between decerebrate and decorticate rigidity.

I. OVERVIEW

▧ brainstem lesions are syndromes most frequently associated with arterial occlusion or circulatory insufficiency that involve the vertebrobasilar system.

II. VASCULAR LESIONS OF THE MEDULLA

▧ result from occlusion of the vertebral artery or its branches (eg, the anterior and posterior spinal arteries and the posterior inferior cerebellar artery [PICA]).

A. Medial medullary syndrome (Figure 12.1A)

▧ results from occlusion of the anterior spinal artery.
▧ includes the following affected **structures** and resultant **deficits**:
   1. **Corticospinal tract**
      ▧ contralateral hemiparesis of the trunk and limbs.
   2. **Medial lemniscus**
      ▧ contralateral loss of conscious proprioception, fine touch, and vibratory sensation from the trunk and limbs.
   3. **Hypoglossal nerve roots (intra-axial fibers)**
      ▧ ipsilateral flaccid paralysis of the tongue.

B. Lateral medullary syndrome (PICA syndrome; Wallenberg syndrome) (see Figure 12.1B)

▧ results from occlusion of the vertebral artery or one of its medullary branches (eg, PICA).
▧ includes the following affected **structures** and resultant **deficits**:
   1. **Vestibular nuclei (medial and inferior)**
      ▧ nystagmus, nausea, vomiting, and vertigo.
   2. **Inferior cerebellar peduncle**
      ▧ ipsilateral cerebellar signs (dystaxia, dysmetria, and dysdiadochokinesia).

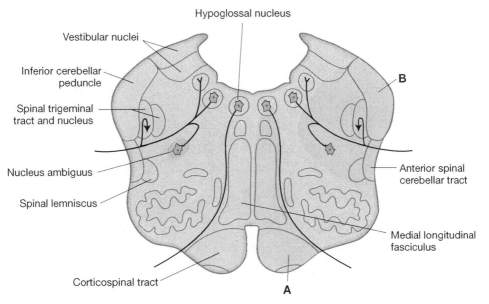

FIGURE 12.1. Vascular lesions of the caudal medulla at the level of the hypoglossal nucleus and the dorsal motor nucleus of CN X. **(A)** Medial medullary syndrome (anterior spinal artery). **(B)** Lateral medullary syndrome (posterior inferior cerebellar artery syndrome).

3. **Nucleus ambiguus**
   - ipsilateral laryngeal, pharyngeal, and palatal paralysis (loss of the gag reflex [efferent limb], dysarthria, dysphagia, and dysphonia).
4. **Glossopharyngeal nerve roots (intra-axial fibers)**
   - loss of the gag reflex (afferent limb).
5. **Vagal nerve roots (intra-axial fibers)**
   - neurologic deficits same as those seen in lesion of the nucleus ambiguus.
6. **Spinothalamic tracts**
   - contralateral loss of pain and temperature sensation from the trunk and limbs.
   - part of the spinal lemniscus at this level.
7. **Spinal trigeminal nucleus and tract**
   - ipsilateral loss of pain and temperature sensation from the face.
8. **Descending sympathetic tract**
   - ipsilateral Horner syndrome (ptosis, miosis, hemianhidrosis, vasodilation, and apparent enophthalmos).

III. VASCULAR LESIONS OF THE PONS

- result from occlusion of the basilar artery or its branches (eg, the anterior inferior cerebellar artery [AICA], transverse pontine arteries, or superior cerebellar artery).

A. Medial inferior pontine syndrome (Figure 12.2A)
- results from occlusion of the paramedian branches of the basilar artery.
- includes the following affected **structures** and resultant **deficits**:
  1. **Abducens nerve roots (intra-axial fibers)**
     - ipsilateral lateral rectus paralysis.
  2. **Corticobulbar tracts**
     - contralateral weakness of the lower face.
  3. **Corticospinal tracts**
     - contralateral hemiparesis of the trunk and limbs.

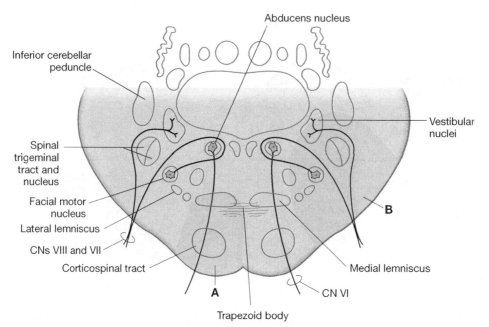

FIGURE 12.2. Vascular lesions of the caudal pons at the level of the abducens nucleus and the facial motor nucleus. **(A)** Medial inferior pontine syndrome. **(B)** Lateral inferior pontine syndrome (anterior inferior cerebellar artery syndrome).

    4. Base of the pons (middle cerebellar peduncle)
- ipsilateral limb and gait ataxia.

    5. Medial lemniscus
- contralateral loss of conscious proprioception, fine touch, and vibration sensation from the trunk and limbs.

B. Lateral inferior pontine syndrome (AICA syndrome) (see Figure 12.2B)
- results from occlusion of a branch of the basilar artery, AICA.
- includes the following affected **structures** and resultant **deficits**:
    1. Facial motor nucleus and intra-axial nerve fibers
- ipsilateral facial paralysis.
- loss of taste from the anterior two-thirds of the tongue.
- loss of the corneal blink and stapedial reflexes.

    2. Cochlear nuclei and intra-axial nerve fibers
- unilateral central nerve deafness.

    3. Vestibular nuclei and intra-axial nerve fibers
- nystagmus, nausea, vomiting, and vertigo.

    4. Spinal trigeminal nucleus and tract
- ipsilateral loss of pain and temperature sensation from the face.

    5. Middle and inferior cerebellar peduncles
- ipsilateral limb and gait dystaxia.

    6. Spinothalamic tracts
- contralateral loss of pain and temperature sensation from the trunk and limbs.
- as part of the spinal lemniscus at this level.

    7. Descending sympathetic tract
- ipsilateral Horner syndrome (ptosis, miosis, hemianhidrosis, vasodilation, and enophthalmos).

C. Lateral midpontine syndrome
- results from occlusion of a circumferential branch of the basilar artery.

    includes the following affected **structures** and resultant **deficits**:
1. **Trigeminal nuclei and nerve root (trigeminal motor and chief sensory nuclei)**
   - **Paralysis of the muscles of mastication.**
   - **Jaw deviation to the paretic side** (owing to unopposed action of the intact lateral pterygoid).
   - **Facial hemianesthesia** (pain, temperature, touch, and proprioception).
   - **Loss of the corneal blink reflex** (afferent limb of CN V_1).
2. **Middle cerebellar peduncle (base of the pons)**
   - ipsilateral limb and gait dystaxia.

D. Lateral superior pontine syndrome
- results from occlusion of a circumferential branch of the basilar artery, the **superior cerebellar artery**.
- includes the following affected **structures** and resultant **deficits**:
  1. **Superior and middle cerebellar peduncles**
     - ipsilateral limb and trunk dystaxia.
  2. **Dentate nucleus**
     - signs similar to those seen with damage to the superior cerebellar peduncle (dystaxia, dysmetria, and intention tremor).
  3. **Spinothalamic and trigeminothalamic tracts (spinal lemniscus)**
     - contralateral loss of pain and temperature sensation from the trunk, limbs, and face.
  4. **Descending sympathetic tract**
     - ipsilateral Horner syndrome (ptosis, miosis, hemianhidrosis, and apparent enophthalmos).
  5. **Medial lemniscus (lateral aspect [gracilis])**
     - contralateral loss of conscious proprioception, fine touch, and vibration sensation from the trunk and lower limb.

E. Locked-in syndrome (pseudocoma)
- results from infarction of the base of the superior part of the pons; infarcted structures include the corticobulbar and corticospinal tracts, resulting in quadriplegia and paralysis of the more inferior cranial nerves.
- may also result from **central pontine myelinolysis**.
- communication occurs only by blinking or moving the eyes vertically.

IV. LESIONS OF THE MIDBRAIN

- result from vascular occlusion of the mesencephalic branches of the posterior cerebral artery.
- may be the outcome of aneurysms of the posterior cerebral arterial circle (of Willis).
- may result from tumors of the pineal gland/region.
- may occur owing to hydrocephalus.

A. Posterior midbrain (Parinaud) syndrome (Figure 12.3A)
- frequently the result of a **pinealoma** or **germinoma** of the pineal region.
- includes the following affected **structures** and resultant **deficits**:
  1. **Superior colliculus and pretectal area**
     - paralysis of upward and downward gaze, pupillary disturbances, and absence of convergence.
  2. **Cerebral aqueduct**
     - noncommunicating hydrocephalus (as a result of compression from a pineal tumor).

B. Paramedian midbrain (Benedikt) syndrome (see Figure 12.3B)
- results from occlusion or hemorrhage of the paramedian midbrain branches of the posterior cerebral artery.

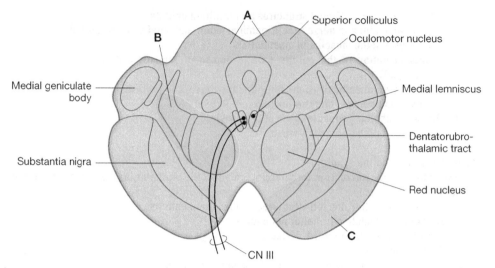

FIGURE 12.3. Lesions of the rostral midbrain at the level of the superior colliculus and oculomotor nucleus. **(A)** Dorsal midbrain (Parinaud) syndrome. **(B)** Paramedian midbrain (Benedikt) syndrome. **(C)** Medial midbrain (Weber) syndrome.

- includes the following affected **structures** and resultant **deficits:**
  1. **Oculomotor nerve roots (intra-axial fibers)**
     - **ipsilateral oculomotor paralysis.**
     - **eye abduction and depression** (ie, down and out) because of the unopposed action of the lateral rectus (CN VI) and the superior oblique (CN IV).
     - ptosis (paralysis of the levator palpebrae superioris).
     - ipsilateral **fixed and dilated pupil** (internal ophthalmoplegia).
  2. **Red nucleus and dentatorubrothalamic tract**
     - contralateral cerebellar dystaxia with intention tremor.
  3. **Medial lemniscus**
     - contralateral loss of conscious proprioception, fine touch, and vibration sensation from trunk and limbs.

C. **Medial midbrain (Weber) syndrome (see Figure 12.3C)**
   - results from occlusion of midbrain branches of the posterior cerebral artery and aneurysms of the cerebral arterial circle (of Willis).
   - includes the following **structures** and resultant **deficits:**
     1. **Oculomotor nerve roots (intra-axial fibers)** (see IV B 1)
     2. **Corticobulbar tracts**
        - contralateral weakness of the lower face (CN VII), tongue (CN XII), and palate (CN X).
     3. **Corticospinal tracts**
        - contralateral hemiparesis of the trunk and limbs.

V. DECEREBRATE AND DECORTICATE RIGIDITY

- Descending vestibulospinal and pontoreticulospinal pathways play an important role in the control of extensor muscle tone.
- Transection of the brainstem or decortication results in a tremendous increase in antigravity tone.

A. **Decerebrate rigidity (posturing)**
   - caused by a lesion that transects the brainstem between the red nucleus and the vestibular nuclei, ie, below the red nucleus.

- results from the tonic activity of the pontine reticular formation and the lateral vestibular nucleus, which activate motor neurons that innervate extensor muscles.
- characterized by **opisthotonos**, which is extension, adduction, and hyperpronation of the arms and extension of the feet with plantarflexion, also known as **gamma rigidity**.
- can be abolished by section of the vestibular nerve, destruction of vestibular nuclei or the vestibulospinal tract, and rhizotomy.

B. Decorticate rigidity (posturing)

- usually results from lesions of the internal capsule or the cerebral hemisphere, ie, above the red nucleus.
- results in posture that consists of flexion of the arm, wrist, and fingers with adduction in the upper limb; with extension, internal rotation, and plantarflexion in the lower limb.
- known as **bilateral spastic hemiplegia**, in the form of bilateral decorticate rigidity.

VI. ACOUSTIC NEUROMA (SCHWANNOMA) (Figure 12.4)

- a benign tumor of the Schwann cells affecting the vestibulocochlear nerve.
- a posterior fossa tumor of the internal auditory meatus and the cerebellopontine (CP) angle.
- frequently compresses the facial nerve, which accompanies CN VIII in the CP angle and internal auditory meatus.
- may impinge on the pons and affect the spinal trigeminal tract (CN V).
- includes the following affected **structures** and resultant **deficits**:

A. Vestibulocochlear nerve (CN VIII)

- unilateral nerve deafness and tinnitus (cochlear part).
- vertigo, nystagmus, nausea, vomiting, and unsteadiness of gait (vestibular part).

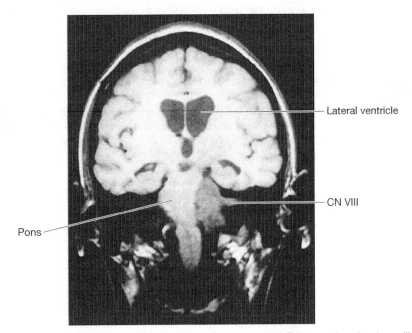

FIGURE 12.4. T$_1$-weighted magnetic resonance image of an acoustic neuroma. This coronal section shows dilation of the ventricles. The vestibulocochlear nerve is visible in the left internal auditory meatus. The tumor indents the lateral pons. Cranial nerve palsies include CNs V, VII, and VIII. (Modified with permission from Fix JD. *High-Yield Neuroanatomy*. 3rd ed. Lippincott Williams & Wilkins; 2005:108.)

B. **Facial nerve (CN VII)**
   - facial weakness and loss of corneal blink reflex (efferent limb).

C. **Spinal trigeminal tract (CN V)**
   - paresthesias and anesthesia of ipsilateral face.
   - loss of the corneal blink reflex (afferent limb).

D. **In advanced cases with large tumors**
   - **Abducens nerve (CN VI)**—diplopia.
   - **Corticospinal tract**—contralateral spastic paresis.

VII. INTERNUCLEAR OPHTHALMOPLEGIA

- also known as medial longitudinal fasciculus (MLF) syndrome, which results from a lesion of the MLF. Lesions occur in the dorsomedial pontine tegmentum and may affect one or both MLFs.
- often seen in multiple sclerosis.
- results in medial rectus palsy on attempted lateral gaze and monocular nystagmus in the abducting eye with normal convergence.
- lesions of the abducens nucleus result in MLF signs and a lateral rectus paralysis with internal strabismus.

VIII. SUBCLAVIAN STEAL SYNDROME

- results from thrombosis of the left subclavian artery proximal to the vertebral artery. Blood is shunted retrogradely down the vertebral artery and into the left subclavian artery.
- leads to the following clinical signs: transient weakness and claudication of the left upper limb on exercise and vertebrobasilar insufficiency (vertigo, dizziness).

CLINICAL CORRELATIONS   **Jugular foramen (Vernet) syndrome** is caused by compression CNs IX, X, and XI as they traverse the jugular foramen. It is most commonly caused by metastatic processes involving the base of the skull. Symptoms include loss of the gag reflex (CNs IX and X), loss of taste (CNs IX and X), laryngeal and palatal paralysis with dysarthria, dysphagia, and weakness of the sternocleidomastoid and trapezius.

Review Test

1. A 20-year-old woman presents to the emergency department after being shot with a 22-caliber bullet in the occiput. Computed tomography shows that the bullet is lodged in the left medullary pyramid. The most prominent neurologic deficit is:

(A) apallesthesia, right side.
(B) exaggerated muscle stretch reflexes, left side.
(C) fasciculations, right side.
(D) hyperreflexia, left side.
(E) plantar reflex extensor, right side.

2. A 70-year-old woman has right-sided hemiparesis. Which of the following signs best localizes the lesion to the brainstem?

(A) Exaggerated muscle stretch reflexes, right side
(B) Lateral strabismus
(C) Loss of kinesthetic and pallesthetic sensation, right side
(D) Lower facial weakness (numbness), right side
(E) Tonic deviation of eyes to the right

3. A 10-year-old boy has right arm and leg dystaxia, nystagmus, hoarseness, along with miosis and ptosis on the right. Bronchoscopy reveals a paretic vocal cord on the right. The lesion site responsible is most likely the:

(A) dorsolateral medulla.
(B) dorsolateral pons.
(C) internal capsule.
(D) left red nucleus.
(E) right dorsal motor nucleus of CN X.

4. Neurologic examination reveals miosis, ptosis, hemianhidrosis, left side; laryngeal and palatal paralysis, left side; facial anesthesia, left side; and loss of pain and temperature sensation from the trunk and limbs, right side. The lesion is in the:

(A) caudal medulla, ventral median zone, right side.
(B) caudal pontine tegmentum, lateral zone, right side.
(C) rostral medulla, lateral zone, left side.
(D) rostral pontine base, left side.
(E) rostral pontine tegmentum, dorsal median zone, left side.

5. Neurologic examination reveals severe ptosis, eye looks down and out, right side; fixed, dilated pupil, right side; spastic hemiparesis, left side; and lower facial weakness, left side. The lesion is in the:

(A) caudal pontine tegmentum, dorsal median zone, left side.
(B) pontine isthmus, dorsal lateral tegmentum, left side.
(C) rostral midbrain, medial basis pedunculi, right side.
(D) rostral midbrain, medial tegmentum, left side.
(E) rostral pontine tegmentum, dorsal lateral zone, right side.

6. Neurologic examination reveals sixth nerve palsy, right side; facial weakness, left side; hemiparesis, left side; and limb and gait dystaxia, right side. The lesion is in the:

(A) caudal medulla, ventral median zone, right side.
(B) caudal pontine base, median zone, right side.
(C) caudal pontine tegmentum, dorsal median zone, left side.
(D) caudal pontine tegmentum, lateral zone, right side.
(E) rostral pontine tegmentum, lateral zone, left side.

7. Neurologic examination reveals paralysis of upward and downward gaze, absence of convergence, and absence of pupillary reaction to light. The lesion is in the:

(A) caudal midbrain tectum.
(B) caudal midbrain tegmentum.
(C) caudal pontine tegmentum.
(D) rostral midbrain tectum.
(E) rostral pontine tegmentum.

8. Neurologic examination reveals bilateral medial rectus paresis on attempted lateral gaze, monocular horizontal nystagmus in the abducting eye, and unimpaired convergence. The lesion is in the:

(A) caudal midbrain tectum.
(B) caudal pontine base.

(C) midpontine tegmentum, dorsomedial zones, bilateral.

(D) rostral midbrain, bases pedunculorum.

(E) rostral midbrain tectum.

9. Neurologic examination reveals ptosis, miosis, and hemianhidrosis, left side; loss of vibration sensation in the right leg; loss of pain and temperature sensation from the trunk, limbs, and face, right side; and severe dystaxia and intention tremor, left arm. The lesion is in the:

(A) caudal medulla, lateral zone, right side.

(B) pontine isthmus, dorsal lateral zone, left side.

(C) rostral medulla, lateral zone, left side.

(D) rostral midbrain tegmentum, right side.

(E) rostral pontine tegmentum, dorsal medial zone, left side.

10. Neurologic examination reveals weakness of the pterygoid and masseter, left side; corneal blink reflex is absent, left side; and facial hemianesthesia, left side. The lesion is in the:

(A) caudal pontine tegmentum, dorsal medial zone, left side.

(B) caudal pontine tegmentum, lateral zone, left side.

(C) foramen ovale, left side.

(D) midpontine base, medial zone, left side.

(E) midpontine tegmentum, lateral zone, left side.

11. Neurologic examination reveals loss of the stapedial reflex, loss of the corneal blink reflex, inability to purse the lips, and loss of taste sensation on the apex of the tongue. The lesion is in the:

(A) basis pedunculi of the midbrain.

(B) caudal lateral pontine tegmentum.

(C) rostral lateral pontine tegmentum.

(D) rostral medulla.

(E) stylomastoid foramen.

12. Which of the following structures is involved in the paramedian infarction of the base of the pons?

(A) Anterior spinocerebellar tract

(B) Descending trigeminal tract

(C) Pyramidal tract

(D) Rubrospinal tract

(E) Trapezoid body

13. A 40-year-old woman presents to her primary care physician with a headache and complaints about her vision. Examination reveals a limited ability to quickly orient her gaze to various objects in the examination room.

The physician initially suspects involvement of which brainstem structure?

(A) Facial motor nucleus

(B) Medial lemniscus

(C) Medial longitudinal fasciculus

(D) Red nucleus

(E) Superior colliculus

14. A 65-year-old woman presents to her primary care physician several months after suffering a stroke of the right vertebral artery that affected the blood supply to the right side of the mid-medulla. The physician explains that the loss of voluntary motor control of the left side of her body is from damage to which of the following structures?

(A) Inferior cerebellar peduncle

(B) Medial lemniscus

(C) Nucleus ambiguus

(D) Pyramids

(E) Spinothalamic tract

Questions 15 to 22

Match the description in items 15 to 22 with the appropriate lettered structure shown in the figure.

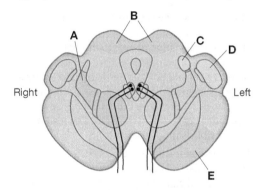

15. Paralysis of upward gaze

16. Loss of pain and temperature on the left side of the body

17. Deviation of the tongue to the left side and the uvula to the right side

18. Intention tremor on the right side

19. Complete third nerve palsy on the right side

20. Loss of vibration sensation in the right limbs

21. Babinski sign on the left side

22. Lesion leads to terminal axonal degeneration in the right superior temporal gyrus (transverse gyrus of Heschl).

Answers and Explanations

1. **E.** The bullet transected the left medullary pyramid, which contains the uncrossed corticospinal tract. This upper motor neuron lesion has produced a right contralateral spastic paresis with pyramidal signs.

2. **B.** Lateral strabismus (exotropia) is seen in midbrain lesions (e.g., Weber syndrome) that transect intra-axial fivers of the oculomotor nerve. The intact lateral rectus pulls the globe laterally.

3. **A.** Lateral medullary syndrome is also called PICA syndrome. The dorsolateral medulla contains the nucleus ambiguus (larynx), hypothalamospinal tract (Horner syndrome), inferior cerebellar peduncle (dystaxia), and vestibular nuclei (nystagmus).

4. **C.** The lesion is a classic Wallenberg syndrome (PICA syndrome) of the lateral medullary zone. Interruption of the descending sympathetic tract produces ipsilateral Horner syndrome. Involvement of the nucleus ambiguus or its exiting intra-axial fibers accounts for lower motor neuron (LMN) paralysis of the larynx and soft palate. The ipsilateral facial anesthesia results from the interruption of the spinal trigeminal tract; the contralateral loss of pain and temperature sensation from the trunk and limbs are the result of transection of the spinothalamic tracts of the anterolateral system. The combination of ipsilateral and contralateral sensory loss is called alternating hemianesthesia. Singultus (hiccup) is frequently seen in this syndrome and is thought to result from irritation of the reticulophrenic pathway.

5. **C.** This constellation of deficits constitutes Weber syndrome, which affects the cerebral peduncles and the exiting intra-axial oculomotor fibers. Severe ptosis, the abducted and depressed (down and out) eyeball, and the internal ophthalmoplegia (fixed, dilated pupil) are oculomotor nerve signs. The contralateral hemiparesis results from interruption of the corticospinal tracts; lower facial weakness is because of the interruption of the corticobulbar tracts. The combination of ipsilateral and contralateral motor deficits is called alternating hemiplegia.

   The corticospinal tract is closely related to three cranial nerve motor nuclei (oculomotor, abducens, and hypoglossal); third nerve signs put the lesion in the midbrain, sixth nerve signs put the lesion in the pons, and 12th nerve signs put the lesion in the medulla. All cranial nerves have ipsilateral signs (the trochlear exhibits contralateral signs if lesioned prior to the decussation of its fibers). Transection of the corticospinal tract rostral to the decussation results in a contralateral spastic hemiparesis. The trochlear nucleus, an exception, gives rise to intra-axial axons that cross the midline and exit just caudal to the frenulum of the superior medullary velum. A lesion of the trochlear nucleus results in a contralateral superior oblique palsy.

6. **B.** These signs point to the base of the pons (medial inferior pontine syndrome) on the right side and include involvement of the exiting intra-axial abducens fibers that pass through the uncrossed corticospinal fibers; this results in an ipsilateral lateral rectus paralysis (LMN lesion) and contralateral hemiparesis. Contralateral facial weakness results from damage to the corticobulbar fibers prior to their decussation. Involvement of the transverse pontine fibers destined for the middle cerebellar peduncle results in cerebellar signs. Furthermore, the involved cranial nerve and pyramidal tract indicate where the lesion must be to account for the deficits. An ipsilateral sixth nerve paralysis and crossed hemiplegia is called the Millard-Gubler syndrome.

7. **D.** These deficits indicate the Parinaud syndrome or dorsal midbrain syndrome. This condition is frequently the result of a tumor in the pineal region (eg, germinoma or pinealoma). A pinealoma compresses the superior colliculus and the underlying accessory oculomotor nuclei that are responsible for upward and downward vertical conjugate gaze. Patients often have pupillary disturbances and absence of convergence.

8. C. The MLF is located in the dorsomedial midpontine tegmentum. MLF syndrome is frequently seen in multiple sclerosis and less often in vascular lesions. Another pontine lesion results in one-and-a-half syndrome; it includes the MLF syndrome and a lesion of the abducens nucleus (see Chapter 16).

9. B. These deficits correspond to a lesion in the dorsolateral zone of the pontine isthmus, lateral superior pontine syndrome. Interruption of the descending sympathetic pathway to the ciliospinal center (of Budge; T1-T2) results in Horner syndrome (ipsilateral). Involvement of the lateral aspect (includes the lower limb fibers) of the medial lemniscus results in a loss of vibratory sense and other posterior column modalities. Damage to the trigeminothalamic and the anterolateral system at this level results in contralateral hemianesthesia of the face and body. Infarction of the superior cerebellar peduncle leads to ipsilateral cerebellar dystaxia.

10. E. These signs indicate lateral midpontine syndrome. This lesion involves the motor and chief sensory nuclei and the intra-axial root fibers of the trigeminal nerve as it passes through the base of the pons. All signs are ipsilateral and refer to CN V. The afferent limb of the corneal blink reflex has been interrupted. This syndrome results from occlusion of the trigeminal artery—a short circumferential branch of the basilar artery.

11. B. These signs constitute lateral inferior pontine syndrome (AICA syndrome). The neurologic findings are signs of a lesion involving the facial nerve. The facial motor nucleus and intra-axial fibers are found in the caudal aspect of the lateral pontine tegmentum. A lesion at the stylomastoid foramen does not include the absence of the stapedial reflex or the loss of taste sensation from the anterior two-thirds of the tongue. The stapedial nerve and the chorda tympani exit the facial canal proximal to the stylomastoid foramen.

12. C. The base of the pons includes the corticospinal (pyramidal), corticobulbar, and corticopontine tracts; pontine nuclei; and transverse pontine fibers. At caudal levels, intra-axial abducens fibers pass through the lateral pyramidal fascicles.

13. E. The superior colliculus, together with the pretectal area, is responsible for searching, tracking, and reflexive movements of the eyes. The facial motor nucleus is not involved in eye movement, just closing via orbicularis oculi. The medial lemniscus is a continuation of the dorsal columns in the brainstem and contains fibers involved with the sensation of fine touch, conscious proprioception, and vibratory sense. The medial longitudinal fasciculus yokes together the brainstem motor nuclei associated with gaze, but it does not "drive" such movement—a lesion here may result in one eye properly orienting and the opposite eye not. The red nucleus is primarily involved in upper limb flexion and relaying signals from the cerebellum to the thalamus.

14. D. The pyramid on the right side of the upper parts of the medulla contains uncrossed descending corticospinal fibers; they will cross in the caudal medulla, thus loss of the pyramid on the right would cause motor loss over the left aspect of the body. Lesion of the inferior cerebellar peduncle damages proprioceptive information entering the cerebellum from the spinal cord and would not lead to loss of voluntary muscle control. The medial lemniscus is a continuation of the dorsal columns in the brainstem and contains fibers involved with the sensation of fine touch, conscious proprioception, and vibratory sense. Nucleus ambiguus is a lower motor neuron nucleus that influences the sternocleidomastoid and trapezius, not the entire side of the body. The spinothalamic tract conveys ascending pain and temperature information and is not related to voluntary motor control.

15. B. Paralysis of upward gaze results from compression of the midbrain tectum by a tumor in the pineal region known as Parinaud syndrome.

16. C. Loss of pain and temperature on the left side of the body is the result of a lesion on the right side of the anterolateral system.

17. E. Deviation of the tongue to the left side results from transection of the right corticobulbar fibers (CN XII) in the medial aspect of the crus cerebri. Deviation of the uvula to the right side results from transection of the right corticobulbar fibers (CN X) in the medial aspect of the crus cerebri.

18. **A.** Transection of the left dentatorubrothalamic tract results in an intention tremor on the right side. The dentatorubrothalamic tract decussates in the caudal midbrain, below the level of this lesion.

19. **E.** Complete third nerve palsy on the right side results from transection of the oculomotor nerve fibers as they pass through the right side of the crus cerebri.

20. **A.** A loss of vibration sense in the right limbs results from destruction of the left medial lemniscus.

21. **E.** A Babinski sign on the left results from transection of the corticospinal tract within the middle three-fifths of the crus cerebri.

22. **D.** Destruction of the right medial geniculate body results in terminal axonal degeneration of the auditory (sublenticular) radiations in the right superior temporal gyrus.

Diencephalon: Thalamus and Hypothalamus

I. OVERVIEW: THE THALAMUS

- largest division of the diencephalon.
- receives precortical input from all sensory systems, except the olfactory system.
- largest input received is from the cerebral cortex.
- projects primarily to the cerebral cortex and to a lesser degree to the basal nuclei and hypothalamus.
- plays an important role in sensory and motor system integration.

II. BOUNDARIES OF THE THALAMUS (Figures 13.1 and 13.2)

A. **Anterior: interventricular foramen**

B. **Posterior: free pole of the pulvinar**

C. **Dorsal: free surface underlying the fornix and the lateral ventricle**

D. **Ventral: plane connecting the hypothalamic sulci**

E. **Medial: third ventricle**

F. **Lateral: posterior limb of the internal capsule**

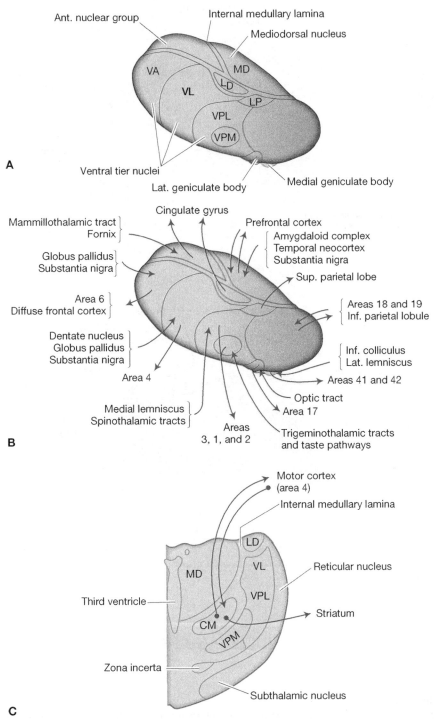

FIGURE 13.1. Major thalamic nuclei and their connections. **(A)** Oblique dorsolateral aspect of the thalamus and major nuclei. **(B)** The major afferent and efferent connections of the thalamus. **(C)** The transverse section of the thalamus showing the major connections of the centromedian nucleus. CM, centromedian nucleus; MD, mediodorsal nucleus; LD, lateral dorsal nucleus; LP, lateral posterior nucleus; VA, ventral anterior nucleus; VL, ventral lateral nucleus; VPL, ventral posterolateral nucleus; VPM, ventral posteromedial nucleus.

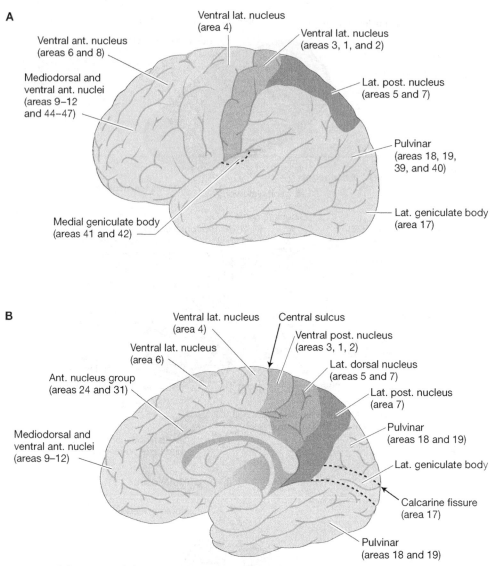

FIGURE 13.2. (A) Lateral and **(B)** medial views of the cerebral hemisphere showing the cortical projection areas of the major thalamic nuclei.

III. PRIMARY THALAMIC NUCLEI AND THEIR MAJOR CONNECTIONS

A. Anterior nucleus
- receives hypothalamic input from the mammillary nucleus via the mammillothalamic tract.
- receives hippocampal input via the fornix.
- projects to the cingulate gyrus.
- part of Papez circuit, a well-described learning and memory circuit.

B. Dorsomedial nucleus (mediodorsal nucleus)
- reciprocally connected to the prefrontal cortex.
- has abundant connections with the intralaminar nuclei.
- receives input from the amygdala, the temporal neocortex, and the substantia nigra.
- part of the limbic and striatal systems.

▨ when destroyed, results in memory loss (Wernicke–Korsakoff syndrome).

▨ plays a role in the expression of affect, emotion, and behavior (limbic function).

C. Intralaminar nuclei

▨ receive input from the brainstem reticular formation, the ascending reticular activating system, and other thalamic nuclei.

▨ receive spinothalamic and trigeminothalamic input via the spinal lemniscus.

▨ project diffusely to the neocortex.

▨ project to the dorsomedial nucleus.

1. Centromedian nucleus

▨ largest of the intralaminar nuclei.

▨ reciprocally connected to the motor cortex (area 4).

▨ receives input from the globus pallidus.

▨ projects to the striatum.

▨ projects diffusely to the neocortex.

▨ plays a role in attention and arousal.

2. Parafascicular nucleus

▨ projects to the striatum and the supplementary motor cortex (area 6).

▨ plays a role in changing patterns of response to stimuli.

D. Dorsal tier nuclei

1. Lateral dorsal nucleus

▨ a posterior extension of the anterior nuclear complex.

▨ receives mammillothalamic input.

▨ projects to the cingulate gyrus.

▨ has reciprocal connections with the limbic system.

▨ plays a role in spatial learning and memory.

2. Lateral posterior nucleus

▨ located between the lateral dorsal nucleus and the pulvinar.

▨ has reciprocal connections with the superior parietal cortex (areas 5 and 7).

▨ plays a role in visual and spatial attention.

▨ often considered with the pulvinar as part of the pulvinar-LP complex.

3. Pulvinar

▨ the largest thalamic nucleus (actually a series of interconnected subnuclei).

▨ has reciprocal connections with the association cortex of the occipital, parietal, and posterior temporal lobes.

▨ receives input from the lateral and medial geniculate bodies (MGBs) and the superior colliculus.

▨ concerned with visual attention and appropriate motor activities in coordination with oculomotor function.

▨ lesions of the dominant side may result in sensory aphasia.

E. Ventral tier nuclei

▨ include primarily specific relay nuclei:

1. Ventral anterior nucleus

▨ receives input from the globus pallidus and the substantia nigra.

▨ projects diffusely to the prefrontal and orbital cortices.

▨ projects to the premotor cortex (area 6).

▨ functions in conjunction with the basal nuclei.

2. Ventral lateral nucleus

▨ receives input from the globus pallidus, substantia nigra, and the cerebellum (dentate nucleus).

▨ projects to the motor cortex (area 4) and to the supplementary motor area (area 6).

▨ influences somatic motor mechanisms via the striatal motor system and the cerebellum.

▨ destruction reduces Parkinsonian tremor.

3. Ventral posterior nucleus

▨ the nucleus of termination of general somatic afferent (pain and temperature) and special visceral afferent (SVA; taste) pathways.

■ contains **three subnuclei**:

a. Ventral posterolateral (VPL) nucleus

■ receives the spinothalamic tracts and the medial lemniscus.

■ projects to the somesthetic (sensory) cortex (areas 3, 1, and 2).

■ lesion results in contralateral loss of pain and temperature sensation as well as loss of tactile discrimination in the trunk and extremities.

b. Ventral posteromedial (VPM) nucleus

■ receives the trigeminothalamic tracts.

■ receives taste from the solitary and parabrachial nuclei.

■ projects to the somesthetic cortex (areas 3, 1, and 2).

■ lesion results in contralateral loss of pain and temperature sensation, and loss of tactile discrimination in the head; results in ipsilateral loss of taste.

c. Ventral posteroinferior nucleus

■ receives vestibulothalamic fibers from the vestibular nuclei.

■ projects to the vestibular area of the somesthetic cortex.

F. Lateral geniculate body (LGB)

■ a visual relay nucleus.

■ receives retinal input via the optic tract.

■ projects to the primary visual cortex (area 17, the lingual gyrus, and the cuneus) via the optic (retrolenticular) radiations.

G. Medial geniculate body

■ an auditory relay nucleus.

■ receives auditory input via the brachium of the inferior colliculus.

■ projects to the primary auditory cortex (areas 41 and 42) via the auditory (sublenticular) radiations.

IV. BLOOD SUPPLY OF THE THALAMUS

A. Posterior communicating artery

■ gives rise to the anterior thalamoperforating arteries.

B. Posterior cerebral artery

■ gives rise to the posterior choroidal arteries.

■ gives rise to the posterior thalamoperforating arteries.

C. Anterior choroidal artery

■ primarily serves the LGB.

V. INTERNAL CAPSULE (Figure 13.3)

■ a layer of white matter (myelinated axons) that separates the caudate nucleus and thalamus medially from the lentiform nucleus laterally.

■ consists of three divisions:

A. Anterior limb

■ located between the caudate nucleus and the lentiform nucleus.

B. Genu

■ contains corticobulbar fibers.

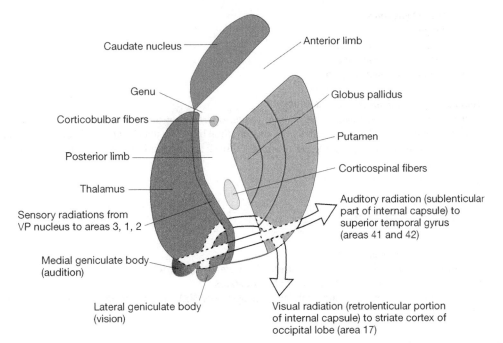

Caudate nucleus

Anterior limb

Genu

Globus pallidus

Corticobulbar fibers

Putamen

Posterior limb

Corticospinal fibers

Thalamus

Sensory radiations from
VP nucleus to areas 3, 1, 2

Auditory radiation (sublenticular
part of internal capsule) to
superior temporal gyrus
(areas 41 and 42)

Medial geniculate body
(audition)

Lateral geniculate body
(vision)

Visual radiation (retrolenticular portion
of internal capsule) to striate cortex of
occipital lobe (area 17)

FIGURE 13.3. Horizontal section of the right internal capsule showing the major fiber projections. Lesions of the internal capsule result in contralateral hemiparesis and contralateral hemianopia. VP, ventral posterior. (Modified with permission from Fix JD. *High-Yield Neuroanatomy.* 3rd ed. Lippincott Williams & Wilkins; 2005:118.)

C. Posterior limb
- located between the thalamus and the lentiform nucleus.
- contains the sensory radiations (pain, temperature, and touch).
- contains the corticospinal fibers.
- includes the retrolenticular (visual) and sublenticular (auditory) radiations.

VI. BLOOD SUPPLY OF THE INTERNAL CAPSULE (See Figure 3.6)

A. Anterior limb
- irrigated by the medial striate branches of the anterior cerebral artery and by the lateral striate branches (lenticulostriate) of the middle cerebral artery.

B. Genu
- perfused either by direct branches from the internal carotid artery or by pallidal branches of the anterior choroidal artery.

C. Posterior limb
- supplied by branches of the anterior choroidal artery and lenticulostriate branches of the middle cerebral arteries.

VII. CLINICAL CONSIDERATIONS

A. Infarction of the internal capsule
- most frequently results from occlusion of the lenticulostriate branches of the middle cerebral artery and results in the following contralateral conditions:

   1. Tactile hypesthesia
   2. Anesthesia
   3. Hemiparesis (with Babinski sign)
   4. Lower facial weakness
   5. Homonymous hemianopia

B. Thalamic syndrome (Dejerine and Roussy)
   - usually caused by occlusion of a posterior thalamoperforating artery.
   - classic signs: contralateral hemiparesis; contralateral hemianesthesia; elevated pain threshold; spontaneous, agonizing, burning pain (hyperpathia); and athetotic posturing of the hand (thalamic hand).

VIII. OVERVIEW: THE HYPOTHALAMUS

- a division of the diencephalon.
- lies within the floor and ventral part of the walls of the third ventricle.
- functions primarily in the **maintenance of homeostasis**.
- subserves three systems: the **autonomic nervous system** (**ANS**), the **endocrine system**, and the **limbic system**.

IX. SURFACE ANATOMY OF THE HYPOTHALAMUS (See Figure 1.5)

- visible only from the inferior aspect of the brain.
- lies between the optic chiasm and the interpeduncular fossa (posterior perforated substance).
- the hypothalamic sulcus forms superior border.
- includes the following **ventral surface structures**:

A. Infundibulum
   - the stalk of the hypophysis.
   - contains the hypophyseal portal vessels.
   - contains the supraopticohypophyseal and tuberohypophyseal tracts.

B. Tuber cinereum
   - the prominence between the infundibulum and the mammillary bodies.
   - includes the **median eminence**, which contains the **arcuate nucleus**.

C. Mammillary bodies
   - contain the mammillary nuclei.

D. Cerebral arterial circle (of Willis)
   - surrounds the inferior surface of the hypothalamus and provides its blood supply.

X. HYPOTHALAMIC REGIONS AND NUCLEI

- the hypothalamus is divided into a lateral area and a medial area separated by the fornix and the mammillothalamic tract.

A. Lateral hypothalamic area
   - traversed by the medial forebrain bundle.

▓ includes two major nuclei:
  1. **Lateral preoptic nucleus**
     ▓ the anterior telencephalic portion.
  2. **Lateral hypothalamic nucleus (Figure 13.4)**
     ▓ when stimulated, induces eating.
     ▓ lesions cause anorexia and starvation.

B. **Medial hypothalamic area (Figure 13.5)**
   ▓ includes the periventricular area that borders the third ventricle.
   ▓ divided into four regions, from anterior to posterior:
     1. **Preoptic region**
        ▓ the anterior telencephalic portion.

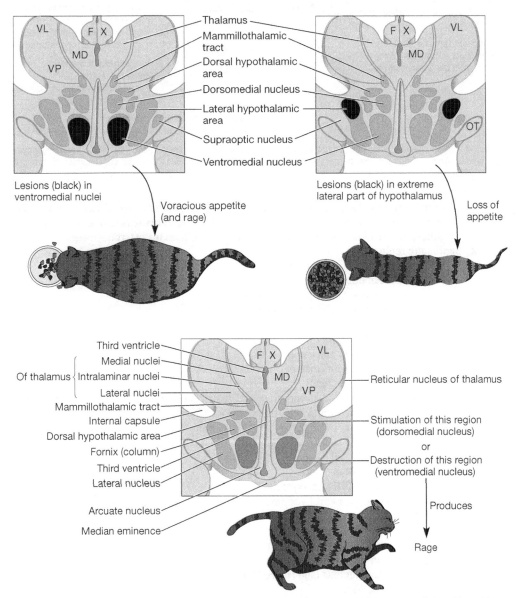

FIGURE 13.4. Coronal section through the hypothalamus at the level of the dorsomedial, ventromedial, and lateral hypothalamic nuclei. The column of the fornix separates the medial from the lateral hypothalamic areas. FX, fornix; MD, medial dorsal nucleus of thalamus; OT, optic tract; VL, ventral lateral nucleus of thalamus; VP, ventral posterior nucleus of thalamus.

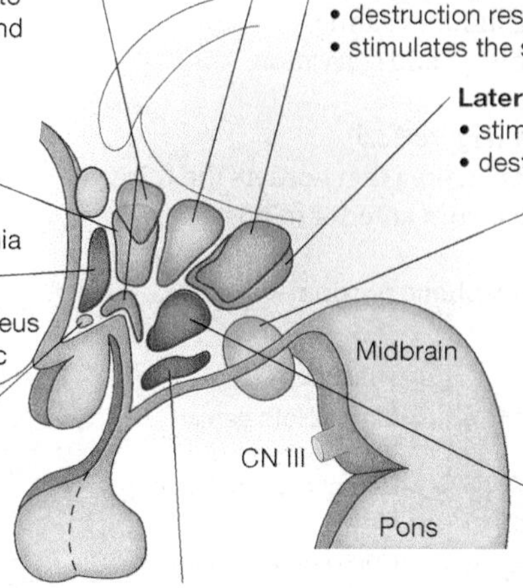

Paraventricular and supraoptic nuclei
- regulate water balance
- produce ADH and oxytocin
- destruction causes diabetes insipidus
- paraventricular nucleus projects to autonomic nuclei of brainstem and spinal cord

Anterior nucleus
- thermal regulation (dissipation of heat)
- stimulates parasympathetic NS
- destruction results in hyperthermia

Preoptic area
- contains sexually dimorphic nucleus
- regulates release of gonadotropic hormones

Suprachiasmatic nucleus
- receives input from retina
- controls circadian rhythms

Dorsomedial nucleus
- stimulation results in obesity and savage behavior

Posterior nucleus
- thermal regulation (conservation of heat)
- destruction results in inability to thermoregulate
- stimulates the sympathetic NS

Lateral nucleus
- stimulation induces eating
- destruction results in starvation

Mammillary body
- receives input from hippocampal formation via fornix
- projects to anterior nucleus of thalamus
- contains hemorrhagic lesions in Wernicke encephalopathy

Midbrain

CN III

Pons

Ventromedial nucleus
- satiety center
- destruction results in obesity and savage behavior

Arcuate nucleus
- produces hypothalamic-releasing factors
- contains DOPA-ergic neurons that inhibit prolactin release

FIGURE 13.5. Major hypothalamic nuclei and their functions. ADH, antidiuretic hormone; DOPA, dihydroxyphenylalanine; NS, nervous system. (Modified with permission from Fix JD. *High-Yield Neuroanatomy.* 3rd ed. Lippincott Williams & Wilkins; 2005:132.)

- contains the **medial preoptic nucleus**, which regulates the release of gonadotropic hormones from the adenohypophysis. The medial preoptic nucleus contains the sexually dimorphic nucleus, whose development is dependent on testosterone levels.

2. **Supraoptic region**
   - lies superior to the optic chiasm.
   a. **Suprachiasmatic nucleus**
      - receives direct input from the retina.
      - plays a role in the **control of circadian rhythms**.
   b. **Anterior nucleus**
      - plays a role in temperature regulation.
      - stimulates the parasympathetic nervous system.
      - destruction results in hyperthermia.
   c. **Paraventricular nucleus**
      - neurosecretory cells synthesize and release antidiuretic hormone (**ADH**), **oxytocin**, and corticotropin-releasing hormone (**CRH**).
      - regulates water balance (conservation of water).
      - gives rise to the supraopticohypophyseal tract, which projects to the neurohypophysis.
      - destruction results in **diabetes insipidus**.
   d. **Supraoptic nucleus**
      - synthesizes **ADH** and **oxytocin**.
      - projects to the neurohypophysis via the supraopticohypophyseal tract.

3. **Tuberal region**
   - lies superior to the tuber cinereum.
   a. **Dorsomedial nucleus (see Figure 13.4)**
      - results in rage when stimulated.
   b. **Ventromedial nucleus (see Figure 13.4)**
      - **satiety center**.
      - when stimulated, inhibits the urge to eat.
      - bilateral destruction involved with hyperphagia, obesity, and savage behavior.
   c. **Arcuate (infundibular) nucleus**
      - located in the tuber cinereum.

- a periventricular nucleus.
- contains neurons that produce **hypothalamic-releasing factors** and gives rise to the tuberohypophyseal tract, which terminates in the hypophyseal portal system of the infundibulum.
- effects, via hypothalamic-releasing factors, the release or nonrelease of adenohypophyseal hormones into the systemic circulation.
- contains dopaminergic neurons; **dopamine** is the **prolactin-inhibiting factor** (**PIF**).

4. Mammillary region

a. Mammillary nuclei

- lies superior to the mammillary bodies.
- receive input from the **hippocampal formation** via the **fornix**.
- receive input from the dorsal and ventral tegmental nuclei and the raphe nuclei via the mammillary peduncle.
- project to the anterior nucleus of the thalamus via the mammillothalamic tract.
- contain hemorrhagic lesions in Wernicke encephalopathy.

b. Posterior nucleus

- plays a role in **thermal regulation** (ie, conservation and increased production of heat).
- lesions result in **poikilothermia**, the inability to thermoregulate.

XI. MAJOR HYPOTHALAMIC CONNECTIONS (Figures 13.6 and 13.7)

- characterized by mostly reciprocal connections.

A. Afferent connections to the hypothalamus

- derive from the following structures:

1. Septal area and nuclei and orbitofrontal cortex

- via the medial forebrain bundle.

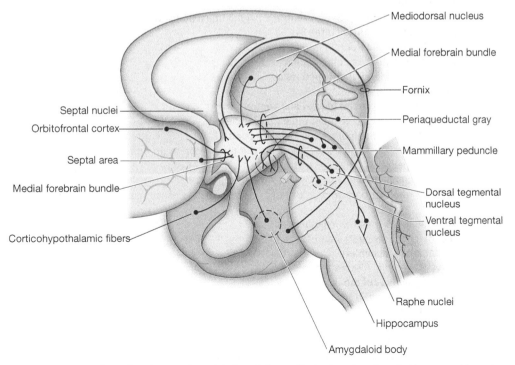

FIGURE 13.6. Major afferent (input) connections of the hypothalamus. The fornix projects from the hippocampal formation to the mammillary bodies. The medial forebrain bundle conducts both afferent and efferent fibers.

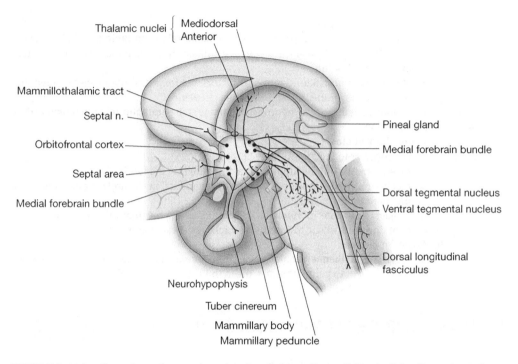

FIGURE 13.7. Major efferent (output) connections of the hypothalamus. The medial forebrain bundle conducts afferent and efferent fibers. The hypothalamus projects directly to the autonomic visceral nuclei of the brainstem and spinal cord.

2. **Hippocampal formation**
   - via the medial forebrain bundle.
   - primarily from the subiculum via the fornix.
3. **Amygdaloid nuclear complex**
   - via the stria terminalis and ventral amygdalofugal pathway.
4. **Primary olfactory cortex (area 34)**
   - via the medial forebrain bundle.
5. **Mediodorsal nucleus of the thalamus**
   - via the inferior thalamic peduncle.
6. **Brainstem nuclei**
   a. **Tegmental nuclei (dorsal and ventral)**
      - project via the mammillary peduncle.
   b. **Raphe nuclei (dorsal and superior central)**
      - project serotonergic fibers via the medial forebrain bundle and the mammillary peduncle (see Figure 21.5).
   c. **Locus ceruleus**
      - projects noradrenergic fibers via the medial forebrain bundle (see Figure 21.4).

B. **Efferent connections from the hypothalamus**
   - **project** to the following structures:
   1. **Septal area and nuclei**
      - via the medial forebrain bundle.
   2. **Anterior nucleus of the thalamus**
      - via the mammillothalamic tract.
   3. **Mediodorsal nucleus of the thalamus**
      - via the inferior thalamic peduncle.
   4. **Amygdaloid nuclear complex**
      - via the stria terminalis and the ventral amygdalopetal pathway.

5. **Brainstem nuclei and spinal cord**
   - via the dorsal longitudinal fasciculus and the medial forebrain bundle.
6. **Adenohypophysis**
   - via the tuberohypophyseal tract and hypophyseal portal system.
7. **Neurohypophysis**
   - via the supraopticohypophyseal tract.

XII. MAJOR FIBER SYSTEMS

A. **Fornix (see Figures 1.4, 1.5, 17.3, and 17.6)**
   - has five parts: the **alveus, fimbria, crus, body**, and **column**.
   - projects from the hippocampal formation to the mammillary nucleus, anterior nucleus of the thalamus, and septal area.
   - the largest projection to the hypothalamus.
   - bilateral transection results in an acute amnestic syndrome.

B. **Medial forebrain bundle (see Figures 13.6 and 13.7)**
   - traverses the lateral hypothalamic area.
   - interconnects the septal area and nuclei, the hypothalamus, and the midbrain tegmentum.

C. **Mammillothalamic tract (see Figure 17.3)**
   - projects from the mammillary nuclei to the anterior nucleus of the thalamus.

D. **Mammillary peduncle (see Figure 13.6)**
   - conducts fibers from the dorsal and ventral tegmental nuclei and the raphe nuclei to the mammillary body.

E. **Mammillotegmental tract (see Figure 13.7)**
   - conducts fibers from the mammillary nuclei to the dorsal and ventral tegmental nuclei.

F. **Stria terminalis (see Figure 17.3)**
   - the most prominent pathway from the amygdaloid nuclear complex.
   - interconnects the septal area, the hypothalamus, and the amygdaloid nuclear complex.
   - lies in the sulcus terminalis between the caudate nucleus and the thalamus.

G. **Ventral amygdalofugal pathway (see Figure 17.3)**
   - interconnects the amygdaloid nuclear complex and the hypothalamus.

H. **Supraopticohypophyseal tract (Figure 13.8)**
   - conducts fibers from the supraoptic and paraventricular nuclei to the **neurohypophysis**.

I. **Tuberohypophyseal (tuberoinfundibular) tract (see Figure 13.8)**
   - conducts fibers from the arcuate nucleus to the hypophyseal portal system of the infundibulum.

J. **Dorsal longitudinal fasciculus (see Figure 13.7)**
   - extends from the hypothalamus to the caudal medulla.
   - projects to the parasympathetic nuclei of the brainstem.

K. **Hypothalamospinal tract**
   - contains direct descending autonomic fibers that influence preganglionic sympathetic neurons of the intermediolateral cell column and preganglionic neurons of the sacral parasympathetic nucleus.
   - interruption above T1 results in Horner syndrome.

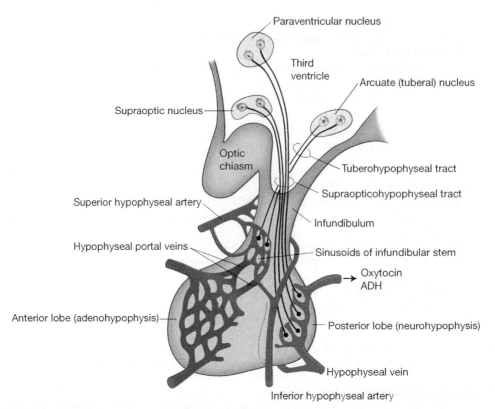

FIGURE 13.8. Hypophyseal portal system. The paraventricular and supraoptic nuclei produce ADH and oxytocin and transport the substances via the supraopticohypophyseal tract to the capillary bed of the neurohypophysis. The arcuate nucleus of the infundibulum transports releasing hormones via the tuberohypophyseal tract to the sinusoids of the infundibular stem, which drain into the secondary capillary plexus in the adenohypophysis. ADH, antidiuretic hormone. (Modified with permission from Fix JD. *High-Yield Neuroanatomy.* 3rd ed. Lippincott Williams & Wilkins; 2005:133.)

XIII. FUNCTIONAL CONSIDERATIONS

A. Autonomic function
1. Anterior hypothalamus
- The ANS is regulated by hypothalamic nuclei.
2. Posterior hypothalamus
- has a stimulatory effect on the parasympathetic nervous system.
- has a stimulatory effect on the sympathetic nervous system.

B. Temperature regulation
1. Anterior hypothalamus
- helps regulate and maintain body temperature.
- destruction causes hyperthermia.
2. Posterior hypothalamus
- helps produce and conserve heat.
- destruction causes the inability to thermoregulate.

C. Water balance regulation
- ADH controls water excretion by the kidneys.

D. **Food intake regulation**
   1. **Ventromedial nucleus**
      - two hypothalamic nuclei play a role in the control of appetite:
         - satiety center.
         - destruction is involved in overeating and obesity.
   2. **Lateral hypothalamic nucleus**
      - the **hunger** or **feeding center**.
      - destruction causes **starvation** and **emaciation**.

E. **Hypothalamic-releasing and release-inhibiting factors**
   - produced in the **arcuate nucleus** of the median eminence.
   - transported via the tuberohypophyseal tract to the hypophyseal portal system.
   - effect the release or nonrelease of adenohypophyseal hormones.
   - with the exception of dopamine, they are all **peptides**, which include:
      1. thyrotropin-releasing hormone.
      2. gonadotropin-releasing hormone.
      3. **somatostatin** (growth hormone–inhibiting hormone).
      4. growth hormone–releasing hormone.
      5. corticotropin-releasing hormone.
      6. prolactin-inhibiting and prolactin-releasing factor.

XIV. CLINICAL CONSIDERATIONS

A. **Craniopharyngioma**
   - originates from embryonic pituitary gland tissue.
   - usually calcified.
   - the most common **supratentorial tumor** found in children.
   - pressure on the optic chiasm results in a **bitemporal hemianopia**. Pressure on the hypothalamus causes **hypothalamic syndrome**, with adiposity, diabetes insipidus, disturbance of temperature regulation, and somnolence.

B. **Pituitary adenoma**
   - constitutes 10% to 20% of all intracranial tumors; 1:10 people will get in lifetime.
   - pressure on the chiasm results in a **bitemporal hemianopia** (most cases show asymmetry of field defects). Pressure on the hypothalamus may cause **hypothalamic syndrome**.

C. **Wernicke encephalopathy**
   - results from thiamine (vitamin **B$_1$**) deficiency.
   - characterized by the triad: **ocular palsies**, **ataxic gait**, and **mental confusion**.
   - lesions are found in the hypothalamus (primarily in the mammillary bodies) and in the periaqueductal gray of the midbrain.

Review Test

1. Which of the following thalamic nuclei has a motor function?

(A) Lateral dorsal
(B) Lateral posterior
(C) Mediodorsal
(D) Ventral lateral
(E) Ventral posterior

2. To which of the following thalamic nuclei do the spinothalamic fibers project?

(A) Anterior nucleus
(B) Pulvinar
(C) Ventral anterior nucleus
(D) VPL nucleus
(E) VPM nucleus

3. To which of the following thalamic nuclei do the cerebellar fibers project?

(A) Anterior nucleus
(B) Lateral dorsal nucleus
(C) Lateral posterior nucleus
(D) Ventral lateral nucleus
(E) VPM nucleus

4. To which set of thalamic nuclei does the globus pallidus project?

(A) Centromedian, lateral dorsal, and lateral ventral nuclei
(B) Centromedian, ventral anterior, and ventral lateral nuclei
(C) Mediodorsal, VPL, and VPM nuclei
(D) Ventral anterior, ventral lateral, and anterior nuclei
(E) Ventral lateral, lateral dorsal, and lateral posterior nuclei

5. Tritiated leucine [(³H)-leucine] is injected into the medial mammillary nucleus for anterograde transport; radioactive label would be found in the:

(A) anterior nucleus thalami.
(B) arcuate nucleus hypothalami.
(C) dorsomedial nucleus thalami.
(D) supraoptic nucleus.
(E) ventral anterior nucleus thalami.

6. Which structure's infarction can give rise to left hypesthesia, left homonymous hemianopia, left facial weakness, tongue deviation to the left side, and plantar extensor on the left side?

(A) Left internal capsule
(B) Left pulvinar
(C) MGB
(D) Right internal capsule
(E) Right pulvinar

7. A capsular stroke is most commonly caused by occlusion of the following artery/arteries:

(A) anterior cerebral artery.
(B) direct branches of the internal carotid artery.
(C) lateral striate arteries.
(D) posterior communicating artery.
(E) recurrent artery of Heubner.

Questions 8 to 13

The response options for items 8 to 13 are the same. Select one answer for each item in the set.

(A) Anterior nucleus
(B) Centromedian nucleus
(C) Lateral geniculate nucleus
(D) Mediodorsal nucleus
(E) Pulvinar
(F) Ventral anterior nucleus
(G) Ventral lateral nucleus
(H) VPL nucleus
(I) VPM nucleus

Match each of the following descriptions with the appropriate thalamic nucleus.

8. Receives input from the ipsilateral central tegmental tract

9. Has reciprocal connections with the inferior parietal lobule

10. Receives input from the contralateral lateral spinothalamic tract

11. Projects to the putamen

12. Receives the dentatorubrothalamic tract

13. Plays a role in the expression of affect, emotion, and behavior (limbic function)

Questions 14 to 18

The response options for items 14 to 18 are the same. Select one answer for each item in the set.

(A) Anterior nucleus
(B) Medial geniculate (nucleus) body
(C) VPL nucleus
(D) VPM nucleus
(E) Ventral lateral nucleus

Match each pathway with the appropriate nucleus to which it gives input.

14. Brachium of the inferior colliculus

15. Thalamic fasciculus (H_1)

16. Mammillothalamic tract

17. Dentatorubrothalamic tract

18. Gustatory (taste) pathway

19. The sexually dimorphic nucleus is located in the:

(A) anterior nucleus.
(B) arcuate nucleus.
(C) medial preoptic nucleus.
(D) posterior nucleus.
(E) ventromedial nucleus.

20. A 40-year-old woman who has taken birth control pills has a 4-month history of amenorrhea and a bitemporal hemianopia that began as a bitemporal quadrantanopia. What is the most likely cause of these deficits?

(A) Aneurysm of the anterior communicating artery
(B) Cavernous sinus meningioma
(C) Optic glioma
(D) Pituitary adenoma
(E) Sella turcica meningioma

21. Which of the following statements concerning the hypothalamus is correct?

(A) It is a division of the subthalamus.
(B) It contains the tuberculum cinereum.
(C) Its suprachiasmatic nucleus receives input from the retina.
(D) It is not related to the limbic system.
(E) Its dorsomedial and the ventromedial nuclei are separated by the striae medullares.

22. Which of the following is a hypothalamic structure?

(A) Alveus
(B) Arcuate
(C) Column
(D) Crus
(E) Fimbria

23. Spring fever is a seasonal change in mood and behavior, coinciding with longer days and more sunshine. One possible anatomical substrate for this phenomenon involves the increased sunlight projecting posteriorly from the retina to which hypothalamic nucleus?

(A) Anterior
(B) Arcuate
(C) Paraventricular
(D) Suprachiasmatic
(E) Ventromedial

24. A 30-year-old woman presents to her primary care physician with a series of concerns, including chronic headaches, visual alterations, irritability, inconsistent menstrual periods, and a recently developed insatiable appetite. Neuroimaging is ordered and a pituitary gland tumor is revealed. Compression of which of the following hypothalamic nuclei may be causing the lack of appetite?

(A) Anterior
(B) Dorsomedial
(C) Mammillary bodies
(D) Supraoptic
(E) Ventromedial

Questions 25 to 31

The response options for items 25 to 31 are the same. Select one answer for each item in the set.

(F) Dorsal longitudinal fasciculus
(G) Fornix
(H) Medial forebrain bundle
(I) Mammillary peduncle
(J) Stria terminalis

Match each description below with the structure it best describes.

25. Extends from the posterior hypothalamic nucleus to the caudal medulla

26. Interconnects the hypothalamus and the amygdaloid nuclear complex

27. Is the largest projection to the hypothalamus

28. Connects the septal area to the midbrain tegmentum

29. Conducts fibers from the hippocampal formation to the mammillary nuclei

30. Lies between the caudate nucleus and the thalamus

31. Separates the medial hypothalamus from the lateral hypothalamus

Questions 32 to 40

The response options for items 32 to 40 are the same. Select one answer for each item in the set.

(A) Anorexia
(B) Craniopharyngioma
(C) Diabetes insipidus
(D) Hyperthermia
(E) Inability to thermoregulate
(F) Obesity and rage
(G) Pituitary adenoma
(H) Wernicke encephalopathy

Match each description below with the appropriate clinical condition.

32. Amenorrhea and galactorrhea

33. Hemorrhagic lesions in the mammillary bodies

34. Associated with the Rathke pouch

35. Destruction of the anterior hypothalamic nuclei

36. Stimulation of the ventromedial nuclei

37. Bilateral lesions of the ventromedial hypothalamic nuclei

38. Bilateral lesions of the posterior hypothalamic nuclei

39. Destruction of the supraoptic and paraventricular nuclei

40. Results from thiamine (vitamin B_1) deficiency

Answers and Explanations

1. **D.** The ventral lateral nucleus receives motor input from the extrapyramidal (striatal) motor system (globus pallidus and substantia nigra) and from the cerebellum (dentate nucleus).

2. **D.** Spinothalamic fibers project to the VPL nucleus, which receives the medial lemniscus.

3. **D.** Cerebellar fibers project to the ventral lateral (primarily) and VPL nuclei, which in turn project to the motor cortex (area 4).

4. **B.** The globus pallidus, a nucleus of the extrapyramidal (striatal) motor system, projects to three thalamic nuclei: the centromedian, the ventral anterior, and the ventral lateral nuclei of the thalamus.

5. **A.** Radioactive label is found in the anterior nucleus of the thalamus, which receives input from the mammillary nuclei via the mammillothalamic tract. The arcuate nucleus of the hypothalamus projects to the portal vessels of the infundibulum via the tuberohypophyseal (tuberoinfundibular) pathway; the ventral anterior nucleus of the thalamus receives input from the globus pallidus and the substantia nigra; the dorsomedial nucleus of the thalamus receives input from the amygdala, temporal neocortex, and substantia nigra; and the supraoptic nucleus of the hypothalamus synthesizes vasopressin and oxytocin and projects to the pituitary gland.

6. **D.** Infarction of the internal capsule gives rise to contralateral symptoms. Thus, infarction to the right internal capsule would result in left-sided symptoms, including tactile hypesthesia, contralateral anesthesia, contralateral hemiparesis (with Babinski sign), contralateral lower facial weakness, and contralateral homonymous hemianopia.

7. **C.** A capsular stroke is most commonly caused by occlusion of the lateral striate branches of the middle cerebral artery.

8. **I.** The VPM nucleus receives taste input via the ipsilateral central tegmental tract. The VPM nucleus receives sensory input from the head and oral cavity.

9. **E.** The pulvinar, the largest thalamic nucleus, has reciprocal connections with the inferior parietal lobule. Pulvinar is often considered as part of the pulvinar–LP system because of the interconnectedness of the nuclei.

10. **H.** The VPL nucleus receives input from the contralateral lateral spinothalamic tract, part of the anterolateral system.

11. **B.** The centromedian nucleus projects to the putamen; this thalamic nucleus also has reciprocal connections with the motor cortex.

12. **G.** The ventral lateral nucleus receives contralateral cerebellar input via the dentatorubrothalamic tract.

13. **D.** The mediodorsal nucleus plays a role in the expression of affect, emotion, and behavior (limbic function). It receives input from the amygdala and has reciprocal connections with the prefrontal cortex. Lesions of the mediodorsal nucleus are found in patients with Korsakoff amnestic state.

14. **B.** The MGB receives auditory input via the brachium of the inferior colliculus.

15. **E.** The ventral lateral nucleus receives input from the globus pallidus via the thalamic fasciculus.

16. **A.** The anterior nucleus receives input from the mammillary nuclei via the mammillothalamic tract. This is a major link in the Papez circuit.

17. **E.** The ventral lateral nucleus receives cerebellar input from the dentate nucleus via the dentatorubrothalamic tract.

18. **D.** The VPM nucleus receives SVA (taste) fibers via the central tegmental tract.

19. C. The sexually dimorphic nucleus is located in the medial preoptic nucleus of the preoptic region.

20. D. A pituitary adenoma is characterized by amenorrhea and visual field defects, specifically a bitemporal hemianopia. The amenorrhea–galactorrhea syndrome includes visual abnormalities, amenorrhea, galactorrhea, and elevated serum prolactin.

21. C. The suprachiasmatic nucleus of the hypothalamus receives direct input from the retina and plays a role in the control of circadian rhythms. The tuberculum cinereum overlies the spinal trigeminal nucleus. The limbic system has reciprocal connections with the hypothalamus. The striae medullares separate the dorsal aspect of the pons from the dorsal aspect of the medulla.

22. B. The arcuate nucleus is a periventricular nucleus in the tuber cinereum. It contains neurons that produce hypothalamic-releasing factors and gives rise to the tuberohypophyseal tract. The alveus, fimbria, crus, body, and column are components of the fornix.

23. D. The retina projects posteriorly to the suprachiasmatic nucleus, which plays a role in circadian rhythms, including activity-related behavior, hormone release, and feeding patterns. The retina does not project to the other nuclei listed.

24. E. An expanding pituitary tumor would most likely affect the inferior/ventral aspects of the hypothalamus first. The ventromedial nucleus is a satiety center, when lesioned—hyperphagia. The other hypothalamic nuclei are not involved with appetite.

25. A. The dorsal longitudinal fasciculus extends from the posterior hypothalamic nucleus to the caudal medulla and projects to autonomic centers of the brainstem. It contains both ascending and descending fibers.

26. E. The amygdaloid nuclear complex is interconnected with the hypothalamus via the stria terminalis and the ventral amygdalofugal pathway.

27. B. The fornix contains 2.7 million fibers and is the largest projection to the hypothalamus.

28. C. The medial forebrain bundle interconnects the septal area, the hypothalamus, and the midbrain tegmentum.

29. B. The fornix projects from the subiculum of the hippocampal formation to the mammillary nucleus of the hypothalamus. The fornix projects to the anterior nucleus of the thalamus, septal nuclei, lateral preoptic region, and the nucleus of the diagonal band of Broca.

30. E. The stria terminalis lies in the sulcus terminalis; it separates the head of the caudate nucleus from the thalamus and interconnects the amygdaloid nuclear complex with the hypothalamus.

31. B. The column of the fornix lies between the medial and lateral hypothalamus.

32. G. Amenorrhea and galactorrhea result from a prolactin-secreting pituitary adenoma, the most common type of pituitary adenoma.

33. H. Hemorrhagic lesions in the mammillary bodies and in the periaqueductal gray of the midbrain are seen in Wernicke encephalopathy.

34. B. Craniopharyngiomas—congenital epidermoid tumors—are derived from Rathke pouch; they are the most common supratentorial tumors found in children.

35. D. Destruction of the anterior hypothalamic nuclei results in hyperthermia.

36. A. Stimulation of the ventromedial nuclei inhibits the urge to eat, resulting in emaciation (cachexia or anorexia). Destruction of these nuclei results in hyperphagia and rage.

37. F. Bilateral lesions of the ventromedial hypothalamic nuclei are involved in hyperphagia and rage.

38. E. Bilateral lesions of the posterior hypothalamic nuclei result in the inability to thermoregulate (poikilothermia). Bilateral destruction of only the posterior aspect of the lateral hypothalamic nucleus results in anorexia and emaciation.

39. C. Destruction of the supraoptic and paraventricular nuclei or the supraopticohypophyseal tract results in diabetes insipidus with polydipsia and polyuria.

40. H. Wernicke encephalopathy results from thiamine (vitamin B_1) deficiency.

14 Auditory System

Objectives

- List three aspects of sounds perceived and how each is accomplished.
- Describe the components of the external, middle, and inner ears.
- Describe the organ of Corti and the scalae.
- Differentiate between inner and outer hair cells.
- Differentiate between perilymph and endolymph.
- Describe the central auditory pathway, including a description of the bilateral nature of the information transmitted.
- Describe the tonotopic organization of the primary auditory cortex.
- Discriminate between conduction and nerve deafness.

I. OVERVIEW

- an exteroceptive special somatic afferent system.
- detects sound frequencies from 20 to 20,000 Hz.
- ordinary conversation ranges between 300 and 3,000 Hz.
- functions over an intensity range of 120 decibels (dB) and can discriminate changes in intensity between 1 and 2 dB.
- characterized by tonotopic (pitch) localization at all levels of the neuraxis.
- there is a loss of high-frequency tones with advanced age.
- three aspects of what we hear, sound:
  - location—a central nervous system comparison involving the superior olivary nuclei.
  - frequency—where along the basilar membrane vibration is the greatest.
  - amplitude—how many CN VIII fibers are recruited to fire.

II. OUTER, MIDDLE, AND INNER EAR

A. Outer ear

- consists of an **auricle** and an external auditory **meatus**.
- separated from the middle ear by the **tympanic membrane**.
- conducts sound waves to the tympanic membrane and functions in sound localization.
- blockage (eg, with cerumen) causes conduction deafness.

B. **Middle ear (tympanic cavity)**
  - located within the petrous part of the temporal bone.
  - serves as an impedance-matching device—the ossicles overcome sound loss caused by transferring vibration from air to liquid in part through transmitting the vibration from the relatively large tympanic membrane to the relatively small footplate of the stapes in the oval window of the inner ear.
  - communicates with the nasopharynx via the auditory (Eustachian, pharyngotympanic) tube.
  - receives sensory innervation from the glossopharyngeal nerve (CN IX).
  - contains the **chorda tympani** of CN VII, which mediates taste sensation and supplies preganglionic parasympathetic innervation of the submandibular ganglion.
  - pathology (eg, ossification of the footplate of the stapes in the oval window) results in conduction deafness.
  - contains the following auditory structures:
    1. **Tympanic membrane**
       - receives airborne sound vibrations and transmits energy to the middle ear ossicles.
    2. **Middle ear ossicles**
       - consist of the **malleus, incus**, and **stapes**.
       - vibration of the tympanic membrane forces the footplate of the stapes into the oval window, creating a traveling wave in the perilymph-filled scala vestibuli.
    3. **Tensor tympani and stapedius**
       - innervated by the trigeminal and facial nerves (CN V and CN VII), respectively.
       - dampen vibrations of the ossicular chain, thus protecting the hair cells of the cochlea from loud sounds (ie, large vibrations), such as our own voice.

C. **Inner ear (membranous labyrinth) (Figure 14.1)**
  - derived from the otic placode of the rhombencephalon.
  - located within the **bony labyrinth** of the temporal bone.
  - receives blood from the labyrinthine artery.
  - contains the **cochlea**, which houses the following structures:
    1. **Scala vestibuli**
       - contains **perilymph**.
       - transmits traveling waves toward the **helicotrema, scala tympani**, and **round window**. Traveling waves spread throughout, but have the most effect on the portion of the basilar membrane that has the same resonant frequency, through the basilar membrane, and via the scala tympani to the round window.
    2. **Cochlear duct (scala media)**
       - contains the organ of Corti.
       - contains **endolymph**.
       - lies between the scala vestibuli and scala tympani.
    3. **Organ of Corti**
       - contains hair cells and the tectorial membrane.
       - rests on and is supported by the basilar membrane.
    4. **Hair cells**
       - auditory receptor cells that have **stereocilia** (microvilli) but no kinocilium. The stereocilia of the outer hair cells are embedded in the overlying tectorial membrane.
       - mechanoreceptors that transduce mechanical (sound) energy into generator potentials.
       - stimulated by vibrations of the basilar membrane.
       - innervated by bipolar neurons of the spiral ganglion.
       - receive efferent input via the olivocochlear bundle.
    5. **Basilar membrane**
       - separates the cochlear duct from the scala tympani.
       - pitch localization along its length: 20 Hz at the apex and 20,000 Hz at the base of the cochlea.
       - vibration results in movement of the endolymph and deformation of the hair cell microvilli against the tectorial membrane; this action serves as the adequate stimulus to produce a generator potential.

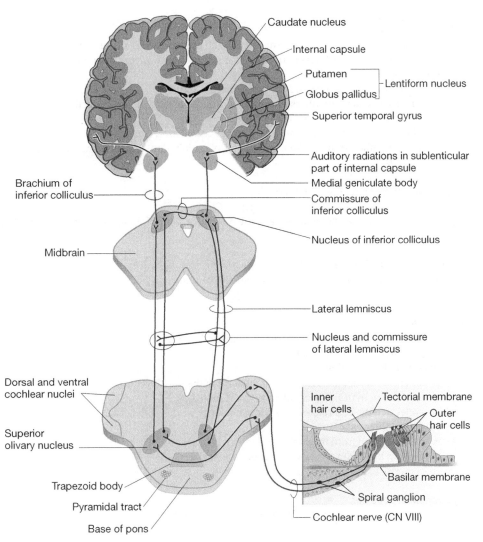

FIGURE 14.1. Peripheral and central connections of the auditory system. This system arises primarily from the inner hair cells of the organ of Corti and terminates in the superior temporal gyrus. It is characterized by bilateral projections and tonotopic localization of sound frequency at all levels beyond the cochlear nuclei. (Modified with permission from Fix JD. *High-Yield Neuroanatomy.* 3rd ed. Lippincott Williams & Wilkins; 2005:83.)

6. Spiral ganglion (of CN VIII)
- located in the **bony modiolus** of the cochlea.
- consists of bipolar neurons of the cochlear division of the vestibulocochlear nerve (CN VIII).

III. AUDITORY PATHWAY (See Figure 14.1)

- characterized by reciprocal connections throughout its caudorostral extent and by multiple decussations at all levels above the cochlear nuclei.
- consists of the following structures:

A. Hair cells of the organ of Corti
- innervated by peripheral processes of bipolar cells of the spiral ganglion.

- consist of two types:
  1. **Inner hair cells**
     - synapse with numerous afferent fibers, each of which makes contact with only one hair cell; the majority of fibers in the cochlear nerve come from the inner hair cells.
  2. **Outer hair cells**
     - contractile and embedded in tectorial membrane.
     - synapse with afferent fibers that contact numerous other outer hair cells.
     - outnumber the inner hair cells in the ratio of 3:1.
     - vibration of the basilar membrane causes contraction leading to movement of the tectorial membrane that causes movement of endolymph, which further stimulates inner ear cells.

B. **Bipolar cells of the spiral (cochlear) ganglion**
  - project peripherally to hair cells of the organ of Corti.
  - project centrally as the **cochlear nerve** to the dorsal and ventral cochlear nuclei at the medullopontine junction.

C. **Cochlear nerve (see Figures 1.1, 9.5, and 14.1)**
  - extends from the spiral ganglion to the cerebellopontine angle, where it enters the brainstem.
  - part of the vestibulocochlear nerve (CN VIII).

D. **Cochlear nuclei**
  - the only auditory nuclei that do not receive binaural input.
  - damage results in unilateral deafness.
  1. **Dorsal cochlear nucleus**
     - underlies the acoustic tubercle of the floor of the fourth ventricle.
     - receives input from the cochlear nerve (CN VIII).
     - projects to the contralateral cochlear nuclei.
  2. **Ventral cochlear nucleus**
     - receives input from the cochlear nerve (CN VIII).
     - projects bilaterally to the superior olivary nuclei.
     - gives rise to the trapezoid body.

E. **Superior olivary nucleus**
  - located in the pons at the level of the facial motor nucleus.
  - receives input from the ventral cochlear nuclei.
  - projects bilaterally to the lateral lemniscus.
  - plays a role in sound localization and binaural processing.
  - gives rise to the efferent olivocochlear bundle, a cochlear feedback pathway.

F. **Trapezoid body**
  - located in the caudal pontine tegmentum at the level of the abducens nucleus.
  - transversed by intra-axial abducens fibers of CN VI.
  - contains decussating fibers from the ventral cochlear nucleus.

G. **Lateral lemniscus**
  - receives input from the contralateral cochlear nuclei.
  - receives input from the superior olivary nuclei.
  - connected to the contralateral lateral lemniscus via commissural fibers.
  - projects to the nucleus of the inferior colliculus.

H. **Nucleus of the inferior colliculus**
  - receives input from the lateral lemniscus.
  - projects via the **brachium of the inferior colliculus** to the medial geniculate body of the thalamus.
  - projects to the superior colliculus to mediate audiovisual reflexes.

I. **Medial geniculate body (see Figures 1.6 and 14.1)**
- receives input from the nucleus of the inferior colliculus.
- projects via the sublenticular portion of the internal capsule (**auditory radiations**) to the primary auditory cortex, the superior temporal gyrus (transverse gyri of Heschl; areas 41 and 42).
- projects to the amygdala.

J. **Superior temporal gyrus (transverse temporal gyri of Heschl) (see Figure 14.1)**
- tonotopic arrangement mirrors basilar membrane.
- contains the primary auditory cortex (areas 41 and 42).
- receives auditory input via the auditory radiations.
- projects to the auditory association cortex (area 22).

IV. EFFERENT COCHLEAR (OLIVOCOCHLEAR) BUNDLE

- a crossed and uncrossed tract that arises from the superior olivary nucleus and projects to the hair cells of the organ of Corti.
- suppresses auditory nerve activity when stimulated.
- plays a role, through inhibition, in "auditory sharpening."

V. HEARING DEFECTS

- may be classified as:

A. **Conduction deafness**
- caused by interruption of the passage of sound waves through the external or middle ear.
- includes the following causes:
    1. **Obstruction by wax (cerumen) or by a foreign body** in the external auditory meatus
    2. **Otosclerosis**
        - produced by neogenesis of the labyrinthine spongy bone around the oval window, resulting in fixation of the stapes.
        - the most frequent cause of progressive conduction deafness.
    3. **Otitis media**
        - an **inflammation of the middle ear.**
        - the most common cause of meningitis (excluding meningococcus) and a common cause of brain abscesses.

B. **Nerve deafness (sensorineural or perceptive deafness)**
- owing to **disease** of the cochlea, cochlear nerve, or central auditory pathway (eg, acoustic neuroma).
- can result from the **action of drugs and toxins** (eg, quinine, aspirin, streptomycin).
- can result from **prolonged exposure to loud noise.**
- can result from **rubella infection in utero**, cytomegalovirus, or syphilis.
- includes the following:
    1. **Presbycusis**
        - **hearing loss occurring with aging.** Results from degenerative disease of the organ of Corti in the first few millimeters of the basal coil of the cochlea (high-frequency loss of 4,000-8,000 Hz).
        - the most common cause of hearing loss.
    2. **Acoustic neuroma** (schwannoma or neurilemmoma) (see Figure 12.4)
        - consists of a peripheral nerve tumor of the vestibulocochlear nerve (CN VIII).
        - located in the internal auditory meatus or in the cerebellopontine angle of the posterior cranial fossa.
        - includes symptoms such as **unilateral deafness** and **tinnitus** (ear ringing).

VI. TUNING FORK TESTS

▨ used to distinguish between conduction deafness and nerve deafness (sensorineural deafness).
▨ compare air conduction with bone conduction.

A. Weber test (Table 14.1)
▨ performed by placing a vibrating tuning fork on the vertex of the skull.
▨ normal subject hears equally on both sides.
▨ patient with unilateral conduction deafness hears the vibration louder in the diseased ear.
▨ patient with unilateral partial nerve deafness hears the vibration louder in the normal ear.

B. Rinne test (see Table 14.1)
▨ compares air and bone conduction.
▨ performed by placing a vibrating tuning fork on the mastoid process until it is no longer heard; then it is held in front of the ear.
▨ normal subject hears vibration in the air after bone conduction is gone.
▨ patient with unilateral conduction deafness fails to hear vibrations in the air after bone conduction is gone.
▨ patient with unilateral partial nerve deafness hears vibrations in the air after bone conduction is gone.

C. Schwabach test
▨ compares bone conduction of a patient with that of a person with normal hearing.
▨ demonstrates bone conduction to be better than normal in cases of conduction deafness.
▨ demonstrates bone conduction to be less than normal in cases of nerve deafness.

VII. BRAINSTEM AUDITORY EVOKED RESPONSE (Figure 14.2)

▨ a noninvasive method used to evaluate the integrity of the auditory pathways.
▨ clicks are delivered to the ear and recorded via scalp electrodes.
▨ seven waves (I-VII) correspond to the auditory nerve, cochlear nuclei, superior olivary nucleus, lateral lemniscus, inferior colliculus, medial geniculate body, and auditory radiations.
▨ used to assess hearing in young children and to diagnose brainstem lesions (eg, multiple sclerosis) and acoustic neuromas of the posterior fossa.

t a b l e **14.1** Tuning Fork Test Results		
Otologic Finding	**Weber Test**	**Rinne Test**
Conduction deafness (left ear)	Lateralizes to left ear	BC > AC on left
		AC > BC on right
Conduction deafness (right ear)	Lateralizes to right ear	BC > AC on right
		AC > BC on left
Nerve deafness (left ear)	Lateralizes to right ear	AC > BC, both ears
Nerve deafness (right ear)	Lateralizes to left ear	AC > BC, both ears
Normal ears	No lateralization	AC > BC, both ears

Conduction deafness, middle ear deafness (eg, otosclerosis, otitis media); nerve deafness, sensorineural deafness (eg, presbycusis). AC, air conduction; BC, bone conduction.

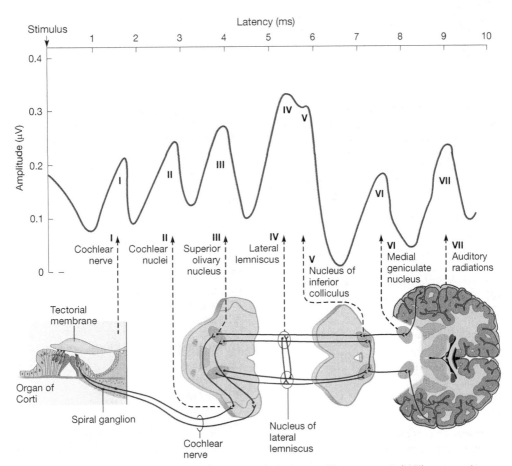

FIGURE 14.2. Graphic representation of brainstem auditory evoked responses. The seven waves (I-VII) correspond to way stations in the auditory pathway. (Adapted from Stockard JJ, Stockard JE, Sharbrough FW. Detection and localization of occult lesions with brainstem auditory responses. *Mayo Clin Proc.* 1977;52(12):761-769. Copyright © 1977 Mayo Foundation for Medical Education and Research. Modified from original drawing by Ellen Grass. With permission.)

Review Test

1. A 70-year-old woman presents to the audiologist for a hearing examination and has the following Weber and Rinne test results:

Test	Left Ear	Right Ear
Weber	No lateralization	Lateralization
Rinne	AC > BC	BC > AC

With which one of the following conditions are the patient's otologic findings most consistent?
(A) Otosclerosis involving the left ear
(B) Otosclerosis involving the right ear
(C) Presbycusis involving the left ear
(D) Presbycusis involving the right ear
(E) A normal examination

2. Frequency is analyzed in the inner ear by the:
(A) organ of Corti.
(B) scala vestibuli.
(C) spiral ganglion.
(D) stapes.
(E) tensor tympani.

3. At what level of the auditory pathway does the abnormal latency of wave V of a brainstem auditory evoked response (BAER) test correspond to a problem in sound transmission?
(A) Cochlear nuclei
(B) Lateral lemniscus
(C) Medial geniculate nucleus
(D) Nucleus of inferior colliculus
(E) Superior olivary nucleus

4. A 2-year-old girl is brought to her pediatrician by her father with congestion and a fever of 102 °F. Her father reports that she has been coughing and occasionally pulls at her right ear. What is the most likely diagnosis?
(A) Acoustic neuroma
(B) Otitis media
(C) Otosclerosis
(D) Presbycusis
(E) Wax obstruction

5. A 35-year-old man presents to his primary care physician with a complaint of worsening hearing loss. He reports that he is a drummer in a heavy metal band. Test results reveal that he senses the vibration from the Weber test louder in his right ear, and his Rinne test is normal. The most likely explanation for his hearing loss is:

(A) conduction deafness caused by obstruction.
(B) conduction deafness caused by otosclerosis.
(C) nerve deafness caused by cochlear nerve disease.
(D) nerve deafness caused by prolonged exposure to noise.
(E) conduction deafness caused by exposure to heavy metal drums.

6. Presbycusis results from degeneration of the:
(A) bipolar cells of the cochlear ganglion.
(B) cochlear nerve.
(C) dorsal cochlear nucleus.
(D) organ of Corti.
(E) ventral cochlear nucleus.

7. One component of the inner ear is the:
(A) auricle.
(B) incus.
(C) meatus.
(D) organ of Corti.
(E) scala vestibuli.

8. A 10-year-old girl is brought to her pediatrician by her mother, subsequent to complaints of an "itchy" and sometimes painful ear. Otoscopic examination reveals a middle ear infection. Which cranial nerve is most likely conveying the pain the patient is experiencing?
(A) Facial
(B) Glossopharyngeal
(C) Trigeminal
(D) Vagus
(E) Vestibulocochlear

9. A 28-year-old woman, who is late in her third trimester, is brought to her OB-Gyn by her spouse, with a chief complaint of a dry, watery eye, drooling, and inability to smile symmetrically. Examination and patient interview reveal hemiparesis of the facial musculature confined to only one side, hyperacusis on the same side, and an altered/diminished sense of taste. What nerve is most likely damaged to lead to hyperacusis in this patient?

(A) Chorda tympani
(B) Facial
(C) Glossopharyngeal
(D) Mandibular
(E) Vestibulocochlear

Answers and Explanations

1. **B.** The woman has otosclerosis involving the right ear. A patient with unilateral conduction deafness hears the vibration more loudly in the affected ear, and bone conduction is greater than air conduction. Otosclerosis is a conduction defect that involves the ossicles of the middle ear; it is the most common type of hearing loss in adults, and it has a strong autosomal dominant inheritance pattern. Presbycusis, the most common cause of sensorineural hearing loss in adults, affects the cochlea or the cochlear nerve (CN VIII).

2. **A.** The organ of Corti, or spiral organ, is a frequency analyzer of the inner ear. It contains hair cells and the tectorial membrane; it rests on and is supported by the basilar membrane. The organ of Corti is contained within the cochlear duct.

3. **D.** Wave V corresponds to the nucleus of the inferior colliculus. Wave I, cochlear nerve; wave II, cochlear nuclei; wave III, superior olivary nucleus; wave IV, lateral lemniscus; wave VI, medial geniculate nucleus; and wave VII, auditory radiations.

4. **B.** The most likely diagnosis is otitis media, commonly known as an ear infection. Acute otitis media is often associated with upper respiratory tract infections. Children are more prone to ear infections because their auditory tubes are shorter and more horizontal than those of adults and are therefore more easily blocked.

5. **D.** The most likely cause of nerve deafness, or sensorineural hearing loss, in this patient is prolonged exposure to loud noise. Because the Rinne test was normal and the Weber test lateralized to his right ear, this patient has nerve deafness in his left ear. Conduction deafness is caused by interruption of the passage of sound waves through the external or middle ear, such as wax obstruction, otosclerosis, or otitis media.

6. **D.** Presbycusis results from degenerative disease of the organ of Corti in the first few millimeters of the basal coil of the cochlea (high-frequency loss of 4,000-8,000 Hz). Presbycusis is hearing loss that occurs as a natural process of aging.

7. **B.** The middle ear contains the incus, which together with the stapes and malleus make up the three middle ear ossicles. The middle ear also contains the tensor tympani and stapedius. Its lateral border is the tympanic membrane.

8. **B.** The glossopharyngeal nerve provides sensory innervation of the middle ear cavity, including pain from a middle ear infection (otitis media). The facial, trigeminal, and vagus nerves do provide some sensory innervation around the external ear, but not the middle ear cavity. The vestibulocochlear conveys special sense innervation from the inner ear apparati; it is also unrelated to the middle ear cavity.

9. **B.** The facial nerve provides motor innervation to the entire ipsilateral face, provides the nerve to stapedius (which causes sound dampening when activated) and taste to the anterior two-thirds of the tongue. Lesion of chorda tympani would cause altered taste, but not hyperacusis or facial paralysis. The glossopharyngeal also provides taste innervation (to the posterior one-third of the tongue), but only innervates one small muscle of the pharynx (stylopharyngeus). The mandibular nerve is a branch of the trigeminal and lesion may lead to hyperacusis, but would not cause facial paralysis. The vestibulocochlear nerve is a purely sensory nerve and, as such, damage would not lead to motor deficits.

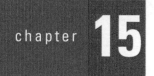

chapter 15 Vestibular System

I. OVERVIEW

- a special somatic afferent proprioceptive system.
- maintains **posture** and **equilibrium** and coordinates **head** and **eye movements**.
- functions in concert with the cerebellum and the visual system.
- contains receptors (hair cells) in the labyrinth of the temporal bone.

II. LABYRINTH (Figure 15.1)

- constitutes the inner ear (**auris interna**) of the temporal bone.

A. Structure
1. **Bony labyrinth**
   - a series of cavities (cochlea, vestibule, and semicircular canals) that house the membranous labyrinth.
   - contains **perilymph**, which fills the space between the bony labyrinth and the membranous labyrinth.
2. **Membranous labyrinth**
   - suspended within the bony labyrinth.
   - filled with **endolymph**.
   - contains receptor (or hair) cells that are bathed in endolymph.

B. Function
1. **Semicircular canal system**

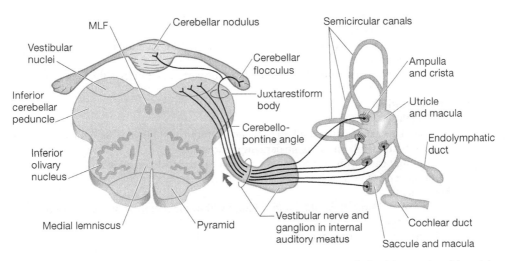

FIGURE 15.1. Connections of the vestibular system. The hair cells of the cristae ampullari and the maculae of the utricle and saccule project through the vestibular nerve to the vestibular nuclei of the medulla and pons and the flocculonodular lobe of the cerebellum (vestibulocerebellum). MLF, medial longitudinal fasciculus. (Modified with permission from Fix JD. *High-Yield Neuroanatomy.* 3rd ed. Lippincott Williams & Wilkins; 2005:85.)

- detects and responds to acceleration and deceleration of the head.
- consists of **three semicircular canals**:
  - anterior, posterior, and horizontally oriented channels that lie in more or less perpendicular planes.
  - each membranous semicircular duct lies within a semicircular canal.
  - contain hair cells.
  a. **Hair cells**
    - embedded in the cupulae of the cristae ampullari.
    - bathed in endolymph.
    - contain one kinocilium and multiple stereocilia.
    - innervated by bipolar cells of the vestibular ganglion (Scarpa ganglion).
    - receive inhibitory input from vestibular nuclei.
    - stimulated by relative endolymphatic movement. Movement toward the kinocilium is excitatory; movement away from the kinocilium is inhibitory.

2. **Utricle and saccule**
   - detect and respond to the position of the head with respect to **gravity**.
   - endolymph-containing dilations of the membranous labyrinth.
   - located within the vestibule of the bony labyrinth.
   - contain hair cells in the maculae of the utricle and the saccule. Both utricle and saccule respond to **head tilt/position**.
   a. **Maculae of the utricle and saccule ("otolith organs")**
     - patches of sensory epithelium.
     - consist of supporting cells and hair cells.
     - exert a tonic influence on the body musculature, reinforce muscle tone, and excite the muscle contractions necessary for the maintenance of equilibrium.
     - essential to the static, postural, tonic neck, and righting reflexes.
     - the utricular macula is disposed in the horizontal plane. It is maximally stimulated when the head is bent forward or backward or side to side.
     - the saccular macula is disposed in the vertical plane. It is maximally stimulated when the head is bent forward or backward or up-and-down.
   b. **Hair cells**
     - structurally similar to those of the cristae ampullari.

▓ embedded in the gelatinous **otolithic membrane**, which contains calcareous otolith crystals.
▓ stimulated by the shearing effect of the otolithic membrane–dependent on position of the head.
▓ receive an efferent innervation from the vestibular nuclei of the brainstem.

C. Fluids of the labyrinth
1. Perilymph
▓ resembles extracellular fluid, plasma, and cerebrospinal fluid (CSF) and surrounds the
  membranous labyrinth (in the perilymphatic space).
▓ communicates with the subarachnoid space via the cochlear aqueduct.
▓ produced from CSF and inner ear blood flow.
2. Endolymph
▓ resembles intracellular fluid and is found within the membranous labyrinth (endolymphatic space).
▓ secreted by the **stria vascularis** of the cochlear duct.

III. VESTIBULAR PATHWAYS (Figures 15.1 and 15.2)

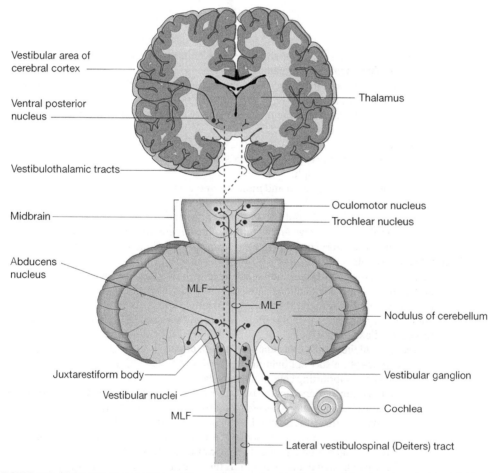

FIGURE 15.2. Major central connections of the vestibular system. Vestibular nuclei project through the medial longitudinal fasciculi (MLFs) to the oculomotor nuclei and subserve vestibulo-ocular reflexes. Vestibular nuclei also project
through the MLFs and the lateral vestibulospinal tracts to the anterior horn of the spinal cord and mediate postural reflexes. (Modified with permission from Fix JD. *High-Yield Neuroanatomy*. 3rd ed. Lippincott Williams & Wilkins; 2005:86.)

A. Bipolar neurons of the vestibular (Scarpa) ganglion (see Figure 15.1)

- located in the lateral end of the internal auditory meatus.
- project, via their peripheral processes, to hair cells.
- project their central processes, as the vestibular nerve (CN VIII), to the vestibular nuclei of the medulla and pons, and via the juxtarestiform body to the flocculonodular lobe of the cerebellum (ie, vestibulocerebellum).

B. Vestibular nuclei (see Figures 9.4 through 9.6)

- include the inferior, medial, superior, and lateral nuclei.

1. Receive input from the following structures:
- Bipolar neurons of the vestibular ganglion
- Cerebellum: flocculonodular lobe and uvula, vermis of the anterior lobe, fastigial nuclei
- Vestibular nuclei of the contralateral side

2. Project fibers to the following structures:
- **Flocculonodular lobe and uvula of the cerebellum**
- **Vestibular nuclei of the contralateral side**
- **Inferior olivary nucleus**
  - a. receives input via the vestibulo-olivary tract.
  - b. mediates vestibular influence to the vermis of the cerebellum.
- **Abducens, trochlear, and oculomotor nuclei**
  - a. receive input via the medial longitudinal fasciculus (**MLF**).
- **Anterior horn motor neurons**
  - a. vestibulospinal tracts (medial and lateral):
    - contain fibers from the ipsilateral lateral vestibular nucleus found at all spinal cord levels.
    - facilitate extensor muscle tone in the antigravity muscles, thus maintaining upright posture.
- **Ventral posterior nuclei of the thalamus**
  - a. receive bilateral input from the vestibular nuclei.
  - b. project to the primary vestibular cortex of the parietal lobe.

IV. EFFERENT VESTIBULAR CONNECTIONS

- arise from neurons in the vestibular nuclei.
- exit the brainstem with CN VIII and innervate hair cells in the cristae ampullari and maculae of the utricle and saccule.
- modulate the firing rate of vestibular nerve fibers.
- activation reduces motion sickness.

V. MEDIAL LONGITUDINAL FASCICULUS

- extends from the sensory decussation of the medulla to the rostral midbrain.
- contains ascending vestibulo-ocular fibers to the motor nuclei of CNs III, IV, and VI.
- mediates adduction of the eyeball in lateral conjugate gaze.
- mediates vestibular nystagmus.
- transection results in medial rectus palsy on attempted lateral gaze.

VI. VESTIBULO-OCULAR REFLEXES

- consist of reflex movement of the eyes to compensate for head movement to keep objects of interest on the center of the retina.
- can be tested in conscious or unconscious subjects by stimulating the semicircular canal system.

▪ afferent limb is CN III.
▪ efferent limb is CNs III, IV, and VI.

A. Oculocephalic reflex (doll's head eye movements) (Figure 15.3)
▪ normally suppressed vestibulo-ocular reflex.
1. Test method
▪ consists of rapid movement of the head in horizontal or vertical planes.
2. Test results
▪ with intact proprioception and brainstem (vestibular nuclei), the eyes move conjugately in the opposite direction.
▪ doll's head eye movements are absent or abnormal when lesions of the vestibular nuclei and MLFs are present.

B. Vestibular nystagmus
▪ consists of involuntary to-and-fro, up-and-down, or rotary movements of one or both eyes.
▪ consists of a slow component, opposite to the direction of head rotation, and a fast compensatory component, in the direction of head rotation.
▪ named after the fast component.
▪ results from the stimulation of hair cells within the semicircular canals on rotation.

C. Postrotational nystagmus
1. Test method
▪ the subject is rotated several times in the same direction and then is suddenly stopped.
2. Test results
▪ the subject with normal labyrinths will have a horizontal nystagmus opposite to the direction of rotation (fast phase).
▪ the subject will past-point and tend to fall in the direction of rotation and experience a sensation of turning (vertigo) to the opposite side.

D. Caloric nystagmus (see Figure 15.3)
▪ induced with cold- or hot-water irrigation of the external auditory meatus.
▪ used to evaluate unconscious patients.
1. Test method (used to stimulate the horizontal semicircular canal)
▪ while sitting erect, the subject tilts the head back 60°, or the recumbent subject elevates the head 30° from a horizontal position.
▪ cold or hot water is syringed into the external auditory meatus.

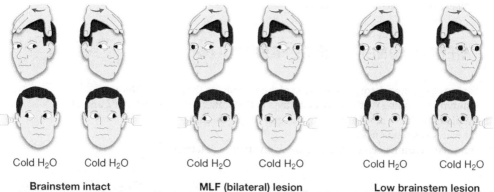

Cold H$_2$O   Cold H$_2$O   Cold H$_2$O   Cold H$_2$O   Cold H$_2$O   Cold H$_2$O

Brainstem intact   **MLF (bilateral) lesion**   **Low brainstem lesion**

FIGURE 15.3. Ocular reflexes in patients who are in coma. The external auditory meatus is irrigated with cold water. If the brainstem is intact, the eyes deviate toward the irrigated side. If the medial longitudinal fasciculi (MLFs) are transected, the eyes deviate toward the side of the abducted eye only. With lower brainstem damage, the eyes do not deviate from the midline. (Adapted with permission of Oxford University Press - Books (US & UK) from Plum F, Posner GB. The pathologic physiology of signs and symptoms of coma. In: The Diagnosis of Stupor and Coma. 3rd ed. New York: Oxford University Press; 1982:55; permission conveyed through Copyright Clearance Center, Inc.)

2. **Test results**
   - cold-water irrigation results in nystagmus to the opposite side and past-pointing and falling to the same side.
   - hot-water irrigation results in the reverse reactions.
   - remember the mnemonic **COWS** = **C**old, **O**pposite; **W**arm, **S**ame.
3. **Test results (in patients who are in coma)**
   - no nystagmus is seen.
   - with the brainstem intact, the eyes deviate to the side of cold irrigation.
   - with bilateral MLF transection, the abducting eye deviates to the side of cold irrigation.
   - with lower brainstem damage to vestibular nuclei, the eyes do not deviate.

VII. CLINICAL CONSIDERATIONS

A. Vertigo
- a sensation of irregular or whirling motion; an **illusion of movement**.

B. Ménière disease
- an inner ear disease associated with an increase in endolymphatic fluid pressure.
- characterized by episodic attacks of vertigo, tinnitus, hearing loss, nausea, vomiting, and a sensation of fullness and pressure in the ear.
- characterized by the presence of horizontal nystagmus during the attack. The fast phase is to the opposite ear; past-pointing and falling occur on the affected side.

C. Labyrinthitis
- characterized by **inflammation of the labyrinth**, which may result from bacterial, viral, or toxic (eg, alcohol, quinine, salicylates) causes.
- exhibits the same symptoms seen in Ménière disease.

D. Labyrinthectomy
1. **Unilateral labyrinthectomy**
   - results in predominantly horizontal nystagmus directed to the opposite side.
2. **Bilateral simultaneous labyrinthectomy**
   - does not give rise to nystagmus.

E. Internuclear ophthalmoplegia (INO)
- consists of medial rectus paresis on attempted lateral gaze.
- associated with monocular horizontal nystagmus in the abducting eye and intact convergence.
- the result of MLF damage, often from a demyelinating plaque as seen in **multiple sclerosis**.

F. Acoustic schwannoma (vestibular schwannoma)
- arises from the vestibular nerve of CN VIII within the internal acoustic meatus.
- usually involves CN V, CN VII, and CN VIII.
- found in the cerebellopontine (CP) angle.
- causes symptoms such as unilateral loss of hearing, tinnitus, and vertigo.
- marked by a lack of response to caloric stimulation—"dead labyrinth."

CLINICAL CORRELATES The most common type of vertigo is **benign paroxysmal positional vertigo (BPPV)**, which is elicited by certain head positions; the paroxysms of vertigo are accompanied by nystagmus. BPPV is not associated with hearing loss or tinnitus. The most common cause is from cuprolithiasis of the posterior semicircular duct (dislocation of utricular macular otoliths). Treatment involves particle repositioning through physical maneuvering of the head (the Epley maneuver).

Review Test

1. A 40-year-old man complains of headaches and inability to control his walking (gait). His physician refers him to a neurologist for further evaluation. The man remembers that 10 years ago he noticed a noise in his right ear that sounded like frying bacon. Neurologic examination reveals the following: loss of hearing on the right side; tinnitus, vertigo, and nausea; wide-based ataxic gait with lurching to the right side; dysphagia; facial weakness on the right side; sensory loss over the face on the right side; loss of the corneal reflex on the right side; absent gag reflex; and diplopia. The lesion site responsible for these neurologic deficits is the:

(A) CP angle.
(B) lateral medulla.
(C) lateral pons.
(D) medial medulla.
(E) medial pons.

2. Tilting the head forward would maximally stimulate the hair cells in the:

(A) crista ampullaris of the anterior semicircular duct.
(B) crista ampullaris of the lateral semicircular duct.
(C) crista ampullaris of the posterior semicircular duct.
(D) macula of the saccule.
(E) macula of the utricle.

3. The head of a patient who is in coma is elevated 30° from the horizontal. Cold water is injected into the left external auditory meatus. If the brainstem is intact, which one of the following ocular reflexes do you expect to see?

(A) Deviation of the eyes to the left
(B) Deviation of the eyes to the right
(C) Horizontal nystagmus to the left
(D) Horizontal nystagmus to the right
(E) Vertical upper nystagmus

4. A 65-year-old woman presents to her primary care physician with the primary concern of dizziness that began about 1 week prior. Patient interview reveals that the bouts of vertigo are short in duration (generally less than a minute) and typically occur when she gets into or out of bed. She reports occasionally being

aware of a similar feeling of dizziness when moving around while in bed. She denies feeling nauseas and reports no issues with hearing. What is the most likely diagnosis in this patient?

(A) Benign positional vertigo
(B) Internuclear ophthalmoplegia
(C) Ménière disease
(D) Nystagmus
(E) Vestibular schwannoma

5. A 20-year-old woman with previously diagnosed multiple sclerosis presents to her primary care physician with a concern about increasingly blurry vision, particularly when looking to one side. Examination reveals horizontal binocular diplopia during lateral gaze to the left, resulting from an adduction deficit of the right eye. Where is the most likely site of the lesion in this patient?

(A) CN II
(B) CN III
(C) CN VIII
(D) MLF
(E) Right semicircular canal

Questions 6 to 10

The response options for items 6 to 10 are the same. Select one answer for each item in the set.

(A) Acoustic schwannoma
(B) Benign positional vertigo
(C) Ménière disease
(D) MLF syndrome
(E) Multiple sclerosis

Match each characteristic with the condition it best describes.

6. Causes symptoms of CN V, CN VII, and CN VIII

7. Is an inner ear disease associated with increased endolymphatic fluid pressure

8. Is the most common cause of INO

9. Results in cuprolithiasis of the posterior semicircular duct

10. Consists of lateral gaze palsy and monocular nystagmus

Answers and Explanations

1. **A.** The acoustic neuroma (acoustic schwannoma) is found in the CP angle. The loss of hearing on the right side and the tinnitus indicate damage to the cochlear nerve. The vertigo and nausea indicate damage to the vestibular nerve. The wide-based ataxic gait with lurching to the right indicates damage to the cerebellum. The dysphagia indicates damage to the glossopharyngeal and vagal nerves. The facial weakness on the right side indicates damage to the facial nerve. The sensory loss over the face on the right side indicates damage to the spinal trigeminal tract of CN V. The loss of the corneal blink reflex on the right side indicates damage to trigeminal (afferent limb) and to facial (efferent limb) nerves. The absent gag reflex indicates damage to glossopharyngeal (afferent limb) and vagal (efferent limb) nerves. The diplopia indicates damage to the abducens nerve. A large tumor can damage the pyramidal tract and the abducens nerve. The differential diagnosis should include other tumors of the CP angle (**S**chwannoma, **A**rachnoid, **M**eningioma, **E**pidermoid; remember SAME).

2. **E.** Tilting the head forward would maximally stimulate the hair cells in the macula of the utricle. Tilting the head to the side would maximally stimulate the hair cells in the macula of the saccule. The utricle and saccule both respond to linear acceleration and the force of gravity.

3. **A.** Nystagmus is not seen in patients who are in coma. In this case, the patient's eyes will deviate toward the side of cold-water injection.

4. **A.** Benign positional vertigo (BPPV) is most common in older (>60 years of age) women. The short duration of her symptoms, particularly acute when horizontal or rising from horizontal, and no hearing loss or nausea, all point to BPPV. Internuclear ophthalmoplegia is most common in patients with multiple sclerosis and does not lead to dizziness. Ménière disease leads to nystagmus, vertigo, tinnitus, hearing loss, and nausea, which the patient does not demonstrate. Nystagmus is a normal eye movement that also manifests in several disease states, but is not related to dizziness per se. Vestibular schwannoma usually involves cranial nerve damage and hearing loss and tinnitus.

5. **5. D.** The MLF conveys fibers from the abducens nucleus across the midline to the contralateral oculomotor nucleus to medial conjugate lateral gaze. Demyelinating lesions, as seen in multiple sclerosis, may occur in the MLF, leading to internuclear ophthalmoplegia. Lesion of CN II would lead to ipsilateral blindness. Lesion of CN III would lead to lateral strabismus during rest and an inability to adduct the affected eye regardless of the direction of gaze. Lesion of CN VIII would produce noticeable issues with balance, as would lesion of the semicircular canal.

6. **A.** The acoustic schwannoma, which is found in the CP angle of the posterior cranial fossa, impinges on CN V, CN VII, and CN VIII. CN V lesions result in loss of pain and temperature sensation on the ipsilateral face and loss of the corneal reflex. CN VII lesions result in a lower motor neuron paralysis of the ipsilateral muscles of facial expression and loss of the corneal reflex. CN VIII lesions result in loss of hearing, nystagmus, tinnitus, nausea, vertigo, and vomiting.

7. **C.** Ménière disease (labyrinthine vertigo) is the most common cause of true vertigo. It is characterized by abrupt attacks of vertigo, nystagmus, nausea, vomiting, tinnitus, fullness in the ear, and hearing loss. This disease is caused by a distension of the endolymphatic system (labyrinthine hydrops). Drugs used to treat motion sickness may be helpful. Destruction (decompression) of the vestibule and an endolymphatic–subarachnoid shunt have proved useful.

8. **E.** The most common cause of INO is multiple sclerosis. Other causes of INO are vascular insults and intraparenchymal tumors (pontine gliomas). Multiple sclerosis, a demyelinating disease of the central nervous system, is characterized by the following deficits: ocular signs (retrobulbar neuritis and INO); brainstem and cerebellar signs (deafness, vertigo, ataxia, and intention tremor); pyramidal tract signs (spastic paresis with Babinski sign); sensory disturbances (paresthesias or dysesthesias); and bladder and rectal incontinence.

9. B. Benign positional vertigo, which is more common than Ménière disease, is characterized by paroxysmal vertigo, oscillopsia, and nystagmus. It occurs as the result of assumption of certain positions of the head (ie, lying down or rolling over in bed). Such vertigo results from cuprolithiasis of the posterior semicircular duct—a dislocation of the otoliths that move freely with movement of the head.

The following procedure is diagnostic. The patient is moved from a sitting to a recumbent position (on an examination table), and the head is tilted 30° down over the edge of the table, then 30° to one side, and then 30° to the other side. The patient has a paroxysm of vertigo (Hallpike maneuver).

10. D. MLF syndrome (INO) consists of medial rectus palsy on attempted lateral gaze. Nystagmus in the abducting eye is evident. Convergence is intact. This syndrome is seen frequently in multiple sclerosis.

Objectives

- Describe the structure of the retina, and include a description of the optic disc, macula lutea, and the fovea centralis.
- List the layers of the retina and the cells found in each.
- Trace the central visual pathway and describe the result of lesions along its course.
- Describe pupillary reflexes—direct versus consensual, dilation, convergence, and accommodation.
- List cortical centers for control of the visual system.
- Describe the retinotopic organization of the visual system pathway.
- Discuss various clinical considerations related to the visual system.

I. THE RETINA

- the innermost tunic of the eye.
- derived from the optic vesicle of the diencephalon.
- contains efferent fibers that give rise to the optic nerve, which is actually a fiber tract of the diencephalon.
- sensitive to wavelengths from 400 to 700 nm.

A. Structures of the ocular fundus—the part of the retina opposite the pupil

1. Optic disc
- located 3.5 mm nasal to the fovea centralis.
- contains unmyelinated axons from the ganglion cell layer of the retina.
- the blind spot (contains no photoreceptors).
- contains a central cup, a peripheral disc margin, and retinal vessels.

2. Macula lutea
- a yellow-pigmented area that surrounds the fovea centralis.

3. Fovea centralis
- located within the macula lutea.
- contains only cones and is the site of the highest visual acuity, with an excellent photoreceptor-to-neuron ratio.
- avascular and receives nutrients by diffusion via the choriocapillaris.
- subserves color or day (photopic) vision.

4. Retinal blood supply
- supplied by the **choriocapillaris** of the choroid layer and the **central artery of the retina**, a branch of the ophthalmic artery.
- occlusion of the central artery of the retina results in blindness, as it is an end artery (ie, it does not anastomose with any other artery).

B. Cells of the retina (Figure 16.1)

▨ constitute a chain of three neurons that project visual impulses via the optic nerve and the lateral geniculate body (LGB) to the visual cortex.

1. Rods and cones

▨ first-order receptor cells that respond directly to light stimulation.

▨ generate graded potentials.

▨ utilize glutamate as a neurotransmitter.

a. Rods (~100 million)

▨ contain **rhodopsin** (visual purple).

▨ sensitive to low-intensity light.

▨ subserve night (scotopic) vision.

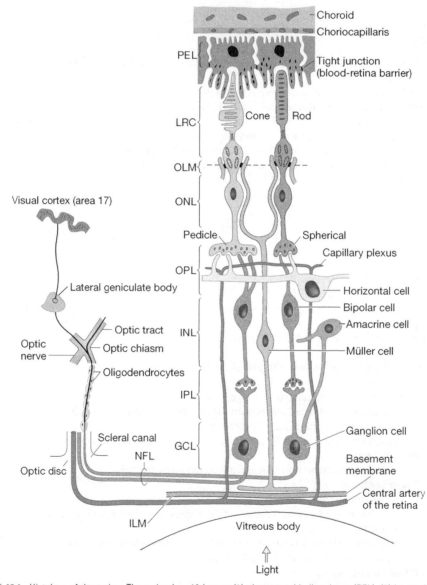

FIGURE 16.1. Histology of the retina. The retina has 10 layers: (1) pigment epithelium layer (PEL), (2) layer of rods and cones (LRC), (3) outer limiting membrane (OLM), (4) outer nuclear layer (ONL), (5) outer plexiform layer (OPL), (6) inner nuclear layer (INL), (7) inner plexiform layer (IPL), (8) ganglion cell layer (GCL), (9) nerve fiber layer (NFL), and (10) inner limiting membrane (ILM). The tight junctions binding the pigment epithelial cells make up the blood-retina barrier. The central artery of the retina perfuses the retina to the outer plexiform layer, and the choriocapillaris supplies the outer five layers of the retina. The Müller cells are radial glial cells that have a support function. (Adapted with permission from Dudek RW. *High-Yield Histology*. 1st ed. Williams & Wilkins; 1997:64.)

    b. Cones (~7 million)
- contain the photopigment **iodopsin**.
- operate only at high illumination levels.
- concentrated in the fovea centralis.
- responsible for day (photopic) vision, color vision, and high visual acuity.

2. Bipolar neurons
- second-order neurons that relay stimuli from the rods and cones to the ganglion cells.
- generate graded potentials.
- utilize glutamate as a neurotransmitter.

3. Ganglion cells
- third-order neurons that form the optic nerve (CN II).
- retinal cells with voltage-gated sodium channels that generate action potentials.
- project directly to the hypothalamus, superior colliculus, pretectal nucleus, and LGB.
- utilize glutamate as a neurotransmitter.

4. Interneurons
- **Horizontal cells**
  - **a.** interconnect photoreceptors and bipolar cells.
  - **b.** inhibit neighboring photoreceptors (lateral inhibition).
  - **c.** generate graded potentials.
  - **d.** utilize gamma-aminobutyric acid (GABA) as a neurotransmitter.
  - **e.** play a role in the differentiation of colors.
- **Amacrine cells**
  - **a.** small cells that have no axons and few dendrites.
  - **b.** receive input from bipolar cells and project inhibitory signals to ganglion cells.
  - **c.** mediate lateral interactions at the bipolar-ganglion cell synapse.
  - **d.** utilize GABA, glycine, dopamine, and acetylcholine as neurotransmitters.

5. Müller cells
- radial glial cells that have a support function similar to that of astrocytes.
- extend from the inner limiting layer to the outer limiting layer.

C. Meridional divisions of the retina
  1. The visual field illustrated in Figure 16.2 is the environment seen by one eye (**monocular field**) or by both eyes (**binocular field**).
  2. The vertical meridian divides the retina into **nasal** and **temporal hemiretinae**; the horizontal meridian divides the retina into upper and lower hemiretinae.
- **Temporal hemiretina**
  - **a.** receives image input from the nasal visual field.
  - **b.** has ganglion cells that project to the ipsilateral LGB layers 2, 3, and 5.
- **Nasal hemiretina**
  - **c.** receives image input from the temporal visual field.
  - **d.** has ganglion cells that project to the contralateral LGB layers 1, 4, and 6.
- **Upper retinal quadrants**
  - **a.** receive image input from the lower visual fields.
  - **b.** have ganglion cells that project via the LGB to the upper banks of the calcarine fissure.
- **Lower retinal quadrants**
  - **a.** receive image input from the upper visual fields.
  - **b.** have ganglion cells that project via the LGB to the lower banks of the calcarine fissure.

D. Concentric divisions of the retina and retinotopy
  1. Macular area
- a small area surrounding the fovea centralis that serves central vision (high visual acuity).
- contains cones.
- predominantly projects to the posterior part of the visual cortex.

  2. Paramacular area
- a large area surrounding the macular area that contains predominantly rods.
- projects to the visual cortex anterior to the macular representation.

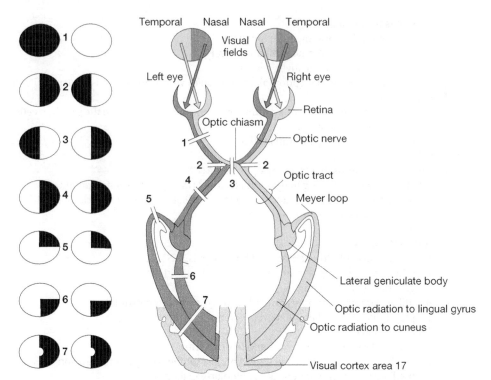

FIGURE 16.2. Visual pathway from the retina to the visual cortex showing visual field defects. (1) Left monocular blindness, (2) binasal hemianopia, (3) bitemporal hemianopia, (4) right hemianopia, (5) right upper quadrantanopia, (6) right lower quadrantanopia, (7) right hemianopia with macular sparing. Homonymous, same visual field from both eyes is lost, resulting from lesions posterior to the optic chiasm; heteronymous, opposite visual field from both eyes is lost, resulting from lesions anterior to the optic chiasm. (Modified with permission from Fix JD. *High-Yield Neuroanatomy.* 3rd ed. Lippincott Williams & Wilkins; 2005:119.)

3. Monocular area
- represents the peripheral monocular field.
- projects to the visual cortex anterior to the paramacular representation.
- lesions result in a contralateral crescentic defect.

II. VISUAL PATHWAY (See Figures 1.2 and 16.2)

- transmits visual impulses from the retina to the LGB and from the LGB to the primary visual cortex (area 17) of the occipital lobe.
- consists of the following structures:

A. Ganglion cells
- constitute the ganglion cell layer of the retina, with axons that form the optic nerve (CN II).
- project from the nasal hemiretina to the contralateral LGB.
- project from the temporal hemiretina to the ipsilateral LGB.

B. Optic nerve (CN II)
- a myelinated tract of the central nervous system (diencephalon)—**not a true nerve**.
- invested by the pia-arachnoid and dura mater and therefore surrounded by the subarachnoid space.
- receives its blood supply from the central artery of the retina, pial arteries, posterior ciliary arteries, and the cerebral arterial circle (of Willis).

▪ compression results in **optic atrophy**.
▪ transection before the optic chiasm results in **ipsilateral blindness**. Transection at the optic chiasm results in a contralateral upper temporal scotoma (**junctional scotoma**).

C. Optic chiasm

▪ part of the diencephalon.
▪ lies dorsal to the hypophysis and diaphragma sellae.
▪ contains decussating fibers from the two nasal hemiretinae.
▪ contains noncrossing fibers from the two temporal hemiretinae.
▪ receives its blood supply from the anterior cerebral and internal carotid arteries.
▪ midsagittal transection or pressure results in **heteronymous bitemporal hemianopia** (pituitary tumor).
▪ bilateral lateral compression results in **heteronymous binasal hemianopia** (calcified internal carotid arteries).

D. Optic tract

▪ contains fibers from the ipsilateral temporal hemiretina and the contralateral nasal hemiretina.
▪ projects to the LGB and via the brachium of the superior colliculus to the pretectal nuclei and superior colliculus.
▪ receives its blood supply from the posterior communicating artery and the anterior choroidal artery.
▪ transection results in **contralateral homonymous hemianopia**.

E. Lateral geniculate body

▪ a thalamic relay nucleus subserving vision.
▪ receives fibers from the ipsilateral temporal hemiretina, which terminate in layers 2, 3, and 5.
▪ receives fibers from the contralateral nasal hemiretina, which terminate in layers 1, 4, and 6.
▪ projects, via the geniculocalcarine tract, the optic radiation to the primary visual cortex (area 17).
▪ irrigated by branches of the posterior cerebral artery and the anterior choroidal artery.
▪ destruction results in a **contralateral homonymous hemianopia**.

F. Geniculocalcarine tract (visual radiation; retrolenticular part of internal capsule) (Figure 16.3)

▪ extends from the LGB to the banks of the calcarine sulcus, the visual cortex (area 17).

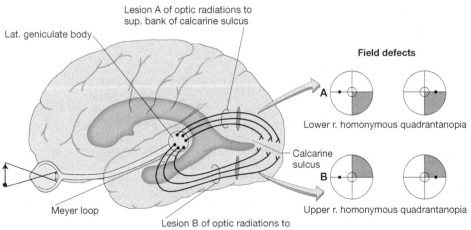

FIGURE 16.3. Relationships of the left upper and left lower divisions of the geniculocalcarine tract to the lateral ventricle and the calcarine sulcus. Transection of the upper division **(A)** results in the right lower homonymous quadrantanopia; transection of the lower division **(B)** results in right upper homonymous quadrantanopia.

- irrigated by branches of the middle cerebral artery, anterior choroidal artery, and calcarine artery (a branch of the posterior cerebral artery).
- transection results in **contralateral homonymous hemianopia**.
- has two divisions (see Figure 16.3):
  1. **Upper division**
     - projects to the upper bank of the calcarine sulcus, the **cuneus**.
     - contains input from the superior retinal quadrants, representing inferior visual field quadrants.
     - transection results in **contralateral lower homonymous quadrantanopia**.
  2. **Lower division**
     - loops from the LGB anteriorly (Meyer loop), then posteriorly to terminate in the lower bank of the calcarine sulcus, the **lingual gyrus**.
     - contains input from the inferior retinal quadrants, representing superior visual field quadrants.
     - transection of Meyer loop results in a **contralateral upper homonymous quadrantanopia**.

G. Visual (striate) cortex (area 17)

- located on the banks of the calcarine sulcus.
- receives retinal input via the ipsilateral LGB.
- receives its blood supply from the calcarine artery, a branch of the posterior cerebral artery; anastomosis with the middle cerebral artery may be substantial and result in **macular sparing**— retention of the macular part of the visual field, even when the adjacent field is lost.
- lesions result in a **contralateral homonymous hemianopia** with macular sparing. Bilateral destruction of both cunei results in a **lower altitudinal hemianopia**, and bilateral destruction of the lingual gyri results in an **upper altitudinal hemianopia**.
- **retinotopic organization** of the visual cortex includes the following:
  1. **Posterior third of the visual cortex**
     - receives macular input (central vision).
  2. **Intermediate area of the visual cortex**
     - receives paramacular input (peripheral input).
  3. **Anterior area of the visual cortex**
     - receives monocular input.

III. PUPILLARY LIGHT REFLEXES AND PATHWAY (Figure 16.4)

A. Pupillary light reflexes

- result when light shined into one eye causes both pupils to constrict.
  1. **Direct pupillary light reflex**
     - the response in the stimulated eye.
  2. **Consensual pupillary light reflex**
     - the response in the unstimulated eye.

B. Pupillary light reflex pathway

- comprises an afferent limb, **CN II**, and an efferent limb, **CN III**.
- consists of the following structures:
  1. **Ganglion cells**
     - project bilaterally to the pretectal nuclei.
  2. **Pretectal nucleus**
     - projects crossed (in the posterior commissure) and uncrossed fibers to the rostral accessory oculomotor nucleus.
  3. **Accessory oculomotor (Edinger-Westphal) nucleus**
     - gives rise to preganglionic parasympathetic fibers, which exit the midbrain as part of the oculomotor nerve (CN III) and synapse with postganglionic parasympathetic neurons of the ciliary ganglion.

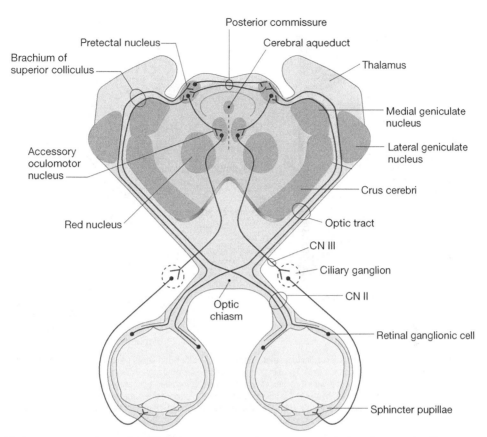

FIGURE 16.4. Diagram of the pupillary light pathway. Light shining into one eye causes both pupils to constrict. The response in the stimulated eye is called the direct pupillary light reflex; the response in the opposite eye is called the consensual pupillary light reflex. (Modified with permission from Fix JD. *High-Yield Neuroanatomy.* 3rd ed. Lippincott Williams & Wilkins; 2005:123.)

4. Ciliary ganglion

- gives rise to postganglionic parasympathetic fibers, which enter the eye via short ciliary nerves.
- innervate the sphincter pupillae of the iris to cause pupillary constriction.

IV. PUPILLARY DILATION PATHWAY

- mediated by the sympathetic division of the autonomic nervous system.
- interruption at any level results in **Horner syndrome**.
- consists of the following structures:

A. Hypothalamus

- contains neurons that project to the ciliospinal center (of Budge; T1-T2) of the intermediolateral cell column (Figure 16.5).

B. Ciliospinal center (of Budge)

- projects preganglionic sympathetic fibers via the sympathetic trunk to the superior cervical ganglion.

C. Superior cervical ganglion

- projects postganglionic sympathetic fibers via the perivascular plexus of the carotid system to the dilator pupillae of the iris to cause pupillary dilation and to the palpebral muscles (of Müller). Postganglionic sympathetic fibers pass through the cavernous sinus and enter the orbit via the superior orbital fissure.

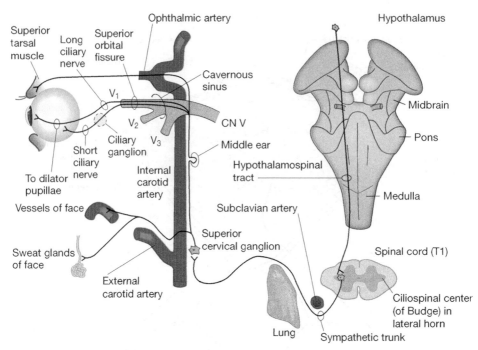

FIGURE 16.5. Pupillary dilation pathway (oculosympathetic pathway). Hypothalamic fibers project to the ciliospinal center (of Budge) of the intermediolateral cell column at T1. The ciliospinal center projects preganglionic sympathetic fibers to the superior cervical ganglion. The superior cervical ganglion projects perivascular postganglionic sympathetic fibers via the tympanic cavity, cavernous sinus, and superior orbital fissure to the dilator pupillae. Interruption of this pathway at any level results in Horner syndrome. (Modified with permission from Fix JD. *High-Yield Neuroanatomy.* 3rd ed. Lippincott Williams & Wilkins; 2005:67.)

V. CONVERGENCE-ACCOMMODATION REFLEX (See Figure 16.5)

▦ essential for visual fixation and acuity at close range.

▦ initiated by conscious visual fixation on a near object or by a blurred retinal image.

A. Reflex changes

▦ with accommodative effort, three reflex changes are evoked:

1. Convergence

▦ occurs as the eyes focus on a near point.

▦ mediated by medial recti innervation via the oculomotor nerve.

2. Accommodation

▦ adjustment of the eyes for various distances.

▦ occurs as contraction of the ciliaris results in a thickening of the lens and an increase in refractive power.

▦ mediated by the accessory oculomotor nucleus via the oculomotor nerve.

3. Pupillary constriction

▦ results in an increase in depth of field and depth of focus.

▦ mediated by the accessory oculomotor nucleus via the oculomotor nerve.

B. The convergence-accommodation pathway (see Figure 16.5)

1. Visual cortex (area 17)

▦ projects to the visual association cortex (area 19).

2. Visual association cortex (area 19)

▦ projects via the corticotectal tract to the pretectal area of the midbrain.

3. Pretectal area

▦ projects to the convergence nucleus (of Perlia).

4. Convergence nucleus (of Perlia)

▦ projects to the accessory oculomotor nuclei and the medial rectus subnuclei of CN III.

▦ anatomically positioned between the oculomotor nuclei to mediate convergence.

VI. CENTERS FOR OCULAR MOTILITY

A. Frontal eye field
- located in the caudal part of the middle frontal gyrus (area 8).
- a cortical center for voluntary eye movements, which are fast, saccadic, searching movements.
- stimulation (irritative lesion) results in **contralateral conjugate deviation of the eyes**.
- destruction (destructive lesion) results in **transient ipsilateral conjugate deviation of the eyes**.

B. Occipital eye fields (areas 18 and 19)
- the cortical centers for involuntary pursuit or tracking movements.
- stimulation results in **contralateral conjugate deviation of the eyes**.
- lesions result in difficulty following a slow-moving object.

C. Subcortical center for vertical conjugate gaze
- located at the level of the posterior commissure.
- includes the **rostral interstitial nucleus** of the **medial longitudinal fasciculus** (**MLF**), which projects to the oculomotor and trochlear nuclei.
- involved in posterior midbrain (**Parinaud syndrome**) (see Chapter 12 IV A).

D. Subcortical center for lateral conjugate gaze (Figure 16.6)
- located in the paramedian pontine reticular formation.
- receives input from the contralateral frontal eye field.
- projects via the contralateral MLF to the medial rectus subnucleus of the oculomotor complex.

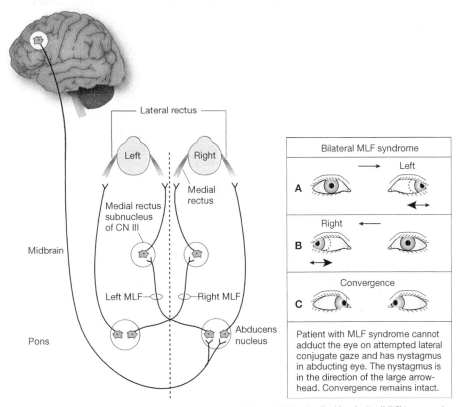

FIGURE 16.6. Connections of the pontine center for lateral gaze. Lesions of the medial longitudinal fasciculus (MLF) between the abducens and oculomotor nuclei result in a medial rectus palsy on attempted lateral conjugate gaze and horizontal nystagmus in the abducting eye. Convergence remains intact (inset). A unilateral MLF lesion would affect the ipsilateral medial rectus only. (Modified with permission from Fix JD. *High-Yield Neuroanatomy*. 3rd ed. Lippincott Williams & Wilkins; 2005:125.)

- projects via abducens nerve to the ipsilateral lateral rectus.
- damage to the MLF between the abducens and oculomotor nuclei results in **medial rectus palsy** (see VII B).

VII. CLINICAL CONSIDERATIONS

A. Anisocoria (unequal pupils)
- a condition where the two pupils are not equal.
- present in 10% of the population.
- seen in **Horner syndrome** and **third nerve palsies**.

B. MLF syndrome (internuclear ophthalmoplegia [INO]) (Figure 16.7; see Figure 16.6)
- a condition in which there is damage (eg, demyelination) to the MLF between the abducens and the oculomotor nuclei.
- results in **medial rectus palsy** on attempted lateral conjugate gaze and **monocular horizontal nystagmus** in the abducting eye.
- convergence is normal.

C. One-and-a-half syndrome
- consists of a bilateral MLF lesion and a unilateral lesion of the abducens nucleus.
- on attempted lateral gaze, the only muscle that functions is the intact lateral rectus.

D. Argyll Robertson pupil (pupillary light-near dissociation) (see Figure 16.7)
- the absence of a miotic reaction to light, both direct and consensual, with preservation of miotic reaction to near stimulus (accommodation-convergence).
- may be present in tertiary **syphilis**, **diabetes mellitus**, and **lupus erythematosus**.

E. Afferent pupil (Marcus Gunn pupil) (see Figure 16.7)
- results from a lesion in the afferent limb of the pupillary light reflex (eg, retrobulbar neuritis of the optic nerve seen in multiple sclerosis).
- can be diagnosed by the swinging flashlight test.
  1. Light shined into the normal eye results in brisk **pupillary constriction** in both the normal eye and the affected eye (consensual reaction).
  2. Light is then immediately shone into the affected eye with the afferent lesion, which results in **dilation of the afferent pupil**. The consensual stimulation of the constrictor pupillae is much greater than the direct stimulation through a defective optic nerve.

F. Transtentorial herniation (uncal herniation) (see Figure 16.7)
- occurs as the result of **increased supratentorial pressure**, commonly owing to a brain tumor or a hematoma (subdural or epidural).
  1. Pressure forces the parahippocampal uncus through the tentorial incisure.
  2. The impacted uncus forces the contralateral crus cerebri against the edge of the tentorial incisure, which increases pressure on the ipsilateral oculomotor nerve and the posterior cerebral artery, resulting in the following neurologic deficits:
     - **ipsilateral hemiparesis** owing to pressure on the corticospinal tract in the crus cerebri.
     - **a fixed and dilated pupil, ptosis, and a down-and-out eye** resulting from pressure on the ipsilateral oculomotor nerve.
     - **contralateral homonymous hemianopia** owing to compression of the ipsilateral posterior cerebral artery, which irrigates the visual cortex.

G. Adie pupil (Holmes-Adie pupil)
- a large tonic pupil that reacts slowly to light but does not react to near stimulus (light-near dissociation).
- associated with damage to the postganglionic innervation of sphincter pupillae.

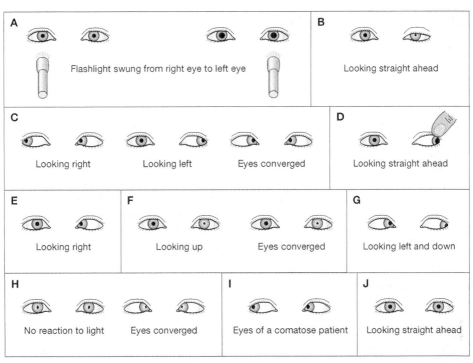

FIGURE 16.7. Ocular motor palsies and pupillary syndromes. **(A)** Relative afferent (Marcus Gunn) pupil, left eye. **(B)** Horner syndrome, left eye. **(C)** Internuclear ophthalmoplegia, right eye. **(D)** Third nerve palsy, left eye. **(E)** Sixth nerve palsy, right eye. **(F)** Paralysis of upward gaze and convergence (Parinaud syndrome). **(G)** Fourth nerve palsy, right eye. **(H)** Argyll Robertson pupil. **(I)** Destructive lesion of the right frontal eye field. **(J)** Third nerve palsy with ptosis, right eye. (Modified with permission from Fix JD. *High-Yield Neuroanatomy.* 3rd ed. Lippincott Williams & Wilkins; 2005:124.)

H. Ptosis (see Figure 16.7)
▦ a drooping eyelid, seen in many syndromes.
1. Oculomotor ptosis
▦ owing to paralysis of the levator palpebrae superioris (eg, transtentorial herniation).
2. Oculosympathetic ptosis
▦ owing to paralysis of the superior tarsal (Müller) muscle as seen in Horner syndrome.
▦ a very slight ptosis or pseudoptosis.
3. Myasthenic ptosis
▦ seen in myasthenia gravis.
▦ usually increases with increasing fatigue.
▦ immediately improves after an injection of a cholinesterase inhibitor.
▦ is usually bilateral and asymmetric.

CLINICAL CORRELATES   **Papilledema** (choked disk) is a noninflammatory congestion of the optic disk caused by increased intracranial pressure. It is most commonly caused by brain tumors, subdural hematoma, and hydrocephalus. Papilledema usually does not alter visual acuity or result in visual field defects. As viewed through an ophthalmoscope, papilloma is bilateral, but usually asymmetric and is greater on the side of the supratentorial pathology.

Review Test

1. Interruption of the MLF at pontine levels:

(A) abolishes accommodation.
(B) abolishes convergence.
(C) results in miosis and ptosis.
(D) results in paralysis of lateral gaze on command.
(E) results in paralysis of upward gaze on command.

2. A 75-year-old woman presents to her primary care provider with a chief complaint of worsening loss of vision. Visual field examination shows visual loss in the upper right quadrant in both visual fields. The lesion would most likely be in the:

(A) left cuneus.
(B) left temporal lobe.
(C) right angular gyrus.
(D) right lingual gyrus.
(E) right occipital pole.

3. An 80-year-old man with a previous diagnosis of Alzheimer disease presents to his primary care physician for issues centered around deteriorating eyesight. Previous tests reveal that he has suffered cell loss in the accessory oculomotor (Edinger-Westphal) nuclear complex. The cell loss is particularly pronounced on the left side. A check of the pupillary light reflex is performed; what would be the expected result of the test when the light is shown in the right eye of this patient?

(A) Both pupils will constrict.
(B) Neither pupil will constrict.
(C) Only the right pupil will constrict.
(D) Only the left pupil will constrict.

4. A 55-year-old woman presents to the emergency department with a chief complaint of a headache and blurred vision. The attending physician observes transient deviation of both eyes to the right during the patient interview. Visual examination reveals normal tracking movement of both eyes, but deficient voluntary gaze to the left. MRI reveals a stroke; based on the patient's symptoms, where is the most likely location of the stroke?

(A) Ciliospinal center (of Budge)
(B) Frontal eye field on the right
(C) Occipital eye field on the left
(D) Pretectal area
(E) Primary visual cortex of the left hemisphere

Questions 5 to 12

The response options for items 5 to 12 are the same. Select one answer for each item in the set.

(A) Binasal hemianopia
(B) Bitemporal hemianopia
(C) Left homonymous hemianopia
(D) Left upper homonymous quadrantanopia
(E) Right lower homonymous quadrantanopia

Match each defect below with the condition it causes.

5. Transection of the right optic tract

6. Transection of the right Meyer loop

7. Midsagittal section of the optic chiasm

8. Tumor of the right LGB

9. Pituitary tumor

10. Tumor of the left cuneus

11. Trauma to the right lingual gyrus

12. Bilateral lateral constriction of the optic chiasm

Questions 13 to 19

The response options for items 13 to 19 are the same. Select one answer for each item in the set.

(A) Anisocoria
(B) Argyll Robertson pupil
(C) Fixed, dilated pupil
(D) Horner syndrome
(E) Marcus Gunn pupil

Match each description below with the syndrome or defect most closely associated with it.

13. Results from interruption of the cervical sympathetic trunk

14. Is present in 10% of the population

15. Is characterized by uncal herniation

16. Is characterized by the absence of the miotic reaction to light but with the presence of the miotic reaction to near stimulus

17. The pupil dilates when light is shone from the normal pupil into the afferent pupil.

18. Is frequently seen in multiple sclerosis

19. Is associated with syphilis

Questions 20 to 25

The response options for items 20 to 25 are the same. Select one answer for each item in the set.

Match the description of the lesion sites in items 20 to 25 with the appropriate visual field defect shown in the figure.

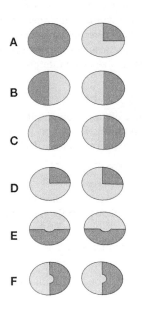

20. Occlusion of the left posterior cerebral artery

21. Transection of the left optic nerve at the chiasm

22. Craniopharyngioma

23. Left temporal lobotomy

24. Bilateral trauma to the cuneate gyri

25. Transection of the left optic tract

Questions 26 to 34

The response options for items 26 to 34 are the same. Select one answer for each item in the set.

Match the description of the lesion sites in items 26 to 34 with the appropriate deficit or pathologic finding shown in the photograph of the base of the brain.

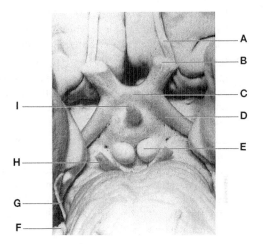

26. Transection results in polyuria and polydipsia.

27. Transection results in ipsilateral ptosis.

28. Transection results in homolateral extortion of the globe.

29. Destruction results in an absent corneal blink reflex on the side of testing.

30. Pathology is seen in Wernicke encephalopathy.

31. Transection results in a contralateral hemianopia.

32. Midsagittal section results in a bitemporal hemianopia.

33. Transection results in total blindness in the left eye.

34. Compression is seen in Foster Kennedy syndrome.

Answers and Explanations

1. **D.** Interruption of the pontine MLF results in a medial rectus palsy on attempted lateral gaze. Convergence remains intact. This syndrome, called INO or MLF syndrome, is commonly seen in multiple sclerosis.

2. **B.** Ablation of the anterior temporal lobe destroys the optic radiations that project to the lower bank of the calcarine sulcus. The field deficit is an upper right homonymous quadrantanopia, which is also called Meyer loop quadrantanopia.

3. **C.** Pupillary constriction is caused by the accessory oculomotor (Edinger-Westphal) nucleus, ipsilaterally on each side. When the light is shown in the right eye, direct (right-sided) constriction is not affected, that is, the right pupil will constrict. The signal will reach the Edinger-Westphal nucleus on the left via the pretectal area, but if cell loss is too great, no indirect pupillary constriction will occur.

4. **B.** The frontal eye field is responsible for voluntary, fast, saccadic eye movements to the contralateral side. Destructive lesions here result in transient deviation of both eyes to the side ipsilateral to the lesion. The ciliospinal center (of Budge) provides sympathetic innervation to the eye and is not involved in eye movement. The occipital eye field is responsible for slow tracking movements of the eyes that are intact in this patient. The pretectal area yokes the eyes together for conjugate reflexive movements. Primary visual cortex is involved with interpretation and perception, not movement of the eyes.

5. **C.** Transection of the right optic tract results in a left homonymous hemianopia.

6. **D.** Transection of the Meyer loop on the right side results in a left upper quadrantanopia ("pie in the sky"). The Meyer loop is the inferior geniculocalcarine pathway, which conveys information from the inferior retinal quadrants to the inferior bank of the calcarine sulcus, the lingual gyrus.

7. **B.** A midsagittal section of the optic chiasm interrupts the decussating fibers from the nasal hemiretinae and results in a bitemporal hemianopia.

8. **C.** A lesion of the right LGB produces a left homonymous hemianopia. A lesion of the optic tract, the LGB, or the visual pathway all produces the same field deficit, a contralateral homonymous hemianopia.

9. **B.** A pituitary tumor most commonly produces a bitemporal hemianopia. The pituitary (hypophysis) gland lies ventral to the optic chiasm.

10. **E.** Destruction of the left cuneus produces a right lower homonymous quadrantanopia. Upper retinal quadrants project to the upper banks of the calcarine sulcus.

11. **D.** Destruction of the right lingual gyrus produces a left upper homonymous quadrantanopia. Lower retinal quadrants project to the lower banks of the calcarine sulcus.

12. **A.** Bilateral constriction of the optic chiasm damages the non-decussating fibers from the temporal hemiretinae and produces a binasal hemianopia.

13. **D.** Horner syndrome results from interruption of the cervical sympathetic trunk.

14. **A.** Anisocoria, unequal pupils, is present in 10% of the population.

15. **C.** In transtentorial herniation, the uncus is forced, by increased pressure (eg, from a brain tumor), through the tentorial incisure. Pressure on the oculomotor nerve (CN III) results in a fixed, dilated pupil and an eye that looks down and out. Pressure on the basis pedunculi, affecting the corticospinal tracts, results in a contralateral hemiparesis.

16. **B.** The Argyll Robertson pupil is characterized by the absence of a miotic reaction to light but with the presence of miotic reaction to a near stimulus.

17. **E.** The Marcus Gunn pupil is an afferent pupil, with a lesion in the afferent limb of the pupillary light pathway.

18. **E.** The Marcus Gunn pupil is commonly seen in multiple sclerosis.

19. **B.** The Argyll Robertson pupil is associated with neurosyphilis.

20. **F.** Occlusion of the left posterior cerebral artery results in a right homonymous hemianopia with macular sparing; macular sparing results from a rich dual blood supply to the visual cortex.

21. **A.** Transection of the left optic nerve at the chiasm results in total blindness on the left side and a scotoma in the right upper temporal quadrant. Fibers from the lower nasal quadrant loop into the contralateral optic nerve before decussating in the optic chiasm. The field defect is called a junctional scotoma.

22. **B.** Craniopharyngiomas and pituitary tumors put pressure on the decussating fibers of the optic chiasm, causing a bitemporal heteronymous hemianopia.

23. **D.** A left temporal lobotomy transects Meyer loop, which projects to the inferior bank of the calcarine sulcus, resulting in a right upper homonymous quadrantanopia.

24. **E.** Bilateral trauma to the cuneate gyri results in a lower altitudinal homonymous hemianopia.

25. **C.** Transection of the left optic tract results in a right homonymous hemianopia with macular sparing.

26. **I.** Transection of the infundibulum interrupts the supraopticohypophyseal tract. This results in diabetes insipidus with polydipsia and polyuria (eg, craniopharyngioma).

27. **H.** Destruction of the oculomotor nerve results in paralysis of the levator palpebrae superioris with a severe ipsilateral ptosis.

28. **G.** The trochlear nerve innervates the superior oblique, which causes intorsion. In fourth nerve palsy, the ipsilateral eye is extorted. The patient's chin points to the side of the lesion. Head tilt is associated with fourth nerve palsy.

29. **F.** The ophthalmic division of the trigeminal nerve mediates the afferent limb of the corneal blink reflex. The efferent limb is mediated by CN VII.

30. **E.** In Wernicke encephalopathy, petechial hemorrhages in the mammillary bodies are commonly found, along with capillary hyperplasia and astrocytic gliosis. Wernicke encephalopathy results from a thiamine (vitamin B_1) deficiency.

31. **D.** Severance of the optic tract results in contralateral hemianopia.

32. **C.** A midsagittal section through the optic chiasm results in bitemporal hemianopia.

33. **B.** Transection of the optic nerve results in total blindness of the ipsilateral eye.

34. **A.** Foster Kennedy syndrome involves the olfactory tract and the optic nerve. This disorder can result from a tumor (eg, an olfactory groove meningioma). The signs are ipsilateral anosmia, ipsilateral optic atrophy, and contralateral papilledema.

Olfactory, Gustatory, and Limbic Systems

Objectives

- Describe the olfactory pathway.
- Describe the gustatory pathway, including a description of taste buds and the primary tastes humans perceive.
- Differentiate between taste and flavor and list various components of flavor.
- List the traditional/main components, connections, and fiber pathways of the limbic system.
- Describe the components and significance of Papez circuit.
- Describe the results of damage to the hippocampus, amygdala, and mammillary bodies.

I. OLFACTORY SYSTEM

- mediates the special visceral afferent (SVA) modality of **smell** via the olfactory nerve (**CN I**).
- the only sensory system that has no precortical relay in the thalamus.
- projects to the thalamus, hypothalamus, amygdala, and hippocampal formation.

A. Olfactory pathway (Figure 17.1; see Figure 1.2)

1. **Olfactory receptor cells (fila olfactoria)**
   - chemoreceptors.
   - number 25 million on each side.
   - replaced throughout life (ie, they are capable of regeneration).
   - found in the nasal mucosa.
   - unmyelinated bipolar neurons whose central processes collectively form CN I.
   - have axons that enter the olfactory bulb and synapse in the olfactory bulbs with **mitral** and **tufted cells**.

2. **Olfactory bulb**
   - lies on the cribriform plate of the ethmoid bone and receives the olfactory nerve.
   - contains **mitral** and **tufted cells** (second-order neurons) that project via the olfactory tract and the lateral olfactory stria to the primary olfactory cortex and the amygdala.

3. **Olfactory tract**
   - contains the anterior olfactory nucleus.
   - gives rise to the medial and lateral olfactory striae.
   - projects to the contralateral olfactory tract via the anterior commissure.

4. **Lateral olfactory stria**
   - projects to the primary olfactory cortex and the amygdala.

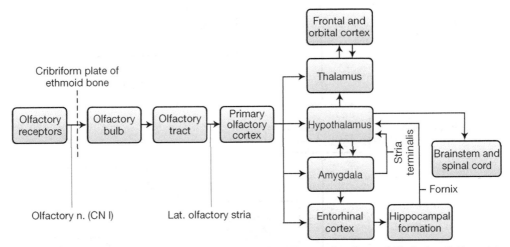

FIGURE 17.1. Pathways of the olfactory system. The olfactory nerve enters the olfactory bulb via the cribriform plate. Mitral and tufted cells of the olfactory bulb project via the lateral olfactory stria to the primary olfactory cortex (prepiriform and periamygdaloid cortices). The primary olfactory cortex projects to the hypothalamus, thalamus, amygdala, and entorhinal area. The olfactory system is the only sensory system that projects directly to the cortex of the telencephalon without a precortical relay in the thalamus.

5. **Primary olfactory cortex**
   - overlies the **uncus** of the parahippocampal gyrus (area 34).
   - receives input from the lateral olfactory stria.
   - consists of **prepiriform** and **periamygdaloid cortices**.
   - projects to the dorsomedial nucleus of the thalamus via the amygdala to the hypothalamus and via the entorhinal cortex (area 28) to the hippocampal formation.
6. **Dorsomedial nucleus of the thalamus**
   - projects to the orbitofrontal cortex, where the conscious perception of smell takes place.

B. **Clinical considerations**
   1. **Anosmia**, the loss of smell, may occur as a result of a lesion of the olfactory nerve.
   2. Olfactory nerves may be damaged by **fractures of the cribriform plate**; by **meningitis, meningiomas**, or **gliomas**; or by abscesses of the frontal lobes.
   3. **Olfactory hallucinations** may be a consequence of lesions of the uncus of the parahippocampal gyrus.
   4. **Foster Kennedy syndrome**
      - results from a space-occupying lesion (most commonly a meningioma) located on the ventral surface of the frontal lobe, which compresses the olfactory tract and the ipsilateral optic nerve.
      - results in ipsilateral anosmia, optic atrophy, and contralateral papilledema.
   5. **Fracture of the cribriform plate of the ethmoid bone** may result in anosmia and cerebrospinal rhinorrhea.

II. GUSTATORY SYSTEM

- mediates the SVA modality of **taste**.
- mediates gustation, which, like smell, is a chemical sense.

A. **Gustatory pathway (Figure 17.2)**
   1. **Taste receptor cells**
      - chemoreceptors.
      - modified epithelial cells.

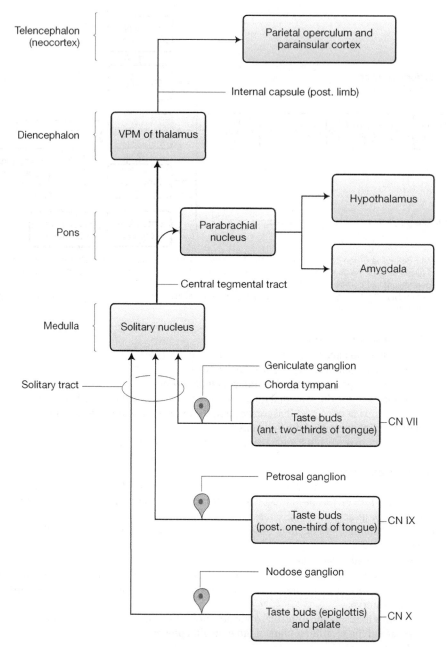

FIGURE 17.2. Gustatory pathway. CN VII, CN IX, and CN X transmit taste (special visceral afferent) information from the anterior two-thirds of the tongue, the posterior third of the tongue, the epiglottis, and the palate to the solitary tract and nucleus; from the solitary nucleus via the central tegmental tract to the medial parabrachial nucleus; and to the ventral posteromedial (VPM) nucleus of the thalamus, hypothalamus, and amygdaloid complex. The gustatory cortex is located in the parietal operculum and in the parainsular cortex.

▓ continuously regenerated.
▓ located in the taste buds of the tongue, epiglottis, and palate.
▓ innervated by SVA fibers of CN VII, CN IX, and CN X.

2. First-order neurons

▓ are **pseudounipolar cells** in the geniculate ganglion of CN VII, in the petrosal ganglion of CN IX, and in the nodose ganglion of CN X.
▓ project centrally, via the solitary tract, to the solitary nucleus.

3. **Solitary nucleus**
   - receives taste input to rostral-most portion, the gustatory nucleus.
   - projects ipsilaterally via the **central tegmental tract** to the ventral posteromedial (VPM) nucleus of the thalamus and the parabrachial nucleus.

4. **Parabrachial nucleus of the pons**
   - receives taste input from the solitary nucleus.
   - projects taste input to the hypothalamus and amygdala.

5. **VPM nucleus**
   - projects to the gustatory cortex of the parietal operculum (area 43) and parainsular cortex.

6. **Gustatory cortex of the insular area (area 43)**
   - projects via the entorhinal cortex (area 28) to the hippocampal formation.

B. **Taste perception**
   1. **Commonly recognized taste receptors** are concentrated:
      - **sweet**—apex of the tongue.
      - **salty**—posterolateral to the apex of the tongue.
      - **bitter**—circumvallate papillae.
      - **sour**—anterior two-thirds of the dorsum of the tongue.

C. **Flavor perception**
   - integrated sensation that combines gustation with olfaction and somatosensation mainly involving the trigeminal nerve.
   - sight, emotional state, and level of satiety are also involved with flavor perception.

CLINICAL CORRELATES **Ageusia** (gustatory anesthesia) is a lack of sense of taste. It is most frequently associated with peripheral lesions of CN VII (Bell palsy and diseases of the middle ear [chorda tympani]) and CN IX. Ageusia is not a life-threatening condition, but it may be an indicator of a more serious underlying cause and can lead to loss of appetite and weight.

III. LIMBIC SYSTEM

- the anatomic substrate underlying behavioral and emotional expression.
- responsible for memory consolidation.
- plays a role in feeling, feeding, fighting, fleeing, and mating.
- expresses itself through the hypothalamus via the autonomic nervous system.

A. **Major components and connections (Figure 17.3)**
   - include structures of the telencephalon, diencephalon, and midbrain.
   1. **Orbitofrontal cortex**
      - mediates the conscious perception of **smell**.
      - has reciprocal connections with the dorsomedial nucleus of the thalamus.
      - interconnected via the medial forebrain bundle with the septal area and hypothalamic nuclei.
   2. **Dorsomedial nucleus of the thalamus**
      - has reciprocal connections with the orbitofrontal and prefrontal cortices and the hypothalamus.
      - receives input from the amygdala.
      - plays a role in **affective behavior** and **memory**.
   3. **Anterior nucleus of the thalamus**
      - receives input from the mammillary nucleus via the mammillothalamic tract and fornix.
      - projects to the cingulate gyrus.
      - a major link in the limbic **circuit of Papez**.

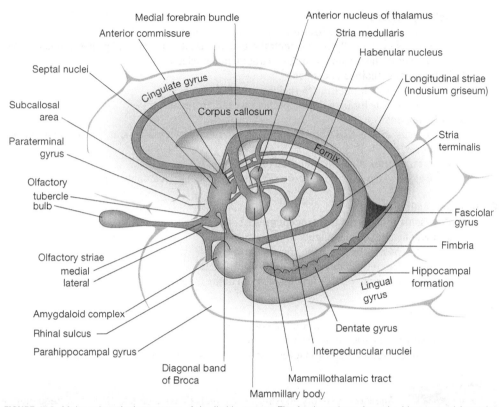

FIGURE 17.3. Major subcortical structures of the limbic system. The fornix projects from the hippocampal formation to the septal nuclei (precommissural fornix) and to the mammillary body (postcommissural fornix). The major pathway from the amygdala is the stria terminalis, which terminates in the septal nuclei and in the hypothalamus. The stria medullaris of the thalamus connects the septal nuclei to the habenula. (Modified with permission from Carpenter MB, Sutlin J. *Human Neuroanatomy.* 8th ed. Williams & Wilkins; 1983:618.)

4. **Septal area** (see Figures 1.4 and 22.1B)
   - consists of a cortical septal area, including the paraterminal gyrus and the subcallosal area.
   - consists of a subcortical septal area (the septal nuclei), which lies between the septum pellucidum and the anterior commissure.
   - has reciprocal connections with the hippocampal formation via the fornix.
   - has reciprocal connections with the hypothalamus via the medial forebrain bundle.
   - projects via the **stria medullaris** (thalami) to the **habenula**—the habenula has a role in motivation and behavior.
5. **Limbic lobe** (see Figure 22.1B)
   - includes the subcallosal area, the paraterminal gyrus, the cingulate gyrus and isthmus, and the parahippocampal gyrus, which includes the uncus (see Figure 1.4).
   - contains, buried in the parahippocampal gyrus, the hippocampal formation and the amygdaloid nuclear complex (amygdala).
6. **Hippocampal formation** (Figure 17.4)
   - functions in learning, memory, and recognition of novelty.
   - major input from the entorhinal cortex.
   - major output via the fornix.
   a. **Major structures of the hippocampal formation**
      - output via the fornix to the septal area and the mammillary nuclei.
      - input via the fornix from the septal area.
      - input from the entorhinal cortex (area 28) as the alveolar pathway to the hippocampus and the perforant pathway to the dentate gyrus.

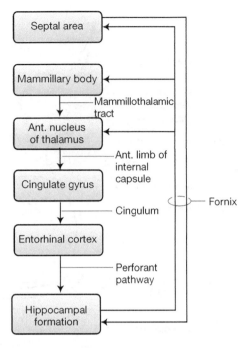

FIGURE 17.4. Limbic connections. Major afferent and efferent connections of the hippocampal formation. The circuit of Papez is hippocampal formation → mammillary nucleus → anterior thalamic nucleus → cingulate gyrus → hippocampal formation. The hippocampal formation consists of three components: the hippocampus proper, the subiculum, and the dentate gyrus. The hippocampus projects to the septal area, the subiculum projects to the mammillary nuclei, whereas the dentate gyrus does not project beyond the hippocampal formation.

(1) Dentate gyrus (see Figure 1.4)
- has a three-layered archicortex.
- contains **granule cells** that receive hippocampal input and project to the pyramidal cells of the hippocampus and subiculum.

(2) Hippocampus (cornu ammonis)
- is a three-layered, archicortex.
- contains **pyramidal cells** that project via the fornix to the septal area and the hypothalamus.
- divided into four cytoarchitectural areas (CA1-CA4).

(3) Subiculum
- receives input via the hippocampal pyramidal cells.
- projects via the fornix to the mammillary nuclei and the anterior nucleus of the thalamus.

  b. Major afferent connections to the hippocampal formation (see Figures 17.4 and 17.5)
- **cerebral association cortices** (areas 19, 22, and 7).
- **septal area.**
- **anterior nucleus of the thalamus** via the cingulate gyrus, cingulum, and entorhinal cortex.

  c. Major efferent connections from the hippocampal formation (see Figures 17.4 and 17.5)
- **mammillary nucleus of the hypothalamus.**
- **septal area.**
- **anterior nucleus of the thalamus.**

7. Amygdala (Figure 17.6)
- may cause rage and aggressive behavior when stimulated.
- divided into a corticomedial group and a basolateral group. The corticomedial group receives olfactory input, and the basolateral group receives cortical input.

  a. Major afferent connections to the amygdala (see Figure 17.6)
- **from** the following structures:

    (1) olfactory bulb and olfactory cortex
    (2) cerebral cortex (limbic and sensory association cortices)
    (3) hypothalamus

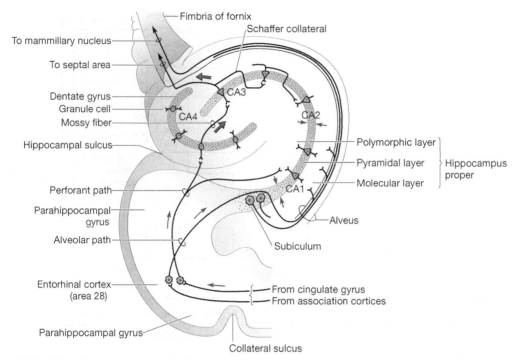

FIGURE 17.5. Major connections of the hippocampal formation. The two major hypothalamic output pathways are (1) granule cell via mossy fiber to pyramidal cell via precommissural fornix to septal nuclei and (2) subicular neuron via postcommissural fornix to the medial mammillary nucleus. The hippocampal formation (HF) plays an important role in learning and memory, and lesions of the HF result in short-term memory defects. In Alzheimer disease, loss of cells in the HF and entorhinal cortex leads to loss of memory and cognitive function. CA, cornu ammonis.

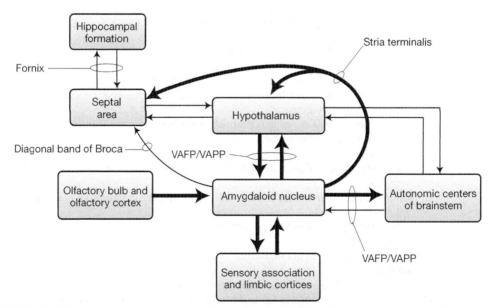

FIGURE 17.6. Major connections of the amygdala. The amygdala receives input from three major sources: the olfactory system, the sensory association and limbic cortices, and the hypothalamus. The major output from the amygdala is via two channels: the stria terminalis that projects to the hypothalamus and the septal area, and the ventral amygdalofugal pathway (VAFP) that projects to the hypothalamus, brainstem, and spinal cord. A smaller efferent bundle, the diagonal band of Broca, projects to the septal area. Afferent fibers from the hypothalamus and brainstem enter the amygdala via the ventral amygdalopetal pathway (VAPP).

   b. **Major efferent connections from the amygdala** (see Figure 17.6)
      ▧ **to** the following structures:
         (1) cerebral cortex (limbic and sensory association cortices)
         (2) hypothalamus
         (3) brainstem and spinal cord

8. **Hypothalamus**
   ▧ functions with the limbic system that projects to the brainstem and spinal cord (see Chapter 13).

9. **Limbic midbrain nuclei project to all limbic structures:**
   ▧ **ventral tegmental area** (see Figure 21.2)—projects dopaminergic fibers.
   ▧ **raphe nuclei of the midbrain** (see Figure 21.5)—project serotonergic fibers.
   ▧ **locus ceruleus** (see Figure 21.4)—projects noradrenergic fibers.

B. Major limbic fiber systems (see Figures 17.3, 17.4, and 17.6)

1. **Fornix** (see Figures 1.4, 1.5, and 17.3)
   ▧ projects from the hippocampal formation to the hypothalamus (mammillary nucleus), the anterior nucleus of the thalamus, and the septal area.
   ▧ projects from the septal area to the hippocampal formation.

2. **Stria terminalis**
   ▧ lies between the thalamus and the caudate nucleus.
   ▧ projects from the amygdala to the hypothalamus and the septal area.

3. **Ventral amygdalofugal pathway**
   ▧ projects from the amygdala to the hypothalamus, thalamus, brainstem, and spinal cord.

4. **Stria medullaris (thalami)**
   ▧ projects from the septal area to the habenula.

5. **Diagonal band of Broca**
   ▧ forms the medial border of the anterior perforated substance.
   ▧ interconnects the amygdala and the septal area.

6. **Habenulointerpeduncular tract-tractus retroflexus**
   ▧ projects from the habenula (part of the epithalamus) to the interpeduncular nucleus of the midbrain.

C. Papez circuit (see Figure 17.4)

   ▧ a circuit that interconnects the major limbic structures.
   ▧ contains the following stations:

1. **Hippocampal formation**
   ▧ projects via the **fornix** to the mammillary nucleus.

2. **Mammillary body**
   ▧ projects via the **mammillothalamic tract** to the anterior nucleus of the thalamus.

3. **Anterior nucleus of the thalamus**
   ▧ projects to the cingulate gyrus.
   ▧ receives the mammillothalamic tract.

4. **Cingulate gyrus**
   ▧ projects via the entorhinal cortex to the hippocampal formation (see Figure 17.5).

D. Functional and clinical considerations

1. **Hippocampus**
   ▧ has a low threshold for seizure activity.
   ▧ involved in learning and memory.
   ▧ bilateral ablation results in the **inability to form long-term memories**.

2. **Cingulate gyrus**
   ▧ lesions result in akinesia, mutism, apathy, and indifference to pain.

3. **Amygdala**
   ▧ modulates hypothalamic and endocrine activities.
   ▧ has the highest concentration of opiate receptors in the brain.

- has a high concentration of estradiol receptors.
- bilateral lesions (eg, from limbic encephalitis or temporal lobe epilepsy) result in **placidity**, with **loss of fear**, **rage**, **and aggression**.

4. **Klüver-Bucy syndrome**
   - results from ablation of the temporal poles, including the amygdalae, the hippocampal formations, and the anterior temporal neocortex.
   - can result from temporal lobe surgery for epilepsy, viral encephalitis (eg, herpes simplex virus affects primarily the temporal lobes), and temporal lobe contusions owing to head trauma.
   - characterized by placidity, hypersexuality, hyperphagia, and psychic blindness (visual agnosia).

5. **Mammillary bodies and the dorsomedial nucleus of the thalamus**
   - damaged by chronic alcoholism and thiamine (vitamin B_1) deficiency, which results in **Korsakoff syndrome** (amnestic-confabulatory syndrome). Clinical signs include memory disturbances (amnesia), confabulation, and temporospatial disorientation.

Review Test

1. Rhinorrhea will most likely result from a fracture of the _____ bone.

(A) ethmoid
(B) frontal
(C) lacrimal
(D) nasal
(E) palatine

2. A patient presents with visual agnosia and is referred to a psychiatric unit. Psychic blindness will most likely result from bilateral lesions of the:

(A) nucleus accumbens.
(B) amygdala.
(C) hippocampus.
(D) subiculum.
(E) superior colliculus.

3. Who wrote the classic paper *A Proposed Mechanism of Emotion* that describes a major pathway of the limbic system?

(A) Brodmann
(B) Klüver and Bucy
(C) Liepmann
(D) Papez
(E) Wernicke and Korsakoff

4. A 40-year-old woman was referred to a psychiatric unit with a previous diagnosis of Klüver-Bucy syndrome, which first appeared after a car accident. The lesion causing her symptoms would most likely be in the:

(A) alveus.
(B) amygdala.
(C) hippocampus.
(D) dentate gyrus.
(E) subiculum.

5. A 40-year-old man was admitted to the hospital and was examined by a staff neurologist. Examination revealed the following: alcohol abuse, paralysis of conjugate gaze, nystagmus, confusion, and memory loss. These symptoms are likely owing to a deficiency in:

(A) niacin.
(B) vitamin A.
(C) vitamin B_1.
(D) vitamin B_6.
(E) vitamin B_{12}.

6. Bilateral ablation of the _____ results in the inability to form long-term memories.

(A) amygdala
(B) cingulate gyrus
(C) hippocampus
(D) hypothalamus
(E) ventral tegmental area

7. A 50-year-old woman presents to her primary care physician with ipsilateral anosmia, optic atrophy, and contralateral papilledema. The syndrome is:

(A) Brown-Séquard.
(B) Edinger-Westphal.
(C) Foster Kennedy.
(D) Klüver-Bucy.
(E) Wernicke-Korsakoff.

8. A 25-year-old woman presents to her primary care physician for evaluation the day after being knocked out in a mixed martial arts bout. Swelling and bruising are evident on her face. She reports that her face is painful to touch, that she has a severe headache, and that her nose will not stop draining a clear liquid. Patient interview reveals that she is also experiencing a loss of smell and altered taste. Imaging on this patient will most likely reveal a fracture of which bony structure to produce the symptoms of cerebrospinal fluid (CSF) leakage, anosmia, and altered taste/flavor.

(A) Cribriform plate
(B) Hard palate
(C) Nasal bone
(D) Orbital margin
(E) Zygomatic arch

9. A 30-year-old woman presents to her primary care physician, subsequent to recent changes in mood, short-term memory problems, sleepiness, and overall feeling cold though her apartment is kept warm. She indicates that she noticed the symptoms about a week prior and that they are getting worse. She is referred to a neurologist who makes a diagnosis of limbic encephalitis, after conducting an electroencephalogram (EEG), imaging and lumbar puncture, and immunosuppressive therapy is started. The changes in the patient's mood are most likely a result of the altered function of which of the following?

(A) Amygdala
(B) Dentate gyrus
(C) Hippocampus
(D) Hypothalamus
(E) Subiculum

Questions 10 to 14

The response options for items 10 to 14 are the same. Select one answer for each item in the set.

(A) Diagonal band of Broca
(B) Medial forebrain bundle
(C) Stria medullaris
(D) Stria terminalis
(E) Tractus retroflexus

Match the characteristic with the structure it best describes.

10. Consists of septohabenular fibers

11. Forms the medial border of the anterior perforated substance

12. Lies between the thalamus and the caudate nucleus

13. Projects from the epithalamus to the midbrain tegmentum

14. Is a major efferent pathway from the amygdala

Questions 15 to 18

The response options for items 15 to 18 are the same. Select one answer for each item in the set.

(A) Amygdala
(B) Hippocampal formation
(C) Both A and B
(D) Neither A nor B

Match each characteristic with the structure it most appropriately describes.

15. Is located in the temporal lobe

16. Is destroyed in Klüver-Bucy syndrome

17. Projects via the stria terminalis

18. Receives direct olfactory input

Answers and Explanations

1. **A.** Rhinorrhea will most likely result from a fracture of the cribriform plate of the ethmoid bone, which can tear the arachnoid membrane and result in a leakage of cerebrospinal fluid into the nasal cavity. Fracture of the frontal bone may produce rhinorrhea, but would also produce more severe deficits and symptoms. Fracture of any of the other three bones would be unlikely to produce rhinorrhea.

2. **B.** Bilateral lesions of the amygdalae result in psychic blindness, the inability to recognize objects visually. Subjects can see objects but do not understand what they see. Bilateral lesions of the hippocampus and subiculum result in memory loss (eg, from viral encephalitis). Lesions of the superior colliculus result in paralysis of upward and downward gaze. Nucleus accumbens is part of the ventral striatum and is part of our motivation and reward systems.

3. **D.** Papez wrote *A Proposed Mechanism of Emotion*; the circuit is hippocampal formation → mammillary body → anterior thalamic nucleus → cingulate gyrus → entorhinal cortex → hippocampal formation (see Figure 17.4). Klüver-Bucy syndrome is characterized by placidity, hypersexuality, hyperphagia, and psychic blindness (visual agnosia). Wernicke-Korsakoff syndrome is characterized by alcohol abuse resulting in thiamine deficiency, conjugate gaze palsies, ataxia, confusion, and memory loss. Liepmann is known for his classic book on ataxias. Brodmann is known for his brain maps called the Brodmann areas.

4. **B.** Bilateral ablation of the inferior temporal cortex results in damage to the amygdala, resulting in hypersexuality, hyperphagia, docility, and psychic blindness (Klüver-Bucy syndrome). Lesion of the hippocampus, dentate gyrus, alveus, and subiculum are all parts or subparts of the memory consolidation system and would be unlikely to produce the symptoms seen in this patient.

5. **C.** Lack of thiamine (vitamin B_1) results in Wernicke-Korsakoff syndrome; the classic clinical triad of Wernicke encephalopathy is confusion, gait ataxia, and ophthalmoplegia. Korsakoff syndrome is profound memory impairment and confabulation. Vitamin A deficiency results in impaired night vision; when ingested in excess, vitamin A may cause pseudotumor cerebri. Pyridoxine (vitamin B_6) is used to prevent isoniazid neuropathy. Vitamin B_{12} deficiency results in anemia and subacute combined degeneration. Niacin (nicotinic acid) is used to prevent pellagra.

6. **C.** Bilateral ablation of the hippocampus results in the inability to form long-term memories. The hippocampus plays a major role in learning and memory. The cingulate gyrus works closely with the hippocampus as part of the limbic lobe, but lesions here may produce a wide variety of symptoms based on lesion location, including higher-order frontal lobe functions and emotional regulation. Lesion of the amygdala results in hypersexuality, hyperphagia, docility, and psychic blindness (Klüver-Bucy syndrome). The ventral tegmental area is involved with reward circuitry. The hypothalamus maintains homeostasis in the body by governing the ANS and the endocrine systems.

7. **C.** Foster Kennedy syndrome includes ipsilateral anosmia, optic atrophy, and contralateral papilledema; pressure on the olfactory tract causes ipsilateral anosmia, whereas pressure on the optic nerve causes ipsilateral optic atrophy and a central scotoma and contralateral papilledema. Edinger and Westphal described this parasympathetic nucleus of the rostral midbrain, more appropriately called the accessory oculomotor nucleus. Brown-Séquard is associated with a spinal cord lesion and spinal cord hemisection. Klüver and Bucy described the limbic lobe syndrome. Wernicke-Korsakoff syndrome consists of Wernicke encephalopathy and Korsakoff psychosis.

8. **A.** The olfactory nerve, which mediates smell, passes through the thin cribriform plate as a series of bipolar neurons—the filia olfactoria. The cribriform plate is often fractured with traumatic impact to the front of the face as in fighting and car accidents. Shearing the filia olfactoria causes anosmia and alters the sense of taste; it often damages the overlying dura mater, leading to

leakage of CSF. Damage to the hard palate may alter taste but would not lead to leakage of CSF or anosmia. Damage to the nasal bone, orbital margin, or zygomatic arch would not produce the symptoms in this patient.

9. **A.** The amygdala is primarily concerned with emotional state (ie, mood); lesions may result in altered emotional states. The amygdala is closely connected to the hippocampus, which functions primarily in short-term memory consolidation. The dentate gyrus and subiculum are parts of the hippocampal formation and are also primarily involved in memory consolidation. The patient's other symptoms of somnolence and hyperthermia are likely attributable to hypothalamic involvement, common in limbic encephalitis.

10. **C.** The stria medullaris (thalami) contains septohabenular fibers (ie, fibers that project from the septal nuclei to the habenula). The stria medullaris (singular) should not be confused with the striae medullares (plural). The striae medullares (rhombencephali) arise from the arcuate nuclei of the medulla and are seen on the floor of the rhomboid fossa.

11. **A.** The diagonal band of Broca is the medial border of the anterior perforated substance. This fiber bundle contains amygdaloseptal and septoamygdalar fibers. The nucleus of the diagonal band projects via the fornix to the hippocampal formation.

12. **D.** The stria terminalis and the vena terminalis lie in the sulcus terminalis between the thalamus and the caudate nucleus.

13. **E.** The tractus retroflexus contains habenulointerpeduncular fibers that project from the habenula of the epithalamus to the interpeduncular nucleus of the midbrain tegmentum.

14. **D.** The stria terminalis is a major efferent pathway from the amygdala. It projects to the septal area and to the bed nucleus of the stria terminalis.

15. **C.** Both the hippocampal formation and the amygdala are found in the parahippocampal gyrus of the temporal lobe.

16. **C.** The hippocampal formation and the amygdala are both involved in Klüver-Bucy syndrome.

17. **A.** The amygdala projects via the stria terminalis and via the ventral amygdalofugal pathway. The stria terminalis is the most prominent projection from the amygdala.

18. **A.** The amygdala receives both direct and indirect olfactory input.

chapter 18

Basal Nuclei and the Extrapyramidal Motor System

I. BASAL NUCLEI (Figure 18.1)

- consist of subcortical nuclei (gray matter) within the cerebral hemispheres.
- historically referred to as **basal ganglia**.
- list of components varies and depends on focus of interest.

A. Four main components

1. **Caudate nucleus**
2. **Putamen**
3. **Globus pallidus**
4. **Amygdala** (see Chapter 17 III A 7)

B. Groupings of the basal nuclei

1. **Striatum (neostriatum)**
   - consists of the **caudate nucleus** and the **putamen**, which are similar in structure and connections and have a common embryologic origin.
2. **Lentiform nucleus**
   - consists of the **putamen** and the **globus pallidus**.
3. **Corpus striatum**
   - consists of the **lentiform nucleus** and the **caudate nucleus**.

II. EXTRAPYRAMIDAL MOTOR SYSTEM (See Figure 18.1)

- also called the striatal motor system.
- plays a role in the initiation and execution of somatic motor activity, in particular of willed movement.

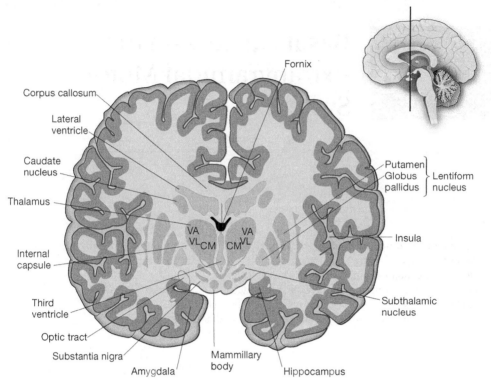

FIGURE 18.1. Coronal section through the mid-thalamus at the level of the mammillary bodies. The basal nuclei are prominent at this level and include the striatum and the lentiform nucleus. The subthalamic nucleus and substantia nigra are important components of the striatal motor system. CM, centromedian; VA, ventral anterior; VL, ventral lateral. (Modified with permission from Fix JD. *High-Yield Neuroanatomy.* 3rd ed. Lippincott Williams & Wilkins; 2005:142.)

- involved in automatic stereotyped motor activity of a postural and reflex nature.
- exerts its influences on motor activities via the thalamus, motor cortex, corticobulbar, and corticospinal systems.

A. Components of the extrapyramidal motor system

- consist of the following nuclei:
    1. **Striatum (caudatoputamen or neostriatum)**
        - caudate nucleus.
        - putamen.
    2. **Globus pallidus (pallidum or paleostriatum)**
        - primary output nuclei of the basal nuclei.
            a. Medial (internal) segment
        - adjacent to the internal capsule.
            b. Lateral (external) segment
    3. **Subthalamic nucleus**
        - adjacent to the putamen.
        - lies between the internal capsule and the thalamus and between the internal capsule and the lenticular fasciculus.
    4. **Thalamus**
        - **Ventral anterior nucleus**
        - **Ventral lateral nucleus**
        - **Centromedian nucleus**

5. **Substantia nigra**
   - **Pars compacta**
     a. contains dopaminergic neurons, which contain the pigment melanin.
   - **Pars reticularis**
     a. contains gamma-aminobutyric acid (GABA)-ergic neurons.
     b. functions as another basal nuclei output.
6. **Pedunculopontine nucleus**
   - lies in the lateral tegmentum of the caudal midbrain.

B. **Major connections of the extrapyramidal system (Figure 18.2)**
   1. **Striatum**
      - receives its largest input from the **neocortex**—from almost all neocortical areas.
      - receives input from the **thalamus** (centromedian nucleus) and from the **substantia nigra**.
      - projects fibers to two major nuclei: the **globus pallidus** and the **substantia nigra** (pars reticularis).
   2. **Globus pallidus** (Figure 18.3)
      - receives input from two major nuclei: the **striatum** and the **subthalamic nucleus**.
      - divided into an external/lateral component (pars externa) adjacent to the putamen and an internal/medial component (pars interna) adjacent to the internal capsule.
      - projects fibers to three major structures: the **subthalamic nucleus**, the **thalamus** (ventral anterior, ventral lateral, and centromedian nuclei), and the **pedunculopontine nucleus**.

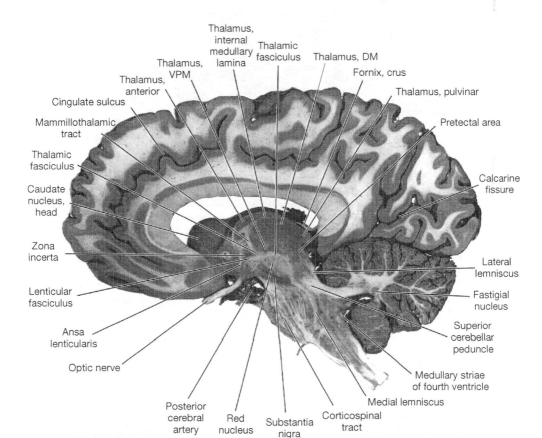

FIGURE 18.2. A parasagittal section through the caudate nucleus and the substantia nigra. DM, dorsomedial; VPM, ventral posteromedial. (Modified from Woolsey TA, Hanaway J, Gado MH. *The Brain Atlas: A Visual Guide to the Human Central Nervous System.* 2nd ed. John Wiley & Sons; 2003:128. Copyright © 2003 by John Wiley & Sons, Inc. Reprinted by permission of John Wiley & Sons, Inc.)

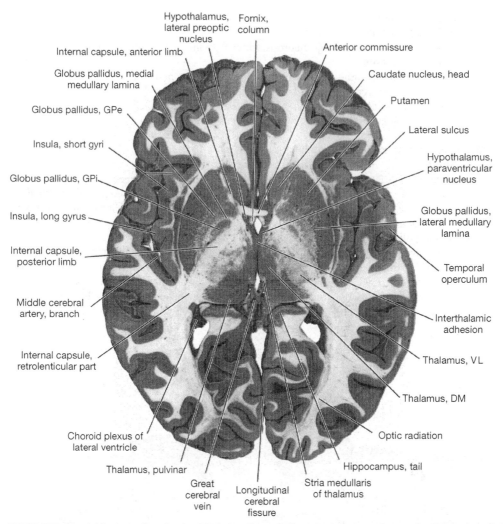

FIGURE 18.3. An axial (horizontal) section through the anterior commissure and the massa intermedia. DM, dorsomedial; GPe, globus pallidus externus; GPi, globus pallidus internus; VL, ventral lateral. (Modified from Woolsey TA, Hanaway J, Gado MH. *The Brain Atlas: A Visual Guide to the Human Central Nervous System.* 2nd ed. John Wiley & Sons; 2003:100. Copyright © 2003 by John Wiley & Sons, Inc. Reprinted by permission of John Wiley & Sons, Inc.)

3. **Subthalamic nucleus**
   - receives input from the **globus pallidus** pars externa and from the **motor cortex**.
   - projects fibers to the globus pallidus pars interna.
4. **Thalamus** (see Figure 13.1)
   - Input to the thalamus
     a. Globus pallidus
        - projects to the ventral anterior, ventral lateral, and centromedian nuclei.
     b. Substantia nigra
        - projects from the pars reticularis to the **ventral anterior**, **ventral lateral**, and the **mediodorsal nuclei** of the thalamus.
   - Projections from the thalamus
     a. Motor cortex (area 4)
        - from the ventral lateral and centromedian nuclei.
     b. Premotor cortex (area 6)
        - from the ventral anterior and ventral lateral nuclei.

    c. Supplementary motor cortex (area 6)
       ▓ from the ventral lateral and ventral anterior nuclei.
    d. Striatum
       ▓ from the centromedian nucleus.
5. Substantia nigra
   ▓ receives input from the **striatum**.
   ▓ projects fibers to the **striatum** and the **thalamus** (ventral anterior, ventral lateral, and dorsomedial nuclei).
6. Pedunculopontine nucleus
   ▓ receives GABA-ergic input from the **globus pallidus**.
   ▓ projects glutaminergic fibers to the **globus pallidus** and to the **substantia nigra**.

C. Major neurotransmitters of the extrapyramidal system (Figure 18.4)
   1. Glutamate-containing neurons (see Figure 21.11)
      ▓ project from the cerebral cortex to the striatum.
      ▓ project from the subthalamic nucleus to the globus pallidus.
      ▓ excite **striatal GABA-ergic** and **cholinergic neurons**.

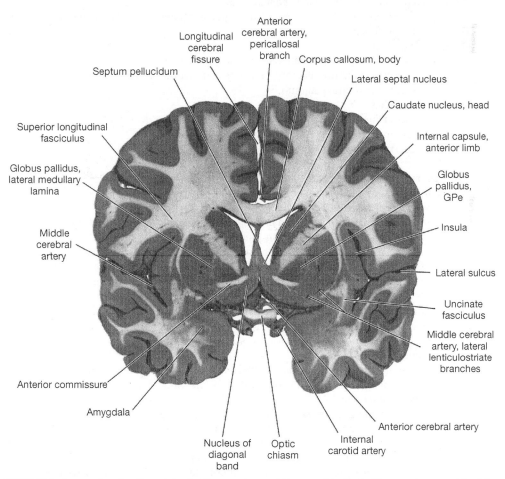

FIGURE 18.4. A coronal section through the lentiform nucleus and the amygdala; the lentiform nucleus consists of the putamen and the globus pallidus. The amygdala appears as a circular profile below the uncus. GPe, globus pallidus externus. (Modified from Woolsey TA, Hanaway J, Gado MH. *The Brain Atlas: A Visual Guide to the Human Central Nervous System*. 2nd ed. John Wiley & Sons; 2003:60. Copyright © 2003 by John Wiley & Sons, Inc. Reprinted by permission of John Wiley & Sons, Inc.)

2. **GABA-containing neurons** (see Figure 21.10)
   - the predominant neurons of the striatal system.
   - found in the striatum, globus pallidus, and substantia nigra (pars reticularis).
   - give rise to the following **GABA-ergic projections**: striatopallidal, striatonigral, pallido-thalamic, and nigrothalamic projections.
   - degenerate in Huntington disease.
3. **Dopamine-containing neurons** (see Figure 21.2)
   - found in the pars compacta of the substantia nigra.
   - give rise to the dopaminergic nigrostriatal projection.
   - degenerate in Parkinson disease.
4. **Neurons containing acetylcholine (ACh)** (see Figure 21.3)
   - local circuit neurons found in the striatum.
5. **Neuropeptide-containing neurons** (see Figures 21.7 and 21.8)
   - include enkephalin, dynorphin, substance P, somatostatin, neurotensin, neuropeptide Y, and cholecystokinin.
   - also found in the basal nuclei.
   - coexist with the major neurotransmitters (eg, GABA and/or enkephalin and GABA and/or substance P).

D. Ventral striatopallidal complex and its connections
   - play a role in initiating movements in response to motivational and emotional activity (eg, limbic functions).
1. **Ventral striatum**
   - consists of the **nucleus accumbens** and the olfactory tubercle.
   - receives input from the olfactory, prefrontal, and hippocampal cortices.
   - projects to the ventral pallidum.
2. **Ventral pallidum**
   - consists of the substantia innominata.
   - receives input from the ventral striatum.
   - projects to the medial dorsal nucleus of the thalamus.

E. Clinical considerations
1. **Progressive supranuclear palsy**
   - mean age of onset is 65 years.
   - associated with **Parkinson disease**. Progressive supranuclear palsy together with Parkinson disease is called the Parkinson-plus syndrome.
   - characterized by supranuclear ophthalmoplegia, gait disturbances, dysarthria, dysphagia, rigidity, and cognitive disturbances. As the disease progresses, the remainder of the motor cranial nerves become involved, resulting in the clinical picture of pseudobulbar palsy (see Glossary).
   - characterized by neuronal cell loss in the globus pallidus, red nucleus, substantia nigra, periaqueductal gray, and dentate nucleus.
   - results in neurofibrillary tangles in the surviving neurons.
2. **Huntington disease (chorea)**
   - an inherited **autosomal dominant movement disorder** associated with severe degeneration of the cholinergic and GABA-ergic neurons, which are located in the caudate nucleus and putamen.
   - usually accompanied by **gyral atrophy** in the frontal and temporal lobes.
   - can be traced to a single gene defect on chromosome 4.
   - characterized by impaired initiation and slowness of saccadic eye movements; patients cannot make a volitional saccade without moving the head.
   - results in clinical manifestations of **choreiform movements** and **progressive dementia**.
   - results in **hydrocephalus ex vacuo** owing to the loss of neurons located in the head of the caudate nucleus, and to a lesser extent in the putamen.
   - prenatal and postnatal diagnosis using DNA techniques is available.

3. **Other choreiform dyskinesias**
   ■ **Sydenham chorea (St. Vitus dance)**
      a. the commonest chorea.
      b. occurs mainly in girls as a sequela to rheumatic fever.
   ■ **Chorea gravidarum**
      a. occurs usually during the second trimester of pregnancy.
      b. in many cases, a history of Sydenham chorea can be obtained.
4. **Ballism and hemiballism**
   ■ extrapyramidal motor disorders most often resulting from a vascular lesion (infarct) of the subthalamic nucleus.
   ■ characterized by **violent flinging** (ballistic) **movements of one or both extremities**; symptoms appear on the contralateral side.
   ■ may be treated with dopamine-blocking drugs or with GABA-mimetic agents.
   ■ may be treated surgically by **ventrolateral thalamotomy**.
5. **Hepatolenticular degeneration (Wilson disease)**
   ■ an autosomal recessive disorder owing to a **defect in the metabolism of copper** (ceruloplasmin).
   ■ has its gene locus on chromosome 13.
   ■ results in clinical manifestations of **tremor, rigidity**, and **choreiform** or **athetotic movements**. Tremor is the commonest neurologic sign.
   ■ has psychiatric symptoms, including psychosis, personality disorders, and dementia.
   ■ results in a **corneal Kayser-Fleischer ring**, which is pathognomonic.
   ■ marked by lesions in the liver (cirrhosis) and in the lentiform nuclei (necrosis and cavitation of the putamen).
   ■ diagnosed by low serum ceruloplasmin, elevated urinary excretion of copper, and increased copper concentration in liver biopsy.
   ■ treated with the copper-chelating agent D-penicillamine and pyridoxine for anemia.
6. **Tardive dyskinesia**
   ■ a syndrome of repetitive choreic movements affecting the face, limbs, and trunk.
   ■ results from treatment with antipsychotic drugs (eg, phenothiazines, butyrophenones, or metoclopramide).
   ■ often reversible with proper pharmacologic manipulations.

CLINICAL CORRELATES   **Parkinson disease** is a condition that is associated with degeneration and depigmentation of neurons in the substantia nigra, resulting in the depletion of dopamine in the caudate nucleus and putamen. The lack of dopamine's modulatory effects in the striatum leads to the clinical manifestations of **bradykinesia** and **hypokinesia** (difficulty in initiating and performing volitional movements), **rigidity** (cog-wheel and lead-pipe rigidity), and **resting tremor** (pill-rolling tremor). Nonmotor manifestations include cognitive dysfunction, mood/ personality disorders, autonomic nervous system disorders, and sleep disturbances. Parkinson disease affects 0.1% to 0.2% of people older than 40 years of age.

Review Test

1. A 6-year-old girl has brief, irregular contractions in her feet; symptoms are suspected to be the result of an untreated strep infection. What is the diagnosis?

(A) Chorea gravidarum
(B) Chorea major
(C) Ballism
(D) Hemiballism
(E) Sydenham chorea

2. Which thalamic nucleus projects to the striatum?

(A) Centromedian
(B) Mediodorsal
(C) Ventral anterior
(D) Ventral lateral
(E) Ventral posterolateral

3. The globus pallidus projects to the thalamus via the:

(A) ansa lenticularis.
(B) ansa peduncularis.
(C) fasciculus retroflexus.
(D) stria medullaris.
(E) stria terminalis.

4. The predominant neurons of the striatal system contain:

(A) acetylcholine.
(B) dopamine.
(C) GABA.
(D) glutamate.
(E) serotonin.

5. An ophthalmologist sees a Kayser-Fleischer ring while examining Descemet membrane with a slit lamp; what trace metal is found in the membrane?

(A) Aluminum
(B) Copper
(C) Iron
(D) Magnesium
(E) Mercury

6. A 50-year-old woman has resting tremor, cog-wheel rigidity, bradykinesia, and shuffling gait. The incidence of this disease in patients older than 50 years of age is:

(A) 1%.
(B) 2%.
(C) 3%.
(D) 4%.
(E) 5%.

7. An 80-year-old man presents to his primary care physician with a chief complaint about increased difficulty eating. The patient was previously diagnosed with Parkinson disease. Patient interview indicates that the eating complaint centers on difficulty chewing and poor coordination of the muscles of mastication. Further, the patient reports a marked increase in falls, which he attributes to his advanced age. Testing reveals increasingly poor cognitive performance. What is the most likely diagnosis, given this patient's symptoms?

(A) Huntington disease
(B) Progressive supranuclear palsy
(C) Sydenham chorea
(D) Tardive dyskinesia
(E) Wilson disease

8. A 60-year-old woman presents to the emergency department subsequent to a stroke for complaints about seizures that seem to be increasing in frequency. Patient interview reveals that the patient suffers from choreiform movements, easily fatigues, and her husband reports that she is "not acting like herself," has trouble focusing, and is more irritable than usual. Imaging reveals atrophy of the gyri and greatly enlarged ventricles. What is the most likely diagnosis in this patient?

(A) Chorea gravidarum
(B) Hydrocephalus ex vacuo
(C) Parkinson disease
(D) Pseudobulbar palsy
(E) Tardive dyskinesia

Questions 9 to 17

The response options for items 9 to 17 are the same. Select one answer for each item in the set.

(A) Chorea gravidarum
(B) Hemiballism
(C) Hepatolenticular degeneration
(D) Huntington disease
(E) Parkinson disease
(F) Sydenham chorea
(G) Tardive dyskinesia

Match each of the characteristics with the appropriate lettered movement disorder.

9. Is the overall commonest cause of chorea

10. Results from a loss of dopaminergic neurons in the pars compacta of the substantia nigra

11. A corneal Kayser-Fleischer ring is pathognomonic for this dyskinesia

12. Results from a lesion of the subthalamic nucleus

13. Is characterized by repetitive choreic movements affecting the face, limbs, and trunk, which result from treatment with antipsychotic drugs

14. Can be traced to a single gene defect on chromosome 4

15. Has its gene locus on chromosome 13

16. Is characterized by cortical atrophy and loss of neurons in the head of the caudate nucleus

17. Central nervous system lesions are characterized by necrosis and cavitation of the putamen.

Answers and Explanations

1. **E.** Sydenham chorea (St. Vitus dance) is the commonest chorea. It occurs mainly in girls as a sequela to rheumatic fever, which may develop after a strep infection. Chorea major (Huntington disease) is an inherited disorder that manifests as choreiform movements and progressive dementia, chorea gravidarum occurs during the second trimester of pregnancy, and ballism and hemiballism are violent flinging movement of one or both extremities as a result of an infarct of the subthalamic nucleus.

2. **A.** The striatum (caudate and putamen) receives thalamic input from the centromedian nucleus—the largest of the intralaminar nuclei. The mediodorsal (dorsomedial) nucleus is most closely related to the limbic system. The ventral anterior and ventral lateral nuclei project primarily to motor cortices. The ventral posterolateral nucleus projects to sensory cortex.

3. **A.** The globus pallidus projects to the thalamus via the lenticular and thalamic fasciculi and via the ansa lenticularis. The ansa peduncularis (part of the inferior thalamic peduncle) interconnects the amygdaloid nucleus and the hypothalamus. It also interconnects the orbitofrontal cortex and the thalamus (mediodorsal nucleus). The fasciculus retroflexus (habenulointerpeduncular tract) interconnects the habenular nucleus and the interpeduncular nucleus. The stria medullaris (thalami) interconnects the septal area (nuclei) and the habenular nuclei. The stria terminalis projects from the amygdaloid complex to the septal area and the hypothalamus.

4. **C.** GABA-containing neurons are the predominant neurons of the striatal system. They are found in the striatum, globus pallidus, and substantia nigra (pars reticularis).

5. **B.** Wilson disease is an autosomal recessive disorder that results from a defect in the metabolism of copper. Wilson disease is diagnosed by low serum ceruloplasmin, elevated urinary excretion of copper, and increased copper concentration in liver biopsy. Tremor is the commonest symptom and is known as the wing-beating tremor.

6. **A.** The incidence of Parkinson disease is 1% of the population past 50 years of age.

7. **B.** Progressive supranuclear palsy is a related form of Parkinson disease that also involves the additional symptoms of cognitive deficits, motor impairment of the cranial nerves, and gait disturbances. Huntington disease is a genetic disorder that manifests in altered eye movement, progressive dementia, and choreiform movements. Sydenham chorea typically manifests in girls aged 5 to 15 years. Tardive dyskinesia is related to antipsychotic drug use. Wilson disease is a genetic disorder that primarily produces movement disorders, such as tremor, and diagnosis is most common in people younger than 35 years of age.

8. **B.** Hydrocephalus ex vacuo may occur subsequent to a stroke, which leads to cell death and atrophy of the gyri. Depending on the location of the stroke, cell death may occur in regions such as the striatum, leading to movement disorders. The atrophy and cell loss lead to hydrocephalus, which is easily seen on imaging. Chorea gravidum refers to chorea that occurs during pregnancy, the patient is 60 years old and so is not likely to be pregnant. Parkinson disease and pseudobulbar palsy are unrelated to a stroke and do not lead to ventricular enlargement. Tardive dyskinesia is related to antipsychotic drug use.

9. **F.** Sydenham chorea (St. Vitus dance) is the commonest cause of chorea overall. Magnetic resonance imaging (MRI) studies show an increased signal in the head of the caudate nucleus with T2-weighted images. Quantitative MRI reveals an increase in the size of the caudate nucleus, putamen, and globus pallidus. In Huntington disease, there is massive loss of neurons in the caudatoputamen.

10. **E.** Parkinson disease results from a loss of dopaminergic neurons in the pars compacta of the substantia nigra.

11. **C.** Hepatolenticular degeneration, Wilson disease, is an autosomal recessive disorder resulting from a defect in the metabolism of copper. The Kayser-Fleischer ring is a green band of pigmentation found around the limbus in Descemet membrane; it is pathognomonic of Wilson disease.

12. **B.** Hemiballism results from a contralateral lesion (usually vascular) of the subthalamic nucleus. It is characterized by violent flinging (ballistic) movements of one or both extremities.

13. **G.** Tardive dyskinesia is a syndrome characterized by repetitive choreic movements affecting the face and trunk, which results from treatment with antipsychotic drugs (eg, phenothiazines, butyrophenones, or metoclopramide).

14. **D.** Huntington disease has its gene locus on chromosome 4 (gene location 4p16.3).

15. **C.** In Wilson disease, the abnormal gene has been assigned to the esterase D locus on chromosome 13.

16. **D.** Huntington disease is characterized by cortical atrophy and loss of neurons in the head of the caudate nucleus, which results in hydrocephalus ex vacuo.

17. **C.** Wilson disease is characterized by necrosis and cavitation of the putamen.

Objectives

■ Describe the external anatomy of the cerebellum.
■ Differentiate between the longitudinal divisions of the cerebellum and the anterior-posterior divisions of the cerebellum and ascribe a general function to each.
■ Describe the cerebellar peduncles.
■ List the layers of the cerebellar cortex and the cells contained within each.
■ List the fiber types of the cerebellum and the cells/systems associated with each.
■ Describe the major cerebellar pathways.
■ Describe the results of cerebellar dysfunction, including hypotonia, disequilibrium, and dyssynergia.
■ Describe the results of cerebellar lesions, including syndromes, tumors, and atrophies.

I. OVERVIEW

▦ develops from the alar plates (rhombic lips) of the metencephalon.
▦ located infratentorially within the posterior cranial fossa; lies between the temporal and occipital lobes and the brainstem.
▦ three primary functions: the **maintenance of posture and balance**, the **maintenance of muscle tone**, and the **coordination of voluntary motor activity**.

II. MAJOR DIVISIONS OF THE CEREBELLUM

▦ consists of a midline **vermis** and two lateral **hemispheres**.
▦ covered by a three-layered **cortex**, formed into folia and fissures.
▦ contains a central medullary core, which is **white matter** that contains myelinated axons and the four cerebellar nuclei (dentate, emboliform, globose, and fastigial). The emboliform and globose nuclei are collectively the interposed nucleus.

A. Cerebellar lobes (Figure 19.1 and see Table 19.1)

▦ phylogenetic and functional divisions.

1. Anterior lobe (spinocerebellum)

▦ lies anterior to the primary fissure.
▦ receives input from stretch receptors (muscle spindles) and Golgi tendon organs via the spinocerebellar tracts.
▦ plays a role in the regulation of muscle tone.

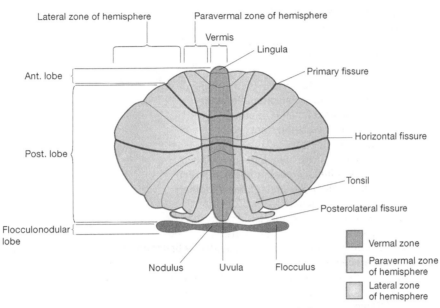

FIGURE 19.1. Schematic diagram of the fissures, lobules, and lobes of the cerebellum.

2. Posterior lobe (neocerebellum)
- lies between the primary fissure and the posterolateral fissure.
- receives input from the neocortex via the corticopontocerebellar fibers.
- plays a role in the coordination of voluntary motor activity.

3. Flocculonodular lobe (vestibulocerebellum)
- consists of the nodulus (of the vermis) and the flocculus.
- receives input from the vestibular system.
- plays a role in the maintenance of posture and balance.

B. Longitudinal organization of the cerebellum (see Figure 19.1 and Table 19.1)
- includes three functional longitudinal zones that are associated with specific cerebellar nuclei and pathways.
  1. Median (vermal) zone
  - projects to the fastigial nucleus.
  2. Paramedian (paravermal) zone
  - projects to the interposed nuclei (emboliform and globose nuclei).
  3. Lateral zone
  - projects to the dentate nucleus.

table **19.1** Divisions of the Cerebellum

Anatomic	Phylogenetic	Functional
Anterior lobe	Paleocerebellum	Spinocerebellum
Primary Fissure		
Posterior lobe	Neocerebellum	Cerebral cerebellum
Posterolateral Fissure		
Flocculonodular lobe	Archicerebellum	Vestibular cerebellum

Archicerebellum (flocculonodular lobe)—sensory information from vestibular system. Functions to maintain equilibrium. Paleocerebellum (spinocerebellum; anterior lobe)—sensory information from muscle, tendon, and spindles via spinal cord tracts. Regulates muscle tone and synergy in trunk musculature and limb girdles, especially for automatic movements (ie, walking, standing, posture). Neocerebellum (lateral hemisphere)—sensory information from motor regions of the cerebral cortex via pontine nuclei and middle cerebellar peduncle. Mostly related to skilled, learned movements with the hands, and hand-eye coordination (especially for voluntary movements).

C. Cerebellar peduncles (see Figure 1.6)
1. **Inferior cerebellar peduncle**
   - connects the cerebellum to the rostral medulla and caudal pons.
   - consists of two divisions:
     a. **Restiform body**
        - an afferent fiber system containing
          (1) **Posterior spinocerebellar tract**
          (2) **Cuneocerebellar tract**
          (3) **Olivocerebellar tract**
     b. **Juxtarestiform body**
        - contains afferent and efferent fibers:
          (1) **Vestibulocerebellar fibers (afferent)**
          (2) **Cerebellovestibular fibers (efferent)**
2. **Middle cerebellar peduncle**
   - the largest cerebellar peduncle.
   - connects the cerebellum to the pons.
   - an afferent fiber system containing **pontocerebellar fibers** to the neocerebellum.
3. **Superior cerebellar peduncle**
   - connects the cerebellum to the rostral pons and caudal midbrain.
   - the major output pathway from the cerebellum.
     a. **Efferent tracts**
        - **Dentatorubrothalamic**
        - **Interpositorubrothalamic**
        - **Fastigiothalamic**
        - **Fastigiovestibular**
     b. **Afferent pathways**
        - **Anterior spinocerebellar tract**
        - **Trigeminocerebellar fibers**
        - **Ceruleocerebellar fibers**

III. CEREBELLAR CORTEX

A. Three-layered cerebellar cortex (Figure 19.2)
1. **Molecular layer**
   - the outer cell-sparse layer that underlies the pia mater.
   - contains dendritic arborizations of Purkinje cells and the parallel fibers of granule cells.
   - contains stellate (outer) cells and basket (inner stellate) cells.
2. **Purkinje cell layer**
   - found between the molecular layer and the granule cell layer.
   - contains Purkinje cell bodies.
3. **Granule cell layer**
   - found between the Purkinje cell layer and the cerebellar white matter.
   - contains granule cells, Golgi cells, and **cerebellar glomeruli**.
   - cerebellar glomeruli: a mass found in the granule cell layer composed of the presynaptic terminals of mossy fibers, surrounded by postsynaptic granule cell dendrites and presynaptic Golgi cell axon terminals.

B. Neurons and fibers of the cerebellum (Figure 19.3; see Figure 19.2)
1. **Purkinje cell**
   - conveys the only output from the cerebellar cortex.
   - projects inhibitory output (gamma-aminobutyric acid [GABA]) to the cerebellar and vestibular nuclei.
   - excited by parallel and climbing fibers.
   - inhibited (GABA) by basket and stellate cells.

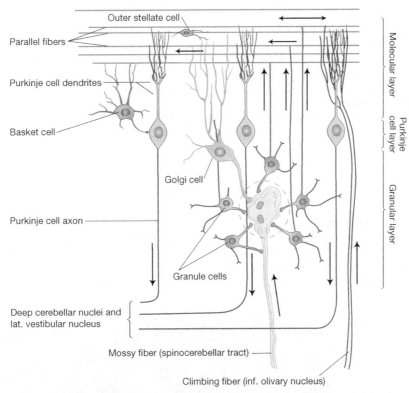

FIGURE 19.2. Schematic diagram of the three-layered cerebellar cortex showing the neuronal elements and their connections. The circular broken line contains a cerebellar glomerulus. Climbing and mossy fibers represent excitatory input. Purkinje cell axons provide the sole output from the cerebellar cortex, which is inhibitory.

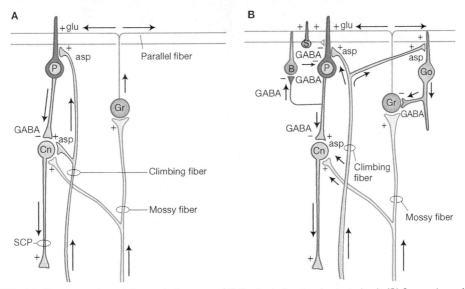

FIGURE 19.3. The connections of the cerebellar cortex. (A) The basic input and output circuit. (B) Connections of the inhibitory interneurons of the cerebellar cortex. Inhibitory neurons of the cerebellum use gamma-aminobutyric acid (GABA). Glutamate is the neurotransmitter used by granule cells. Aspartate (asp) is the neurotransmitter of the climbing fibers, whereas glutamate is the neurotransmitter of the mossy fibers. Excitatory synapses are indicated by a plus sign (+); inhibitory synapses are indicated by a minus sign (−). B, basket cell; Cn, neuron of the cerebellar nuclei; Gr, granule cell; glu, glutamate; Go, Golgi cell; P, Purkinje cell; S, stellate cell; SCP, superior cerebellar peduncle.

2. **Granule cell**
   - excites (glutamate) Purkinje, basket, stellate, and Golgi cells via parallel fibers.
   - inhibited by Golgi cells.
   - excited by mossy fibers.
3. **Mossy fibers**
   - the afferent excitatory fibers of the spinocerebellar and pontocerebellar tracts.
   - terminate as mossy fibers on granule cells.
   - excite granule cells to discharge via their parallel fibers.
4. **Climbing fibers**
   - the afferent excitatory fibers of the **olivocerebellar tract**.
   - terminate on neurons of the cerebellar nuclei and on dendrites of Purkinje cells.

IV. MAJOR CEREBELLAR PATHWAYS (Figure 19.4)

A. Vestibulocerebellar pathway
- plays a role in the maintenance of posture, balance, and the coordination of eye movements.
- receives its major input from the vestibular receptors of the kinetic and static labyrinths.
1. **Semicircular ducts and otolith organs**
   - project to the flocculonodular lobe and the vestibular nuclei.

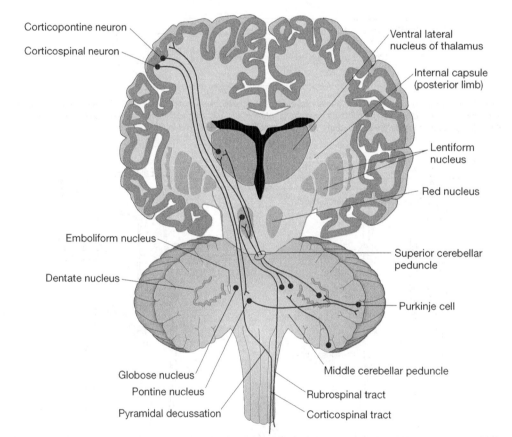

FIGURE 19.4. The principal cerebellar connections. The major efferent pathway is the dentatothalamocortical tract. The cerebellum receives input from the cerebral cortex through the corticopontocerebellar tract. (Modified with permission from Fix JD. *High-Yield Neuroanatomy*. 3rd ed. Lippincott Williams & Wilkins; 2005:112.)

2. **Flocculonodular lobe**
    - receives visual input from the superior colliculus and the striate cortex.
    - projects to the vestibular nuclei.
3. **Vestibular nuclei**
    - project via the medial longitudinal fasciculi to the ocular motor nuclei of CN III, CN IV, and CN VI to coordinate eye movements.
    - project via the medial and lateral vestibulospinal tracts to the spinal cord to regulate neck and antigravity muscles, respectively.

B. **Vermal spinocerebellar pathway**
- maintains muscle tone and postural control over truncal (axial) and proximal (limb girdle) muscles.
    1. **Vermis**
        - receives spinocerebellar and labyrinthine input.
        - projects to the fastigial nucleus.
    2. **Fastigial nucleus**
        - has excitatory output.
        - projects via the vestibular nuclei to the spinal cord.
        - projects to the ventral lateral nucleus of the thalamus.
    3. **Ventral lateral nucleus of the thalamus**
        - receives input from the fastigial nucleus.
        - projects to the trunk area of the precentral gyrus.
    4. **Precentral gyrus**
        - gives rise to the **anterior corticospinal tract**, which regulates muscle tone of the truncal and proximal muscles.

C. **Paravermal spinocerebellar pathway**
- maintains muscle tone and postural control over distal muscle groups.
    1. **Paravermis**
        - receives spinocerebellar input from distal muscles.
        - projects to the interposed nuclei.
    2. **Interposed nuclei (emboliform and globose)**
        - have excitatory output.
        - project to:
        a. **Ventral lateral nucleus**
            - projects to the extremities area of the precentral gyrus. The precentral gyrus gives rise to the **lateral corticospinal tract**, which regulates distal muscle groups.
        b. **Red nucleus**
            - gives rise to the crossed **rubrospinal tract**, which mediates control over distal muscles.
            - receives input from the contralateral nucleus interpositus and bilateral input from the motor and premotor cortices.

D. **Lateral hemispheric cerebellar pathway (see Figure 19.4)**
- also called the neocerebellar or pontocerebellar pathway.
- regulates the initiation, planning, and timing of volitional motor activity.
    1. **Cerebellar hemisphere**
        - receives input from the contralateral motor and sensory cortex via the **corticopontocerebellar tract**.
        - projects via Purkinje cell axons to the dentate nucleus.
    2. **Dentate nucleus**
        - has excitatory output.
        - projects via the superior cerebellar peduncle to the contralateral red nucleus, ventral lateral nucleus of the thalamus, and the inferior olivary nucleus.

   a. **Red nucleus pathway**
      - The **red nucleus** projects to the inferior olivary nucleus.
      - The **inferior olivary nucleus** projects via the contralateral inferior cerebellar peduncle to the cerebellum.
   b. **Ventral lateral nucleus pathway**
      - The **ventral lateral nucleus** of the thalamus projects to the motor (4) and premotor (6) cortices.
      - The **motor and premotor cortices** give rise to the following tracts:
        (1) Corticobulbar tract
           - innervates cranial nerve nuclei.
        (2) Lateral corticospinal tract
           - regulates volitional synergistic motor activity.
        (3) Corticopontocerebellar tracts
           - regulate the output of the neocerebellum.
   c. **Inferior olivary nucleus pathway**
      - The inferior olivary nucleus **receives direct input from the dentate nucleus** via the crossed descending fibers of the superior cerebellar peduncle.
      - The inferior olivary nucleus **projects directly to the dentate nucleus** via the contralateral inferior cerebellar peduncle.

V. CEREBELLAR DYSFUNCTION

- characterized by hypotonia, disequilibrium, and dyssynergia.

A. Hypotonia
- a loss of the resistance normally offered by muscles to palpation or to passive manipulation.
- results from the loss of cerebellar facilitation of the motor cortex via tonic firing of the cerebellar nuclei.
- results in a floppy, loose-jointed, rag-doll appearance with pendular reflexes; the patient appears inebriated.

B. Disequilibrium
- refers to loss of balance, characterized by gait and trunk dystaxia.

C. Dyssynergia
- a loss of coordinated muscle activity and includes the following:
  1. **Dysarthria**
     - slurred or scanning speech.
  2. **Dystaxia**
     - a lack of coordination in the execution of voluntary movement (eg, gait, trunk, and limb dystaxia).
  3. **Dysmetria**
     - the inability to arrest muscular movement at the desired point (past-pointing).
  4. **Intention tremor**
     - a type of dysmetria that occurs during a voluntary movement.
  5. **Dysdiadochokinesia**
     - the inability to perform rapid alternating movements (eg, rapid supination and pronation of the hands).
  6. **Nystagmus**
     - a form of dystaxia consisting of to-and-fro eye movements (ocular dysmetria).
  7. **Decomposition of movement (by-the-numbers phenomenon)**
     - consists of breaking down a smooth muscle act into a number of jerky awkward component parts.

8. **Rebound or lack of check**
   - results from the inability to adjust to changes in muscle tension.
   - caused by loss of the cerebellar component of the stretch reflex.
   - may be tested for by having the patient flex the forearm at the elbow against resistance; sudden release results in the forearm striking the patient's chest.

VI. CEREBELLAR LESIONS

A. **Anterior vermis syndrome**
   - involves the lower limb region of the anterior lobe.
   - results from atrophy of the rostral vermis—commonly caused by alcohol abuse.
   - results in gait, trunk, and lower limb dystaxia.

B. **Posterior vermis syndrome**
   - involves the flocculonodular lobe.
   - usually the result of brain tumors in children.
   - most frequently caused by medulloblastomas or ependymomas.
   - results in truncal dystaxia.

C. **Hemispheric syndrome**
   - usually involves one cerebellar hemisphere.
   - frequently the result of a brain tumor or an abscess.
   - results in limb, trunk, and gait dystaxia.
   - results in cerebellar signs that are ipsilateral to the lesion.

D. **Phenytoin (antiepileptic drug) intoxication**
   - may cause ataxia, nystagmus, gait disturbances, and dysarthric speech.

E. **Tumors of the cerebellum**
   1. **Astrocytomas**
      - cystic.
      - high mortality rate.
      - low-grade most common in children, high-grade most common in adults.
      - after a surgical removal, survival for many years is common.
   2. **Medulloblastomas**
      - most common primary brain tumor in children, boys more than girls.
      - occur most frequently in the cerebellum.
      - may obstruct passage of cerebrospinal fluid (CSF) and cause hydrocephalus.
      - may disseminate throughout the CSF.
   3. **Ependymomas**
      - arise from ependymal cells.
      - found intracranially in children and most often in the spinal cord in adults.
      - occur most frequently in the fourth ventricle.
      - may obstruct passage of CSF and cause hydrocephalus.

F. **Cerebellar atrophies**
   - inherited disorders.
   1. **Cerebello-olivary degeneration (Holmes disease)**
      - has an autosomal dominant mode of inheritance.
      - results in a loss of Purkinje and granule cells, followed by a loss of neurons in the inferior olivary nuclei.
      - results in gait ataxia, dysarthria, and intention tremor.

2. Olivopontocerebellar degeneration (Dejerine-Thomas syndrome)

- has an autosomal dominant mode of inheritance.
- results in a loss of Purkinje cells, neurons of the inferior olivary nucleus, and neurons in the pontine nuclei; results in demyelination of the posterior columns and the spinocerebellar tracts.
- frequently results in a loss of neurons in the substantia nigra and basal nuclei.
- results in gait ataxia, dysarthria, and intention tremor; may show parkinsonian signs (rigidity and akinesia).

CLINICAL CORRELATES   The most common hereditary ataxia is **Friedreich ataxia**. Friedreich ataxia has an autosomal recessive mode of inheritance. It involves the posterior columns, corticospinal tracts, spinocerebellar tracts, and dentate nuclei. Friedreich ataxia has the same spinal cord pathology as **subacute combined degeneration** (see Chapter 8 VI G) and is frequently associated with chronic myocarditis.

Review Test

1. A 30-year-old woman complains of unsteadiness while standing and walking. She tends to deviate to the right. Neurologic examination reveals the following signs: dysmetria on the right, dysdiadochokinesia, and a nystagmus that is more marked when she looks to the right side. The lesion is most likely found in the:

(A) cerebellar hemisphere, left side.
(B) cerebellar hemisphere, right side.
(C) globus pallidus, left side.
(D) globus pallidus, right side.
(E) primary motor cortex.

2. To which of the following nuclei do the Purkinje cells of the cerebellum project inhibitory axons?

(A) Arcuate
(B) Fastigial
(C) Inferior olivary
(D) Superior olivary
(E) Ventral lateral

3. The most common cause of anterior vermis syndrome is _____.

(A) alcohol abuse
(B) an abscess
(C) a tumor
(D) lead intoxication
(E) vascular occlusion

4. A child with the diagnosis of hydrocephalus resulting from a cerebellar tumor that spreads via the CSF most likely has a(n):

(A) astrocytoma.
(B) ependymoma.
(C) glioblastoma.
(D) medulloblastoma.
(E) oligodendrocytoma.

5. A tumor that is derived from the external granular layer of the cerebellar cortex is a(n) _____.

(A) astrocytoma
(B) chordoma
(C) ependymoma
(D) germinoma
(E) medulloblastoma

6. A 10-year-old boy has a headache, early-morning vomiting, staggering gait, dysdiadochokinesia, finger-to-nose sign, heel-to-shin sign, bilateral Babinski sign, choked disk, abducens palsy, and scanning speech, as in "I DID not GIVE any TOYSTO my son for CHRISTmas." What is the most likely diagnosis?

(A) Brown-Séquard syndrome
(B) Olivopontocerebellar degeneration
(C) Posterior vermis syndrome
(D) Sturge-Weber syndrome
(E) Tabes dorsalis

7. An 8-year-old girl is examined by a neurologist who finds the followings deficits: ataxia, marked sensory hypesthesias, kyphoscoliosis, pes cavus, myocarditis, and retinitis pigmentosa inherited as autosomal recessive trait. What is the name of this disease?

(A) Amyotrophic lateral sclerosis
(B) Brown-Séquard syndrome
(C) Friedrich ataxia
(D) Subacute combined degeneration
(E) Werdnig-Hoffmann disease

8. A 60-year-old man presents to his occupational therapist to begin therapy subsequent to a stroke. The man's symptoms include right hemiataxia, difficulty standing from a seated position, and problems in walking. Based on the symptoms, where does the therapist localize this patient's stroke?

(A) Basal nuclei
(B) Left cerebral cortex
(C) Left cerebellar hemisphere
(D) Right cerebral cortex
(E) Right cerebellar hemisphere

9. A 5-year-old boy is brought to his pediatrician by his parents, who are concerned because he complains about morning headaches, which are becoming almost a daily occurrence. They convey that more recently he has been increasingly nauseous and seems "in a daze," like he is tired throughout the day. Further, they report that he has begun to regress with regard to daily tasks such as brushing his teeth, dressing himself (eg, buttoning his shirt and tying his shoes), and using utensils at the dinner table. Physical examination confirms dysmetria. Imaging reveals a noncystic, paramedian, posterior cranial fossa tumor with enlargement of the fourth ventricle. What is the most likely diagnosis at this point in the examination?

(A) Anterior vermis syndrome
(B) Cerebello-olivary degeneration
(C) Dejerine-Thomas syndrome
(D) Medulloblastoma
(E) Subacute combined degeneration

Answers and Explanations

1. **B.** Dysmetria, dysdiadochokinesia, intention tremor, and nystagmus are classic cerebellar signs. In the finger-to-nose test, the patient past-points on the side of the lesion. The globus pallidus is atrophied in Huntington disease and in Wilson disease and would produce movement disorders differing from the above, for example, ballistic or choreiform movements. Primary motor cortex is involved in the initiation of movement.

2. **B.** Purkinje cells project inhibitory axons to all cerebellar nuclei: fastigial, globose, emboliform, and dentate. In addition, they project to all vestibular nuclei: lateral, superior, medial, and inferior. The superior olivary nucleus is an auditory relay nucleus, and the inferior olivary nucleus is a cerebellar relay nucleus. The arcuate nucleus is an ectopic pontine nucleus that lies next to the pyramidal tract; it functions in control of respiratory rate. The ventral lateral thalamic nucleus receives input from the dentate nucleus.

3. **A.** Anterior vermis syndrome is a result of chronic alcohol abuse. Patients have dystaxia of the lower limb and trunk. Posterior vermis syndrome involves the flocculonodular lobe; it is most frequently caused by an ependymoma or a medulloblastoma. Patients have truncal dystaxia. Hemispheric syndrome usually is the result of a tumor (astrocytoma) or abscess; patients have limb, trunk, and gait dystaxia.

4. **D.** Medulloblastoma is the most common primary brain tumor in children, typically occurring in the cerebellum and often disseminated via the CSF.

5. **E.** Medulloblastomas are derived from the external granular layer of the cerebellar cortex. Medulloblastomas give rise to posterior vermis syndrome.

6. **C.** Posterior vermis syndrome is generally indicative of brain tumors in children, frequently a medulloblastoma. Symptoms include vomiting, morning headache, stumbling gait, frequent falls, diplopia, papilledema, and sixth nerve palsy. Tabes dorsalis is posterior column syndrome that results from untreated syphilis. Olivopontocerebellar degeneration has an autosomal dominant mode of inheritance and results in gait ataxia, dysarthria, intention tremor, and possibly parkinsonian signs (rigidity and akinesia). Sturge-Weber syndrome is a neurocutaneous congenital disorder caused by an arteriovenous malformation in the telencephalon. Brown-Séquard syndrome is paralysis, ataxia, and loss of sensation as a result of a spinal cord hemisection.

7. **C.** Friedreich ataxia is the most common hereditary ataxia, with an autosomal recessive mode of inheritance. It is often associated with chronic myocarditis; other symptoms include muscle weakness, loss of coordination, vision impairment, hearing loss, slurred speech, and curvature of the spine (kyphoscoliosis). Friedreich ataxia has the same spinal cord pathology (posterior column syndrome) as subacute combined degeneration, which is caused by a vitamin B_{12} deficiency. Symptoms include loss of tactile discrimination; loss of joint and vibratory sensation; stereoanesthesia; sensory dystaxia; paresthesias and pain; hyporeflexia or areflexia; urinary incontinence, constipation, and impotence; and Romberg sign. Subacute combined degeneration includes both sensory and motor deficits; amyotrophic lateral sclerosis is a pure motor syndrome; Werdnig-Hoffmann disease is a heredofamilial degenerative disease of infants that affects only lower motor neurons; and Brown-Séquard syndrome is paralysis, ataxia, and loss of sensation as a result of spinal cord hemisection (see Chapter 8).

8. **E.** There is no issue with executing/initiating movement in this patient, which points to a cerebellar lesion. Cerebellar control of the body is ipsilateral, unlike the cerebrum—so a right cerebellar lesion would lead to issues such as lack of coordinated movement concentrated on the right side. Lesion of the basal nuclei would produce movement issues, but those would not involve a lack of coordinated movement.

9. **D.** Medulloblastomas are the most common primary brain tumor in children, with a prevalence in boys over girls. They are most commonly found in the cerebellum and cause progressive symptoms, including worsening headache and altered mental states. The patient's symptoms point to a laterally displaced tumor that is compressing the cerebellar lateral hemisphere causing dysmetria. Anterior vermis syndrome involves gait issues from damage to the cerebellar vermis, not present in this patient. Cerebello-olivary degeneration/atrophy (Holmes disease) also results in gait disturbances and a tremor. Dejerine-Thomas syndrome (olivopontocerebellar degeneration) results in symptoms similar to Holmes disease and may include Parkinson disease symptoms as well if there is cell loss in the substantia nigra. Subacute combined degeneration involves the spinal cord and leads to both gait and upper limb ataxia and is typically seen in individuals who are anemic.

Autonomic Nervous System

Objectives

■ Differentiate between the sympathetic and the parasympathetic nervous systems—include cell locations, neurotransmitters, and functions.
■ Describe visceral afferents and their relationship to the motor fibers.
■ Describe autonomic influence on the eye, heart, blood vessels, and bladder.

I. OVERVIEW

▓ general visceral efferent (**GVE**) motor system that controls and regulates smooth muscle, cardiac muscle, and glands.
▓ two divisions: **sympathetic** and **parasympathetic**. The **enteric** nervous system of the gut will also be presented here because of its close relationship to the autonomic nervous system (ANS) and because of its relative level of independence from the central nervous system (CNS).
▓ consists of **preganglionic neurons** and **postganglionic neurons**.
▓ general visceral afferent (GVA) fibers run with GVE fibers.
▓ all sympathetic fibers in the head are postganglionic and run on branches of CN V to reach their target.

II. DIVISIONS OF THE AUTONOMIC NERVOUS SYSTEM

A. Sympathetic division (Figure 20.1; Table 20.1)
▓ also called the thoracolumbar or adrenergic system.
▓ stimulates activities that are mobilized during more energy-requiring, emergency-type situations, the fight, fright, and flight responses, which include increased heart rate and force of contraction and increased blood pressure.
1. Preganglionic neurons (see Figures 6.2 and 6.3)
▓ located in the intermediolateral cell column (T1-L2).
▓ project via anterior roots and white communicating rami to the sympathetic trunk, where they synapse or pass through via splanchnic nerves to prevertebral (collateral) ganglia, where they synapse.
2. Postganglionic neurons (see Figures 6.2 and 6.3)
▓ located in the sympathetic trunk (paravertebral ganglia) and in prevertebral (collateral) ganglia.
▓ in the sympathetic trunk, project via gray communicating rami to spinal nerves and innervate body wall targets (ie, blood vessels, arrector pili muscles, and sweat glands), or

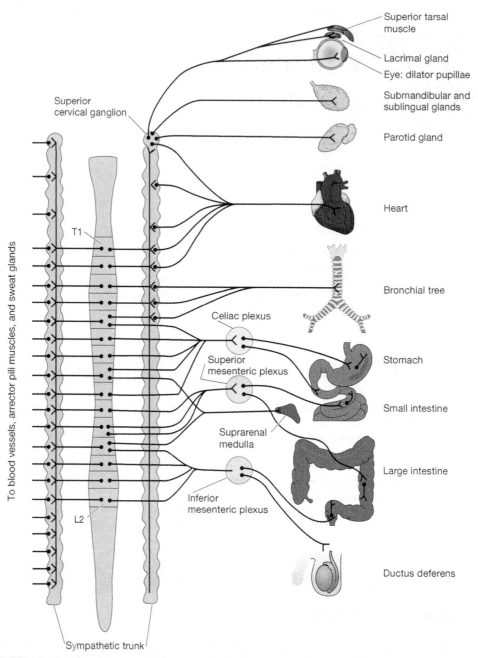

FIGURE 20.1. Schematic diagram showing the sympathetic (thoracolumbar) innervation of the autonomic nervous system. The entire sympathetic innervation of the head is via the superior cervical ganglion. Gray communicating rami are found at all spinal cord levels, whereas white communicating rami are found only in spinal segments T1 to L2. (Modified with permission from Fix JD. *High-Yield Neuroanatomy*. 3rd ed. Lippincott Williams & Wilkins; 2005:128.)

ride blood vessels to targets in the head, or pass through splanchnic nerves to the organs of the pelvis.

- in prevertebral ganglia, project to abdominal and pelvic viscera on periarterial plexuses.

3. Interneurons

- small intensely fluorescent (SIF) cells.
- located in sympathetic ganglia.
- dopaminergic and inhibitory.

table 20.1	Sympathetic and Parasympathetic Activity on Organ Systems	
Structure	**Sympathetic Function**	**Parasympathetic Function**
Eye		
Radial muscle of iris (dilator pupillae) Circular muscle of iris (sphincter pupillae) Ciliaris	Dilates pupil (mydriasis)	Constricts pupil (miosis) Contracts for near vision (accommodation)
Lacrimal gland		Stimulates secretion
Salivary glands	Viscous secretion	Watery secretion
Sweat glands Thermoregulatory Apocrine (stress)	Increases Increases	
Heart Sinoatrial node Atrioventricular node Contractility	Accelerates Increases conduction velocity Increases	Decelerates (vagal arrest) Decreases conduction velocity Decreases (atria)
Vascular smooth muscle Skin, splanchnic vessels Skeletal muscle vessels	Contracts Relaxes	
Bronchiolar smooth muscle	Relaxes	Contracts
Gastrointestinal tract Smooth muscle Walls Sphincters Secretion and motility	Relaxes Contracts Decreases	Contracts Relaxes Increases
Genitourinary tract Smooth muscle Bladder wall Sphincter Penis, seminal vesicles	Little or no effect Contracts Ejaculation	Contracts Relaxes Erection
Suprarenal medulla	Secretes epinephrine and norepinephrine	
Metabolic functions Liver Fat cells Kidney	Gluconeogenesis and glycogenolysis Lipolysis Renin release	

4. **Neurotransmitters**
   - **Acetylcholine** (ACh)
     a. the neurotransmitter of **preganglionic neurons**.
   - **Norepinephrine**
     a. the neurotransmitter of all **postganglionic sympathetic neurons**, with the exception of sweat glands and some blood vessels that receive cholinergic sympathetic innervation.
   - **Epinephrine**
     a. produced by the chromaffin cells of the suprarenal medulla.

B. **Parasympathetic division (Figure 20.2; see Table 20.1)**
   - **craniosacral** or **cholinergic system**.
   - stimulates activities that conserve energy and restore body resources, including reduction of heart rate and increase in digestion and absorption of food.
   - **uses ACh** as the neurotransmitter for both preganglionic and postganglionic synapses.
   1. **Cranial division**
      - associated with four cranial nerves.
      - preganglionic fibers are found within the cranial nerves (III, VII, IX, and X) at the point of attachment to the brainstem and so are considered part of the nerve.

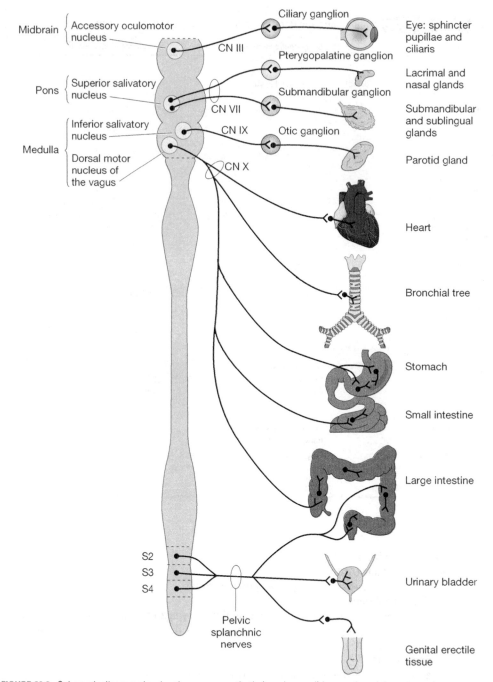

FIGURE 20.2. Schematic diagram showing the parasympathetic (craniosacral) innervation of the autonomic nervous system. Sacral outflow includes segments S2 to S4. Cranial outflow is mediated via four cranial nerves: CN III, CN VII, CN IX, and CN X. (Modified with permission from Fix JD. *High-Yield Neuroanatomy*. 3rd ed. Lippincott Williams & Wilkins; 2005:129.)

    ▪ all postganglionic fibers in the head "hitch a ride" on branches of CN V to reach their target.

        a. Oculomotor nerve (CN III) (see IV A 2; Figure 16.4)

            ▪ **Accessory oculomotor (Edinger-Westphal) nucleus**

                (1) projects preganglionic fibers to ciliary ganglion.

      ▪ **Ciliary ganglion**

            (1) projects postganglionic fibers to sphincter pupillae and ciliaris.

   b. **Facial nerve (CN VII)** (see Figure 10.6)
      - **Superior salivatory nucleus**
         (1) projects preganglionic fibers to the pterygopalatine and submandibular ganglia.
      - **Pterygopalatine ganglion**
         (1) projects postganglionic fibers to the lacrimal gland and to the mucosa of the nasal cavity and palate.
      - **Submandibular ganglion**
         (1) projects postganglionic fibers to the submandibular and sublingual glands.
   c. **Glossopharyngeal nerve (CN IX)** (see Figure 9.5)
      - **Inferior salivatory nucleus**
         (1) projects preganglionic fibers to the otic ganglion.
      - **Otic ganglion**
         (2) projects postganglionic fibers to the parotid gland.
   d. **Vagus nerve (CN X)** (see Figures 9.3 and 9.4)
      - **Dorsal motor nucleus**
         (1) projects preganglionic fibers to intramural (terminal) ganglia within or adjacent to visceral organs.
      - **Intramural (terminal) ganglia**
         (1) innervate, via short postganglionic fibers, viscera of the thorax and abdomen as far as the mid-transverse colon.
   2. **Sacral division**
      - originates from the sacral parasympathetic nucleus of sacral segments S2 to S4.
      - postganglionic neurons lie near or on the wall of the innervated viscus.
      - innervates via pelvic splanchnic nerves the lower abdomen and pelvic viscera, including the colon distal to the mid-transverse colon, urinary bladder, and genital viscera.
      - involved with **micturition, defecation**, and **erection**.

C. **Enteric division**
   - consists of intramural (enteric) ganglia and plexuses of the gastrointestinal tract, including the submucosal (Meissner) plexus and the myenteric (Auerbach) plexus.
   - influenced by postganglionic adrenergic sympathetic and preganglionic cholinergic parasympathetic input.
   - functions independently when deprived of CNS innervation.
   - plays a major role in the control of **gastrointestinal motility**.
   - primary source of serotonin in the body.

III. VISCERAL AFFERENT FIBERS AND PAIN

- visceral afferent fibers ride with sympathetic and parasympathetic fiber-containing nerves.

A. **GVA fibers and innervated structures**
   1. **GVA cell bodies**
      - found in spinal ganglia, inferior ganglia of the glossopharyngeal nerve (CN IX) and the vagus nerve (CN X), and the geniculate ganglion of the facial nerve (CN VII).
   2. **GVA pain fibers**
      - found in the white communicating rami.
      - accompany nerves carrying sympathetic fibers.
      - have their cell bodies in the spinal ganglia of the thoracolumbar region (T1-L2).
   3. **GVA reflex fibers**
      - accompany both sympathetic and parasympathetic fibers.
      - terminate centrally in the solitary nucleus.
   4. **Carotid sinus**
      - a dilation of the common carotid artery at its bifurcation. It contains baroreceptors; when stimulated, the receptors cause bradycardia and a decrease in blood pressure.
      - innervated by GVA fibers from CN IX.

5. Carotid body

- a small structure just above the bifurcation of the common carotid artery; it contains chemoreceptors that respond to carbon dioxide, oxygen, and pH levels in the blood.
- innervated by GVA fibers from CN IX and CN X.

B. Visceral pain

- results from the following conditions:
  1. **Distension**
  2. **Spasms or strong contractions**
  3. **Mechanical stimulation**
  4. **Ischemia**

C. Referred pain

- pain seeming to arise from a region or site other than its origin.
- multiple types:
  1. visceral-somatic: visceral origin that is conveyed to the somatic dermatome of the same spinal cord segment (eg, pain from myocardial infarction radiating down the left upper limb). May occur when an inflamed viscus irritates the overlying parietal peritoneum.
  2. embryologic: pain is referred to the embryologic origin of the affected organ (eg, inflammation of the pleura is referred to the neck and shoulder region).
  3. proximal-distal: pain from a proximal injury is referred distally (eg, pain from a lumbar disk herniation is referred down the lower limb).

IV. AUTONOMIC INNERVATION OF SELECTED ORGANS (See Table 20.1)

A. Eye

1. Sympathetic input

- **hypothalamic neurons** project to the intermediolateral cell column at T1 and T2, the ciliospinal center (of Budge).
- the **intermediolateral cell column** (T1-T2) projects preganglionic fibers via the sympathetic trunk to the superior cervical ganglion.
- the **superior cervical ganglion** projects postganglionic fibers via the internal carotid artery to the cavernous sinus.
- pupillodilator fibers reach the dilator pupillae muscle of the iris via the superior orbital fissure and via the nasociliary and ciliary nerves (CN V; long and short). Some pupillodilator fibers accompany the caroticotympanic nerves prior to entering the orbit; this explains Horner syndrome (ptosis, enophthalmos, miosis, flushing, and hemianhidrosis) with otitis media.
- fibers to the superior tarsal muscle (of **Müller**) reach the upper eyelid via the **ophthalmic artery**.
- interruption of sympathetic input to the eye at any level results in **Horner syndrome**.

2. Parasympathetic input (see Figure 16.4)

- the accessory oculomotor **nucleus** projects preganglionic fibers via the oculomotor nerve (CN III) to the ciliary ganglion.
- the **ciliary ganglion** projects postganglionic fibers via the short ciliary nerves (CN V_1) to the sphincter pupillae (which acts to constrict the pupil) and ciliaris (which allows the lens to "round up" for accommodation).
- **postganglionic fibers** mediate the efferent limb of the pupillary light reflex.
- interruption of the parasympathetic input results in **internal ophthalmoplegia** (a fixed [unresponsive] and dilated pupil) and cycloplegia (paralysis of accommodation).

B. Blood vessels

- receive their innervation from the **sympathetic** division of the ANS.
  ### 1. Arteries and arterioles
  - constriction of cutaneous and splanchnic blood vessels results from sympathetic stimulation of alpha-receptors.
  - dilation of skeletal muscle arteries results from sympathetic stimulation of beta-receptors.
  - parasympathetic stimulation leads to dilation of the erectile tissues of the genitals.
  ### 2. Large veins and venules
  - only moderately innervated.
  ### 3. Cerebral blood vessels
  - respond to circulating metabolites (carbon dioxide and oxygen).

C. Heart

1. Sympathetic input
- the **intermediolateral cell column** (T1-T5) projects preganglionic fibers to the upper thoracic ganglia and to the three cervical ganglia of the sympathetic trunk.
- the **rostral sympathetic trunk** projects postganglionic fibers via cardiac nerves to the ventricular and atrial walls and the pacemaker tissue.
- **stimulation of cardiac nerves** results in an increase in heart rate and in the force of cardiac contractility.

2. Parasympathetic input
- the **dorsal motor nucleus of the vagus** projects preganglionic fibers via the vagus nerve to the intramural ganglia of the atria and the sinoatrial node.
- **postganglionic fibers** from the intramural ganglia innervate the heart.
- **vagal stimulation** lowers the strength and rate of cardiac contraction.

D. Bladder

1. Sympathetic input
- control is predominantly parasympathetic.
- from T12 to L2 via the inferior mesenteric plexus and via the inferior hypogastric plexus to the detrusor and the internal urethral sphincter.
- damage to sympathetic fibers has little effect on bladder function.

2. Parasympathetic input
- from S2 to S3 via the pelvic splanchnic nerves to the detrusor and the internal urethral sphincter.
- stimulation results in emptying the bladder.
- paralysis produces an atonic bladder, with no reflex or voluntary control.

3. Somatomotor input
- from S2 to S4 via the pudendal nerves to the external urethral sphincter.

4. Sensory input to spinal cord
- via hypogastric, pelvic, and pudendal nerves.
- damage results in an atonic bladder with overflow incontinence.

5. Ascending pathway for bladder sensation
- controls the urge to void.
- found with sacral fibers of the anterolateral system.
- transection results in loss of the urge to void and overflow incontinence.

6. Upper motor neuron input
- controls volitional micturition primarily through maintenance of an inhibitory tone.
- from the paracentral lobule via the corticosacral tract (between the denticulate ligament and the lateral horn).
- bilateral transection results in an uninhibited neurogenic bladder. Sensation is normal, but the patient has no control over voiding; the bladder fills and suddenly empties without cortical control.

V. CLINICAL CONSIDERATIONS

A. Megacolon (Hirschsprung disease)
- also called **congenital aganglionic megacolon**.
- most common in males.
- characterized by extreme dilation and hypertrophy of the colon with fecal retention and by the absence of ganglion cells in the myenteric plexus.
- results from the **failure of neural crest cells to migrate into the colon**.

B. Familial dysautonomia (Riley-Day syndrome)
- an **autosomal recessive trait** characterized by abnormal sweating, blood pressure instability (orthostatic hypotension), difficulty in feeding owing to inadequate muscle tone in the gastrointestinal tract, and progressive sensory loss.
- results from a **loss of neurons in autonomic** and **sensory ganglia**.

C. Raynaud disease
- a painful disorder of the terminal arteries of the extremities.
- characterized by idiopathic paroxysmal bilateral cyanosis of the digits owing to arterial and arteriolar contraction caused by cold or emotion.
- may be treated by **preganglionic sympathectomy**.

D. Peptic ulcer
- results from **excessive production of hydrochloric acid** because of increased parasympathetic (tone) stimulation.

E. Botulism
- occurs when *Clostridium botulinum* toxin blocks the release of ACh from presynaptic vesicles in motor end plates and in synapses of autonomic ganglia.
- leads to paralysis of striated muscles.
- dry eyes and mouth and gastrointestinal ileus are the autonomic deficits.
- characterized by the absence of sensory impairment.

Review Test

1. Postganglionic sympathetic cholinergic fibers innervate the: _____.

(A) detrusor
(B) ductus deferens
(C) lacrimal gland
(D) sweat glands
(E) trigone of the urinary bladder

2. Which of the following ganglia does not contain postganglionic parasympathetic neurons?

(A) Celiac
(B) Ciliary
(C) Otic
(D) Pterygopalatine
(E) Submandibular

3. Which one of the following deficits results from the destruction of the ciliary ganglion?

(A) Loss of corneal reflex
(B) Loss of direct pupillary reflex
(C) Loss of lacrimation
(D) Miosis
(E) Severe ptosis

4. A 55-year-old woman, who is a lifelong smoker, undergoes a surgical procedure to remove a cancerous lung tumor from the posterior wall of her thorax. During the operation, her right paravertebral chain was severed near the T1 vertebral level. Which of the following functions/actions would be *most* affected by this event?

(A) Constriction of the pupil
(B) Contraction of the diaphragm
(C) Flexion of the biceps brachii
(D) Peripheral vasoconstriction
(E) Peristalsis

5. A 48-year-old man suffers from chronic heart burn. The parietal cells of the stomach release acid in a process that is largely controlled by the vagus nerve; therefore, he chooses to undergo an elective vagotomy to reduce his stomach acid. What other effects would you anticipate this patient to have as a result of the vagotomy? Reduced:

(A) cardiac output.
(B) constriction of the greater omental artery.

(C) peristalsis in the jejunum.
(D) excitation of the suprarenal medulla.
(E) tone of the pyloric sphincter.

6. A 23-year-old woman presents to her primary care physician with a chief complaint of cold and painful fingers and toes. Patient interview reveals that her symptoms have been progressing and she didn't think it was unusual because she lives in a very cold climate. She decided to seek help because her fingers and toes now turn white and then blue after she is outside in the cold. When she comes back into a heated space, they turn red and prickly after about 15 minutes. The physician orders blood work to rule out an autoimmune disorder, but suspects the patient may be suffering from which of the following disorders?

(A) Hirschsprung disease
(B) Ménière disease
(C) Parkinson disease
(D) Raynaud disease
(E) Riley-Day syndrome

7. A new mother presents to her baby's pediatrician 4 days after the birth with a chief concern that the baby has not passed their first stool yet (meconium). The mother relates that her new baby boy has been extremely fussy and has vomited several times. Examination reveals a swollen abdomen. The pediatrician refers the baby for a rectal biopsy and suspects the baby has which of the following disorders?

(A) Botulism
(B) Hirschsprung disease
(C) Peptic ulcer
(D) Raynaud disease
(E) Riley-Day syndrome

Questions 8 to 12

The response options for items 8 to 12 are the same. Select one answer for each item in the set.

(A) Hirschsprung disease
(B) Horner syndrome
(C) Peptic ulcer disease
(D) Raynaud disease
(E) Riley-Day syndrome

Match each of the characteristics below with the condition it best describes.

8. Results from increased parasympathetic stimulation

9. Is a painful vasospastic disorder affecting the digits

10. Is an autosomal recessive trait characterized by abnormal sweating and blood pressure instability

11. Results from congenital absence of ganglion cells in the myenteric plexus

12. Consists of anisocoria and lack of sweating

Questions 13 to 18

The response options for items 13 to 18 are the same. Select one answer for each item in the set.
(A) Ach
(B) Dopamine
(C) Nitric oxide
(D) Norepinephrine
(E) Vasoactive intestinal peptide (VIP)

Match the characteristics below with the appropriate neurotransmitter.

13. Is a vasodilator

14. Is the neurotransmitter of the SIF cells

15. Innervates apocrine sweat glands

16. Innervates eccrine (merocrine) sweat glands

17. Is the transmitter responsible for penile erection

18. Is the neurotransmitter of the arrector pili

Answers and Explanations

1. **D.** Postganglionic sympathetic cholinergic fibers innervate the eccrine (merocrine) sweat glands and some blood vessels; blood vessels, however, are predominantly innervated by postganglionic sympathetic adrenergic fibers. Apocrine sweat glands of the axilla are innervated by adrenergic fibers; these glands secrete in response to mental stress.

2. **A.** The celiac ganglion is a sympathetic prevertebral/preaortic (collateral) ganglion that contains postganglionic neurons. The other four ganglia listed are the postganglionic parasympathetic ganglia of the head.

3. **B.** Destruction of the ciliary ganglion interrupts postganglionic parasympathetic fibers, which innervate the sphincter pupillae and ciliaris; this results in mydriasis and loss of accommodation. In addition, postganglionic sympathetic vasomotor fibers are interrupted, resulting in a hyperemic globe. Postganglionic sympathetic pupillodilator fibers reach the iris via the nasociliary and long ciliary nerves. Severe ptosis results from an oculomotor paralysis involving the fibers that innervate the levator palpebrae superioris. Mild ptosis results from a lesion of the oculosympathetic fibers, which innervate the superior tarsal muscle (Horner syndrome).

4. **D.** Destruction of the sympathetic chain would affect body wall targets, which include blood vessels, sweat glands, and erector pili muscles. Both pupillary constriction and peristalsis are parasympathetically controlled. Both the diaphragm and biceps brachii are skeletal muscles and as such are not controlled by the ANS.

5. **C.** The vagus influences peristalsis through parasympathetic influence on the smooth muscle of the gut. The vagus slows heart rate, so a vagotomy would lead to an increase in heart rate because of the unopposed actions of the sympathetic nervous system. Peripheral vasoconstriction is controlled by the sympathetic nervous system. The suprarenal medulla is essentially a postganglionic sympathetic ganglion. Sphincter tone is controlled largely by sympathetics.

6. **D.** Raynaud disease/syndrome is a disease of the peripheral arterioles caused by spasmodic contraction of the vessels, leading to cyanosis and pain, primarily in the digits. It is most common in women between 15 and 30 years of age. Hirschsprung disease (megacolon) has to do with fecal retention, not the digits. Ménière disease leads to nystagmus, vertigo, tinnitus, hearing loss, and nausea, which the patient does not demonstrate. Parkinson disease is a disorder of the dopaminergic system and unrelated to the blood supply of the peripheral digits. Riley-Day syndrome (familial dysautonomia) is characterized by orthostatic hypertension, progressive sensory loss, and GI disturbances, which this patient does not demonstrate.

7. **B.** Hirschsprung disease results from a failure of neural crest migration into the colon, resulting in fecal retention. It most commonly manifests in newborn, male babies, in the first few days of life, characterized by irritability and lack of a first bowel movement. Botulism and peptic ulcer are related to the GI tract, but would be much less likely in a newborn. Raynaud disease/syndrome is a disease of the peripheral arterioles caused by spasmodic contraction of the vessels, leading to cyanosis and pain, primarily in the digits. It is most common in women between 15 and 30 years of age. Riley-Day syndrome (familial dysautonomia) is characterized by orthostatic hypertension, progressive sensory loss, and GI disturbances.

8. **C.** Peptic ulcer disease results from increased parasympathetic tone.

9. **D.** Raynaud disease is a benign symmetric disease characterized by painful vasospasms affecting the digits.

10. **E.** Riley-Day syndrome—familial dysautonomia—is an autosomal recessive trait characterized by abnormal sweating and blood pressure instability.

11. **A.** Congenital aganglionic megacolon (Hirschsprung disease) results from failure of the neural crest cells to migrate into the wall of the distal colon (sigmoid colon and rectum) and form the myenteric plexus. It is characterized by extreme dilation and hypertrophy of the colon, with fecal retention.

12. **B.** Anisocoria (unequal pupils) and hemianhidrosis (lack of sweating on half of the face) are consistent with Horner syndrome, which also involves ptosis, miosis, and hemianhidrosis.

13. **E.** VIP is a vasodilator found in postganglionic parasympathetic fibers, colocalized with ACh.

14. **B.** Dopamine is the neurotransmitter of the SIF cells.

15. **D.** Norepinephrine innervates apocrine sweat glands; these glands of the axilla and anal region respond to emotional stress.

16. **A.** ACh innervates eccrine (merocrine) sweat glands, which respond to heat stress.

17. **C.** Nitric oxide is the transmitter responsible for penile erection.

18. **D.** Norepinephrine is the neurotransmitter of the erector pili.

21 Neurotransmitters and Pathways

Objectives

- List the various types of pathways as characterized by their neurotransmitter.
- Describe the major pathways, function, and characteristics of acetylcholine, dopamine, norepinephrine, serotonin, opioid and nonopioid peptides, and amino acids.
- Describe endogenous pain control pathways.

I. OVERVIEW

A. Neurotransmitters

- substances released on excitation, typically from presynaptic neurons (can be reversed, eg, nitric oxide). They produce the effects of nerve stimulation in postsynaptic neurons or in receptor cells.

B. Neurochemical pathways and loci

- classified based on the chemical composition of their neurotransmitters.

  1. **Monoaminergic pathways**
     - make use of **monoamines** as neurotransmitters; they contain one amine group. Monoamines include **dopamine**, **norepinephrine**, **epinephrine**, and **serotonin**.
       a. **Catecholaminergic pathways** (Figure 21.1)
          - make use of a monoamine that contains a catechol nucleus. Catecholamines include **dopamine**, **norepinephrine**, and **epinephrine**.
          - include dopaminergic, noradrenergic (norepinephrinergic), and adrenergic (epinephrinergic) pathways.
       b. **Indolaminergic pathways**
          - make use of a monoamine that contains an indole nucleus. **Serotonin** is an indolamine.
          - include serotonergic pathways.
  2. **Cholinergic pathways**: use **acetylcholine** (ACh) as a neurotransmitter
  3. **Peptidergic pathways**: use **peptides** as neurotransmitters
  4. **Gamma-aminobutyric acid (GABA)-ergic pathways**: use **GABA** as a neurotransmitter
  5. **Glutamatergic pathways**: use **glutamate** as a neurotransmitter
  6. **Glycinergic pathways**: use **glycine** as a neurotransmitter
  7. **L-Arginine-nitric oxide pathway**: use the gaseous neurotransmitter **nitric oxide**

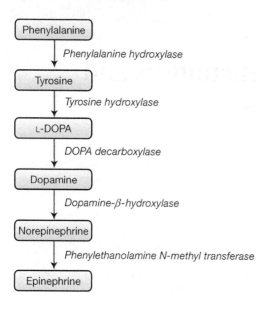

FIGURE 21.1. Synthesis of catecholamines from phenylalanine. Epinephrine, which is derived from norepinephrine, is found primarily in the suprarenal medulla. DOPA, dihydroxyphenylalanine; L-DOPA, levodopa.

II. DOPAMINE

A. Characteristics

- a catecholamine.
- role in cognitive, motor, and neuroendocrine functions.
- **depleted in Parkinson disease.**
- has **increased production in schizophrenia**.
- only found in the central nervous system (CNS).

B. Major dopaminergic pathways (Figure 21.2)

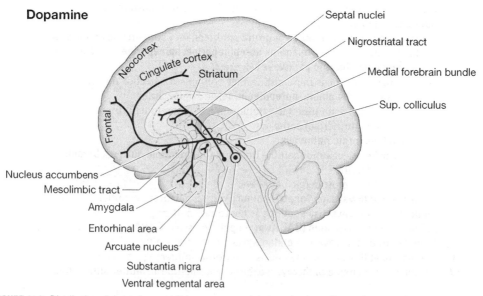

FIGURE 21.2. Distribution of dopamine-containing neurons and their projections. Two major ascending dopamine pathways arise in the midbrain: the nigrostriatal tract from the substantia nigra and the mesolimbic tract from the ventral tegmental area. In Parkinson disease, loss of dopaminergic neurons occurs in the substantia nigra pars compacta and in the ventral tegmental area.

1. **Nigrostriatal pathway**
   - the substantia nigra projects to the striatum.
   - destruction of dopaminergic nigral neurons results in **parkinsonism**.
2. **Mesolimbic pathway**
   - the ventral tegmental area projects widely to the structures of the limbic system.
   - linked to behavior and schizophrenia.
3. **Mesocortical pathway**
   - the ventral tegmental area projects to the prefrontal cortex.
   - linked to motivation and emotional response.
4. **Tuberohypophyseal (tuberoinfundibular) pathway**
   - the arcuate nucleus of the hypothalamus projects to the portal vessels of the infundibulum.
   - released dopamine inhibits the release of **prolactin** from the adenohypophysis.

III. ACETYLCHOLINE

A. Characteristics
- the major neurotransmitter of the peripheral nervous system, neuromuscular junction, parasympathetic nervous system, preganglionic sympathetic fibers, and postganglionic sympathetic fibers to the sweat glands.
- found in neurons of the somatic and visceral motor nuclei in the brainstem and spinal cord.
- receptors are muscarinic (metabotropic; postganglionic parasympathetics and sweat glands) or nicotinic (ionotropic; preganglionic sympathetic and parasympathetic, by all alpha, beta, and gamma motor neurons).

B. Major cholinergic pathways (Figure 21.3)
1. **Septal nuclei**
   - project via the fornix to the hippocampal formation.
2. **Basal nucleus of Meynert**
   - located in the substantia innominata of the basal forebrain, between the globus pallidus and the anterior perforated substance.
   - projects to the entire neocortex.

Acetylcholine

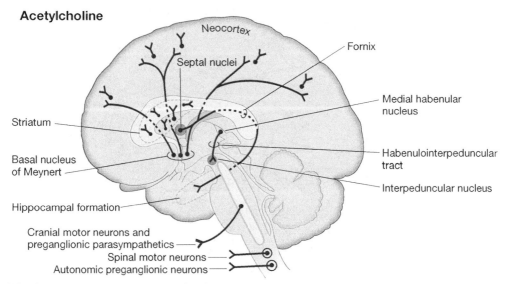

FIGURE 21.3. Distribution of acetylcholine (ACh)-containing neurons and their axonal projections. The basal nucleus of Meynert projects to the entire cortex; this nucleus degenerates in Alzheimer disease. Striatal Ach-local circuit neurons degenerate in Huntington disease.

- receives input from the locus ceruleus, raphe nuclei, substantia nigra, amygdala, and orbitofrontal and temporal cortices.
- degenerates in **Alzheimer disease**.

3. Striatum

- contains ACh in its local circuit neurons.
- has cholinergic neurons that degenerate in **Huntington disease** and **Alzheimer disease**.

4. Neocortex

- contains ACh in its local circuit neurons.

IV. NOREPINEPHRINE (NORADRENALINE)

A. Characteristics

- a catecholamine.
- the transmitter of the postganglionic sympathetic neurons.
- may play a role in the genesis and maintenance of **mood**. The catecholamine hypothesis of affective disorders states that reduced norepinephrine activity is related to **depression** and that increased norepinephrine activity is related to **mania**.

B. Noradrenergic pathways (Figure 21.4)

1. Locus ceruleus

- contains the largest concentration of noradrenergic neurons in the CNS.
- located in the pons and midbrain.
- projects to all parts of the CNS.
- receives input from the cortex, limbic system, reticular formation, raphe nuclei, cerebellum, and spinal cord.

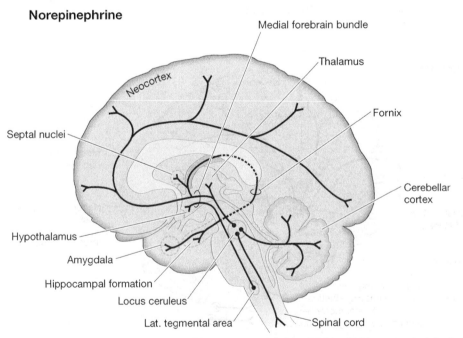

FIGURE 21.4. Distribution of norepinephrine-containing neurons and their projections. The locus ceruleus, located in the pons and midbrain, is the chief source of noradrenergic fibers. The locus ceruleus projects to all parts of the central nervous system.

- shows a significant loss of neurons in Alzheimer and Parkinson diseases.
- modulates levels of arousal, upregulated in threatening/stressful events, has a role in **anxiety** and **panic disorders** in situations of chronic stress.

2. **Lateral tegmental area**
   - located in the medulla and pons.
   - projects via the central tegmental tract and the medial forebrain bundle to the hypothalamus and thalamus.

V. SEROTONIN (5-HYDROXYTRYPTAMINE)

A. Characteristics
- mostly localized to gastrointestinal (GI) tract where it regulates GI motility.
- found in the raphe nuclei of the brainstem—plays a role in pain modulation.
- role in influencing arousal, sensory perception, emotion, mental status (eg, anxiety and mood), and higher cognitive functions.
- tricyclic antidepressants and fluoxetine increase 5-hydroxytryptamine (5-HT) availability by reducing its reuptake.

B. Major serotonergic pathways (Figure 21.5)
- 5-HT neurons are found in the **raphe nuclei** of the brainstem. Raphe nuclei project diffusely to the entire CNS (Figure 21.4).

   1. **Raphe nuclei of the medulla**
      - project to the posterior horns of the spinal cord.
   2. **Raphe nuclei of the pons**
      - project to the spinal cord and cerebellum.
   3. **Raphe nuclei of the midbrain**
      - project to widespread areas of the diencephalon and the telencephalon, including the striatum.

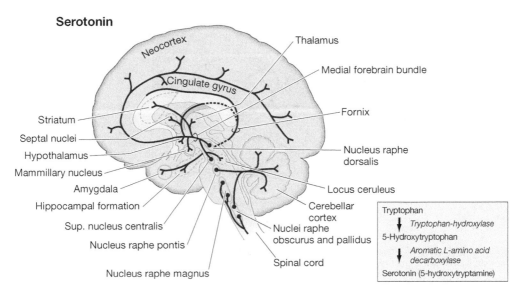

FIGURE 21.5. Distribution of 5-hydroxytryptamine (serotonin)-containing neurons and their projections. Serotonin-containing neurons are found in nuclei of the raphe. They project widely to the forebrain, cerebellum, and spinal cord. The inset shows the synthetic pathway of serotonin.

C. Pineal gland (epiphysis cerebri)

- ▓ contains the highest concentration of 5-HT in the CNS; however, the vast majority (85%–90%) is found in the gut.
- ▓ contains pinealocytes, which convert 5-HT to melatonin.

VI. OPIOID PEPTIDES

A. Endorphins (Figure 21.6)

- ▓ derived from three peptide precursors: (1) **pro-opiomelanocortin**, the precursor of adrenocorticotropic hormone; (2) **proenkephalin**; and (3) **prodynorphin**.
- ▓ include beta-endorphin, the major endorphin found in the brain.
- ▓ endorphinergic neurons are found primarily in the **hypothalamus** (arcuate and premammillary nuclei). These neurons project to the hippocampus, amygdala, nucleus accumbens, septal area, thalamus, and locus ceruleus (midbrain and pons).
- ▓ major role in endocrine function.

B. Enkephalins (Figure 21.7)

- ▓ all three peptide precursors produce enkephalin.
- ▓ the most widely distributed and abundant opioid peptides.
- ▓ found in highest concentrations in the **globus pallidus**.
- ▓ synthesized in striatal neurons, which project to the globus pallidus.
- ▓ located mainly in local circuits of the limbic and striatal systems.
- ▓ coexist with dopamine, norepinephrine, ACh, and GABA.
- ▓ role in **pain suppression** in the posterior horn of the spinal cord.

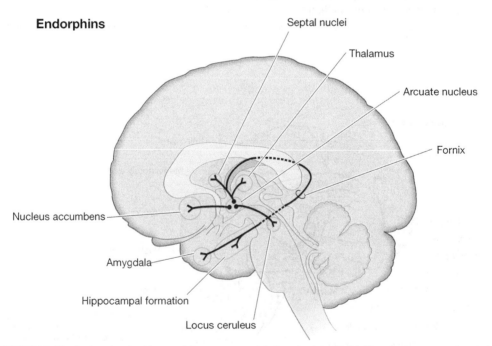

FIGURE 21.6. Distribution of endorphin-containing neurons and their projections. Endorphinergic neurons are found almost exclusively in the hypothalamus (arcuate nucleus).

Enkephalins

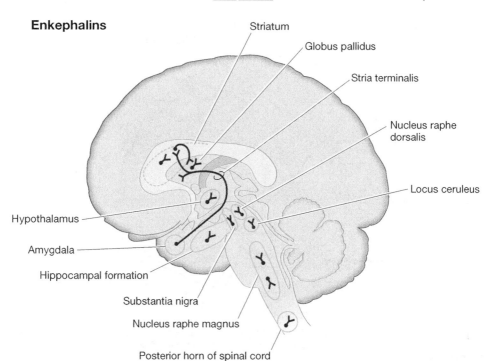

FIGURE 21.7. Distribution of enkephalin-containing neurons and their projections. Enkephalinergic neurons are found primarily in local circuits of the limbic and striatal systems. Enkephalinergic neurons of the brainstem and spinal cord play a role in pain suppression mechanisms.

C. Dynorphins
- derived from **prodynorphin**.
- follow, in general, the distribution map for enkephalin.
- found in high concentrations in the limbic system and **hypothalamus**.

VII. NONOPIOID NEUROPEPTIDES

A. Substance P (Figure 21.8)
- a modulatory neurotransmitter.
- found in spinal ganglion cells, which project to the substantia gelatinosa.
- role in **pain transmission** (in A-delta and C fibers) and inflammatory processes.
- synthesized in striatal neurons, which project to the globus pallidus and the substantia nigra.

B. Somatostatin (Figure 21.9)
- also called somatotropin release-inhibiting factor.
- somatostatinergic neurons are found in the anterior hypothalamus and in the preoptic region, striatum, amygdala, cerebral cortex, and in spinal ganglion cells.
- somatostatinergic neurons from the anterior hypothalamus project their axons to the median eminence.
- involved in endocrine system regulation—somatostatin enters the hypophyseal portal system and regulates the release of growth hormone and thyroid-stimulating hormone.

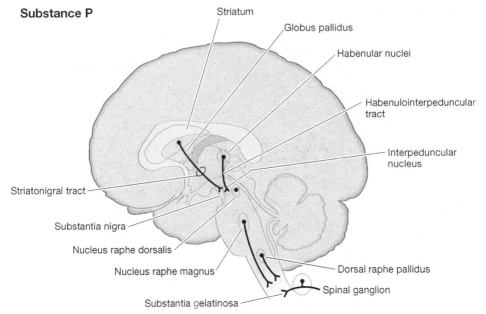

FIGURE 21.8. Distribution of substance P-containing neurons and their projections. Substance P is the neurotransmitter for nociceptive neurons of the spinal ganglia. Striatal substance P neurons project via the striatonigral tract to the substantia nigra.

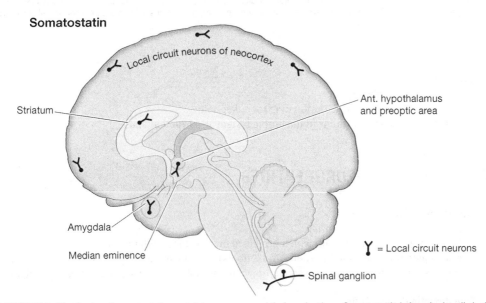

FIGURE 21.9. Distribution of somatostatin-containing neurons and their projections. Somatostatin is found primarily in the anterior hypothalamus and preoptic area. Somatostatinergic neurons project to the hypophyseal portal system and thus regulate the release of growth hormone.

VIII. AMINO ACIDS

A. Inhibitory amino acid transmitters

1. GABA (Figure 21.10)

- can be localized by the marker glutamic acid decarboxylase.
- the major inhibitory neurotransmitter of the brain.

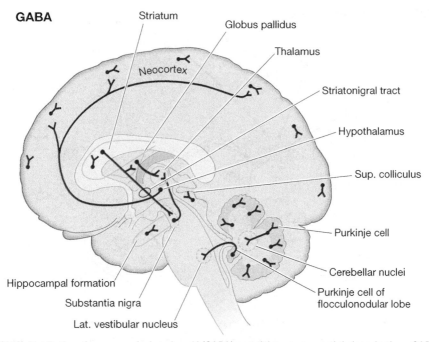

FIGURE 21.10. Distribution of gamma-aminobutyric acid (GABA)-containing neurons and their projections. GABA-ergic neurons are the major inhibitory cells of the central nervous system. GABA local circuit neurons are found in the neocortex, allocortex, and in the cerebellar cortex (Purkinje cells). Striatal GABA-ergic neurons project to the globus pallidus and the substantia nigra. Pallidal GABA-ergic neurons project to the thalamus and the subthalamic nucleus.

- coexists with substance P and with enkephalin.
- Purkinje, stellate, basket, and Golgi cells of the cerebellar cortex are GABA-ergic (see Figure 19.3).
- GABA-ergic striatal neurons project to the globus pallidus and the substantia nigra.
- GABA-ergic pallidal neurons project to the thalamus.
- GABA-ergic nigral neurons project to the thalamus.

2. Glycine
- the major inhibitory neurotransmitter of the spinal cord.
- used by the Renshaw cells of the spinal cord.
- its inhibitory action is blocked by strychnine.

B. Excitatory amino acid neurotransmitters

1. Glutamate (Figure 21.11)
- major excitatory neurotransmitter of the brain; 60% of brain synapses are glutamatergic.
- the neurotransmitter of the cerebellar granule cell.
- used by the corticobulbar and corticospinal tracts.
- used by spinal ganglion cells.
- believed to be involved in long-term potentiation of hippocampal neurons via N-methyl-D-aspartate receptors.
- role in kindling-induced seizures.
- role in **pain transmission** (in A-delta and C fibers).
- neocortical glutamatergic neurons project to the striatum, the subthalamic nucleus, and the thalamus. The subthalamic nucleus projects glutamatergic fibers to the globus pallidus.

2. Aspartate (see Figure 21.11)
- a major excitatory neurotransmitter of the brain.
- neurotransmitter of the climbing fibers of the cerebellum.

Glutamate and aspartate

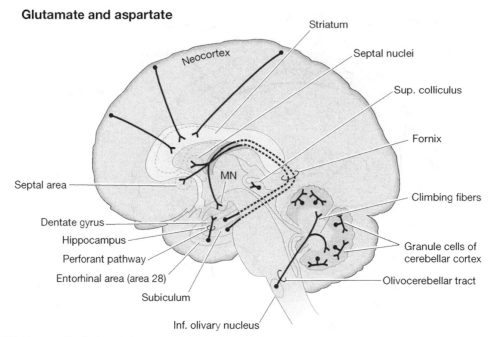

FIGURE 21.11. Distribution of glutamate- and aspartate-containing neurons and their projections. Glutamate is considered the major excitatory transmitter of the central nervous system. Cortical glutamatergic neurons project to the striatum; hippocampal and subicular glutamatergic neurons project via the fornix to the septal area and hypothalamus. Neurons of the inferior olivary nucleus project aspartatergic fibers to the cerebellum. The granule cells of the cerebellum are glutamatergic. MN, mammillary nucleus.

IX. NITRIC OXIDE

▦ a gaseous neurotransmitter that is produced when nitric oxide synthase converts arginine to citrulline.
▦ located in the olfactory system, striatum, cortex, hippocampal formation, supraoptic nucleus of the hypothalamus, and cerebellum.
▦ responsible for the smooth muscle relaxation of the corpus cavernosum and thus penile erection.
▦ believed to play a role in memory formation (long-term potentiation in the hippocampal formation).

X. FUNCTIONAL AND CLINICAL CONSIDERATIONS

A. Endogenous pain control system
1. Ascending pathway
▦ spinoreticular pain impulses project to the periaqueductal gray of the midbrain.
2. Descending raphespinal pathway
▦ excitatory neurons of the periaqueductal gray project to the nucleus raphe magnus of the pons.
▦ excitatory neurons of the nucleus raphe magnus project serotonergic fibers to enkephalinergic inhibitory neurons of the substantia gelatinosa.
▦ enkephalinergic neurons of the substantia gelatinosa inhibit afferent pain fibers (substance P) and tract neurons that give rise to the spinoreticular and spinothalamic tracts.

3. **Descending ceruleospinal pathway**
   - projects from the locus ceruleus to the spinal cord.
   - inhibits tract neurons that give rise to ascending pain pathways.

B. **Parkinson disease**
   - results from **degeneration of dopaminergic neurons** found in the pars compacta of the substantia nigra, which results in **reduction of dopamine** in the striatum and in the substantia nigra.
   - results in resting tremor, bradykinesia, postural instability (shuffling gait), and rigidity.

C. **Huntington disease (Huntington chorea)**
   - results from **loss of ACh- and GABA-containing neurons** in the striatum (caudatoputamen).
   - results in **loss of GABA** in the striatum and substantia nigra.

D. **Lambert-Eaton myasthenic syndrome**
   - caused by a presynaptic defect of ACh release.
   - results in weakness in the limb muscles but not in the bulbar muscles. Muscle strength improves with use, unlike in myasthenia gravis, where muscle use results in fatigue.
   - associated with neoplasms (eg, lung, breast, prostate) in 50% of cases.
   - leads to autonomic dysfunction, with dry mouth, constipation, impotence, and urinary incontinence.

CLINICAL CORRELATES Alzheimer disease is the most common type of dementia, affecting approximately 6 million individuals in the United States, most of whom are older than 65 years. It is a progressive disease characterized primarily by memory problems and cognitive impairment. Caused by a combination of factors, including age-related changes in the brain (eg, amyloid plaques, neurofibrillary and tau tangles, and the degeneration of neurons in the basal nucleus of Meynert) and genetic and environmental factors.

CLINICAL CORRELATES Myasthenia gravis is an autoimmune disease that occurs in the presence of antibodies to the nicotinic ACh receptor. It is caused by the action of antibodies that reduce the number of receptors in the neuromuscular junction resulting in muscle paresis. Myasthenia gravis is most common in women younger than 40 years and men older than 60 years. It involves the extraocular and eyelid muscles (eg, in diplopia, ptosis) and bulbar muscles (eg, in nasal speech, jaw fatigue) and leads to weaker limbs proximally and stronger limbs distally. It may be diagnosed with intravenous edrophonium and can be effectively treated with thymectomy, followed by corticosteroid therapy.

Review Test

Questions 1 to 19

The response options for items 1 to 19 are the same. Select one answer for each item in the set.

(A) Ach
(B) Aspartate
(C) Beta-endorphin
(D) Dopamine
(E) Endorphin
(F) Enkephalin
(G) Epinephrine
(H) GABA
(I) Glutamate
(J) Glycine
(K) Nitric oxide
(L) Norepinephrine
(M) Serotonin
(N) Somatostatin
(O) Substance P

Match each of the statements with the neurotransmitter it best describes.

1. Its highest CNS concentration is found in the pineal gland

2. Is found in pseudounipolar ganglion cells and in the substantia gelatinosa

3. Is responsible for the smooth muscle relaxation of the corpus cavernosum and thus penile erection

4. Is produced by neurons found in the locus ceruleus

5. Is the neurotransmitter of the corticostriatal pathway

6. Is produced by neurons of the raphe nuclei

7. Is the neurotransmitter of the climbing fibers of the cerebellum

8. Low levels are associated with severe depression and insomnia.

9. Is produced by neurons found in the basal nucleus of Meynert

10. Is produced almost exclusively in the hypothalamus

11. A reduction of postsynaptic receptor sites for this neurotransmitter causes myasthenia gravis.

12. Is the neurotransmitter of the Renshaw cells

13. Striatal levels of this neurotransmitter are reduced in Huntington disease.

14. Is the neurotransmitter of the Purkinje cells

15. Is the neurotransmitter of the cerebellar granule cell

16. Is found in high concentration in the pars compacta of the substantia nigra and in the ventral tegmental area of the mesencephalon

17. Is the neurotransmitter of the mesolimbic pathway

18. Inhibits the release of prolactin from the adenohypophysis

19. Is the main neurotransmitter of the pallido-thalamic and nigrothalamic tracts

Questions 20 to 24

The response options for items 20 to 24 are the same. Select one answer for each item in the set.

(A) Alzheimer disease
(B) Huntington disease
(C) Lambert-Eaton myasthenic syndrome
(D) Myasthenia gravis
(E) Parkinson disease

Match each of the cases with the disorder it best describes.

20. A 60-year-old man presents to his primary care physician for ongoing evaluation of a resting tremor in his right upper limb that has progressively worsened over the past 3 years. He recently had a positron emission tomography scan using a radioactive marker, which showed a reduction of levodopa metabolism. This reduction was likely caused by dopaminergic neuronal death. What is the most likely diagnosis for this patient?

21. A 25-year-old woman presents to her primary care physician with a chief complaint of difficulty swallowing and weakness in her hands and fingers. A blood test reveals antibodies to the nicotinic ACh receptor. What is the most likely diagnosis for this patient?

22. A brain autopsy of an 85-year-old woman reveals neurofibrillary tangles and neuritic plaques. What is the most likely diagnosis for this patient?

23. A 53-year-old man presents to his primary care physician with a complaint of weakness in his arms and legs but notes that his muscle strength seems to improve when exercising. He is a long-time smoker and also complains of dry mouth and constipation. A chest radiograph reveals a mass in the left lung. What is the most likely diagnosis for this patient?

24. A 45-year-old man presents to his primary care physician with a chief complaint that he has been experiencing jerky, uncontrollable movements. He reports having noticed similar symptoms for the past few years but notes that the symptoms seem to be getting worse. His family history reveals that his father had some of the same symptoms prior to his death in an automobile accident. The magnetic resonance imaging scan shows cell loss in the caudatoputamen. What is the most likely diagnosis for this patient?

25. A 78-year-old woman presents to her primary care physician with progressively worsening symptoms of Alzheimer disease, particularly memory loss. Previous imaging revealed degeneration of the basal nucleus of Meynert, leading to low levels of which neurotransmitter in this patient?

(A) Acetylcholine
(B) Dopamine
(C) Glutamate
(D) Norepinephrine
(E) Serotonin

26. A 30-year-old woman with previously diagnosed multiple sclerosis presents to her primary care physician to address new and worsening symptoms. Patient interview reveals that the patient has been feeling more depressed and lethargic as of late and reports feeling dizzy when standing from a seated position. Based on the patient's symptoms, imaging is most likely to reveal a sclerotic plaque affecting which of the following?

(A) Basal nucleus of Meynert
(B) Globus pallidus
(C) Locus ceruleus
(D) Pontine raphe nuclei
(E) Substantia nigra

27. _____ is the major excitatory neurotransmitter in the brain.

(A) Ach
(B) Aspartate
(C) GABA
(D) Glutamate
(E) Glycine

28. The major inhibitory neurotransmitter in the brain is _____.

(A) GABA
(B) nitric oxide
(C) serotonin
(D) somatostatin
(E) substance P

Answers and Explanations

1. **M.** The highest concentration of serotonin in the CNS is found in the pineal body (epiphysis cerebri). Pinealocytes convert 5-HT to melatonin. The vast majority of serotonin in the body is found in the gut.

2. **O.** Substance P is the neurotransmitter of pain fibers and is found in pseudounipolar ganglion cells and in the substantia gelatinosa of the spinal cord. Substance P is also found in the caudal part of the spinal trigeminal tract.

3. **K.** Nitric oxide is responsible for the smooth muscle relaxation of the corpus cavernosum and thus penile erection.

4. **L.** The highest concentration of norepinephrinergic neurons is found in the locus ceruleus.

5. **I.** Glutamate is the neurotransmitter of the corticostriatal pathway.

6. **M.** Serotonin is produced by neurons of the raphe nuclei of the brainstem.

7. **B.** Aspartate is the neurotransmitter of the climbing fibers of the cerebellum.

8. **M.** Low levels of 5-HT are associated with severe depression and insomnia.

9. **A.** ACh is found in highest concentration in the basal nucleus of Meynert, between the anterior perforated substance and the globus pallidus, a forebrain nucleus.

10. **E.** Endorphin is produced almost exclusively in the hypothalamus (arcuate nucleus).

11. **A.** In myasthenia gravis, there is a reduced ACh receptor concentration in the motor end plate owing to an autoimmune reaction directed against the receptor proteins.

12. **J.** Glycine is the major inhibitory neurotransmitter of the spinal cord; glycine is used by Renshaw cells, inhibitory interneurons driven by axon collaterals of lower motor neurons.

13. **H.** Striatal levels of GABA are greatly reduced in Huntington disease. This attrition of GABA-ergic neurons in the head of the caudate nucleus results in hydrocephalus ex vacuo.

14. **H.** GABA is the neurotransmitter of the Purkinje cells.

15. **I.** Glutamate is the neurotransmitter of the cerebellar granule cells.

16. **D.** Dopamine is found in high concentration in the pars compacta of the substantia nigra and in the ventral tegmental area of the mesencephalon.

17. **D.** Dopamine is the neurotransmitter of the mesolimbic pathway. This pathway is linked to behavior and schizophrenia.

18. **D.** Dopamine inhibits the release of prolactin from the adenohypophysis. Dopaminergic neurons are found in the arcuate nucleus of the hypothalamus.

19. **H.** GABA, the most common inhibitory neurotransmitter of the brain, is the main neurotransmitter of the pallidothalamic and nigrothalamic tracts.

20. **E.** Parkinson disease results from degeneration of dopaminergic neurons found in the pars compacta of the substantia nigra. Although Parkinson disease is typically diagnosed based on neurologic symptoms, a positron emission tomography scan with radioactive labeling can sometimes be used as a diagnostic tool.

21. **D.** Myasthenia gravis is an autoimmune syndrome whose symptoms usually include the presence of antibodies to the nicotinic ACh receptor. Other symptoms include muscle paresis, diplopia, ptosis, jaw fatigue, and weak proximal limbs.

22. **A.** Alzheimer disease is characterized histologically by the presence of neurofibrillary tangles, senile (neuritic) plaques, granulovacuolar degeneration, and Hirano bodies. This disease results from the degeneration of cortical neurons and cholinergic neurons found in the basal nucleus of Meynert. It is also associated with a 60% to 90% loss of choline acetyltransferase in the cerebral cortex.

23. **C.** Lambert-Eaton myasthenic syndrome is an autoimmune syndrome caused by a presynaptic defect of ACh release. It results in weakness in limb muscles, and muscle strength improves with use. It is associated with neoplasms (eg, lung, breast, prostate) in 50% of cases.

24. **B.** Huntington disease is a hereditary disorder that results from a loss of ACh- and GABA-containing neurons in the striatum. Some symptoms include jerky, random, uncontrollable, rapid (choreiform) movements; slowness of saccadic eye movements; and progressive dementia.

25. **A.** The basal nucleus of Meynert produces acetylcholine, low levels of which are associated with Alzheimer disease. Dopamine is produced in the substantia nigra and ventral tegmental areas of the brain. Glutamate is produced through a recycling process involving the glial cells of the brain. Norepinephrine is primarily produced by the locus ceruleus in the brain. In the brain, serotonin is produced in the raphe nuclei; however, most serotonin in the body is produced in the gut.

26. **C.** Low norepinephrine would explain the lethargy and blood pressure/dizziness in this patient. A sclerotic plaque affecting the locus ceruleus would cause depressed levels of norepinephrine. The basal nucleus of Meynert produces acetylcholine, and the lack of acetylcholine would not produce the symptoms seen in this patient. The globus pallidus does contain high concentrations of enkephalin, but that is mostly involved with pain suppression. The raphe nuclei are serotonin producers and are also involved with pain suppression. The substantia nigra produces dopamine, the lack of which produces movement symptoms, such as Parkinson disease.

27. **D.** Glutamate is the major excitatory neurotransmitter; 60% of brain synapses are glutamatergic.

28. **A.** GABA is the major inhibitory neurotransmitter and can be localized by using glutamic acid decarboxylase as a marker.

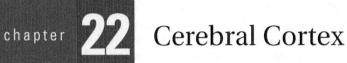

Objectives

- Differentiate between neocortex and allocortex.
- List the six layers of neocortex and the characterizing feature of each.
- List the major functional areas of the cerebral cortex with their Brodmann areas, including sensory areas, motor areas, and higher association areas.
- Describe cortical dominance.
- Describe the blood flow to the major cortical areas.
- Define the various types of apraxia, aphasia, and dysprosodies.

I. OVERVIEW

- contains 20 billion nerve cells.
- consists of the neocortex (90%) and the allocortex (10%).

A. Neocortex (isocortex; homogenetic cortex)
- six-layered cortex.

B. Allocortex (heterogenetic cortex)
1. Archicortex
   - three-layered, includes two types:
2. Paleocortex
   - includes the hippocampus and the dentate gyrus.
   - includes the olfactory cortex.

II. NEOCORTEX

- the six layers of neocortex are expressed as roman numerals I through VI.

A. Molecular layer (I)
- the superficial layer deep to the pia mater.

B. External granular layer (II)

C. External pyramidal layer (III)
- gives rise to association and commissural fibers.

D. Internal granular layer (IV)

- receives thalamocortical fibers from the thalamic nuclei of the ventral tier (eg, ventral postero-lateral [VPL] and ventral posteromedial [VPM] nuclei).
- in the striate cortex (area 17), receives input from the lateral geniculate body.
- myelinated fibers of this layer form the line (stria) of Gennari—visible to the naked eye.

E. Internal pyramidal layer (V)

- gives rise to corticobulbar, corticospinal, and corticostriatal fibers.
- contains the giant cells of Betz that are found only in the motor cortex (area 4) of the precentral gyrus and the anterior paracentral lobule.

F. Multiform layer (VI)

- the deepest layer of the cortex. It gives rise to projection, commissural, and association fibers.
- the major source of corticothalamic fibers.

III. FUNCTIONAL AREAS OF THE CEREBRAL CORTEX (FIGURE 22.1)

- divided into 47 cytoarchitectural areas, the **Brodmann areas**.

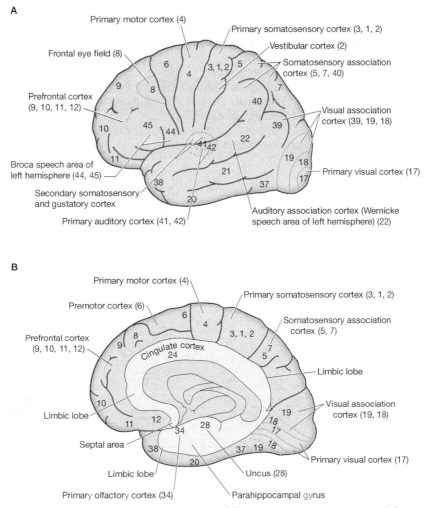

FIGURE 22.1. Motor and sensory areas of the cerebral cortex. **(A)** Lateral surface of the hemisphere. **(B)** Medial surface of the hemisphere. The numbers refer to the Brodmann areas.

A. Sensory areas

1. Primary somatosensory cortex (areas 3, 1, and 2)

- located in the **postcentral gyrus** and in the posterior part of the **paracentral lobule**.
- receives input from the ventral posterior nuclei of the thalamus.
- somatotopically organized as the **sensory homunculus** (Figure 22.2A).
- stimulation results in contralateral numbness and tingling (paresthesia).
- destruction results in a contralateral loss of tactile discrimination (**hypesthesia** and **astereognosis**) and a loss of ability to localize sensation.

2. Secondary somatosensory cortex

- lies ventral to the primary somatosensory area along the superior bank of the lateral sulcus.

3. Somatosensory association cortex

- Superior parietal lobule (areas 5 and 7)
    - **a.** receives input from areas 3, 1, and 2. Area 7 receives visual input from area 19.
    - **b.** destruction results in **contralateral loss of tactile discrimination**, **stereognosis** (the ability to recognize form), and **statognosis** (the ability to recognize the position of body parts in space). Destruction also leads to neglect of events occurring in the contralateral portion of the external world.
- Supramarginal gyrus (area 40)
    - **a.** interrelates somatosensory, auditory, and visual input (multimodal sensory stimuli).
    - **b.** destruction in the dominant hemisphere may result in the following deficits:
        - Ideomotor or "classic" apraxia
            - **(1)** the inability to button one's clothes or comb one's hair when asked.
            - **(2)** the inability to manipulate tools, with retention of the ability to explain their use.
        - Ideational or sensory apraxia
            - **(1)** characterized by the inability to formulate the ideational plan for executing the several components of a complex multistep act (eg, performing the steps of tying a shoe when asked to do so).
            - **(2)** occurs most frequently in diffuse cerebral degenerating disease, Alzheimer disease, and multi-infarct dementia.

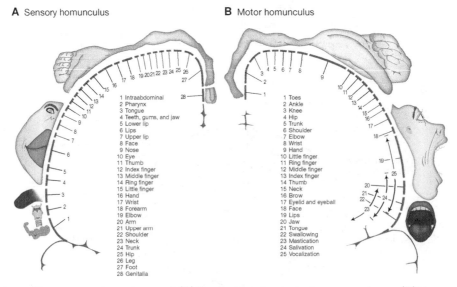

A Sensory homunculus

B Motor homunculus

1	Intraabdominal
2	Pharynx
3	Tongue
4	Teeth, gums, and jaw
5	Lower lip
6	Lips
7	Upper lip
8	Face
9	Nose
10	Eye
11	Thumb
12	Index finger
13	Middle finger
14	Ring finger
15	Little finger
16	Hand
17	Wrist
18	Forearm
19	Elbow
20	Arm
21	Upper arm
22	Shoulder
23	Neck
24	Trunk
25	Hip
26	Leg
27	Foot
28	Genitalia

1	Toes
2	Ankle
3	Knee
4	Hip
5	Trunk
6	Shoulder
7	Elbow
8	Wrist
9	Hand
10	Little finger
11	Ring finger
12	Middle finger
13	Index finger
14	Thumb
15	Neck
16	Brow
17	Eyelid and eyeball
18	Face
19	Lips
20	Jaw
21	Tongue
22	Swallowing
23	Mastication
24	Salivation
25	Vocalization

FIGURE 22.2. The sensory and motor homunculi. **(A)** Sensory representation in the postcentral gyrus. **(B)** Motor representation in the precentral gyrus. (Modified from Penfield W, Rasmussen T. *The Cerebral Cortex of Man*. Hafner Publishing; 1968:44, 57.)

▣ Facial apraxia

(1) the inability to perform facial-oral movements on command (eg, lick the lips); the most common apraxia.

▣ Conduction aphasia

(1) associated with poor repetition of spoken language (results from interruption of the arcuate fasciculus; see III C 4).

4. **Primary visual cortex (area 17)**
   ▣ located in the occipital lobe along both banks of the calcarine sulcus.
   ▣ receives input from the lateral geniculate body.
   ▣ destruction results in **visual field deficits** (eg, contralateral homonymous hemianopia) (see Figure 16.2).

5. **Secondary and tertiary visual cortices**
   ▣ include areas 18 and 19 of the occipital lobe.
   ▣ lesions may result in **visual hallucinations**.

6. **Visual association cortex (angular gyrus [area 39])**
   ▣ receives input from areas 18 and 19.
   ▣ destruction of the underlying optic radiation (retrolenticular fasciculus of the internal capsule) results in **contralateral homonymous hemianopia** or **lower quadrantanopia**.
   ▣ destruction in the dominant hemisphere results in **Gerstmann syndrome** with the following deficits:
   a. Right-left confusion
   b. Finger agnosia (inability to recognize, name, or select one's own or another's fingers)
   c. Agraphia (inability to express thoughts in writing with possible retention of the ability to copy written or printed words; often coexists with alexia)
   d. Dyscalculia (difficulty with arithmetic)

7. **Primary auditory cortex (areas 41 and 42)**
   ▣ located in the superior temporal gyrus on the transverse gyrus (of Heschl).
   ▣ receives input from the medial geniculate body.
   ▣ unilateral destruction results in only **partial deafness** (owing to bilateral cochlear representation).

8. **Auditory association cortex (area 22)**
   ▣ located in the posterior part of the superior temporal gyrus.
   ▣ includes the sensory **speech area**.
   ▣ includes the **planum temporale** (part of the sensory speech area), which is larger in the dominant hemisphere.
   ▣ lesion in the dominant hemisphere results in **sensory aphasia**.
   ▣ lesion in the nondominant hemisphere results in **sensory dysprosody** (inability to perceive the pitch or rhythm of speech).

9. **Gustatory cortex (area 43)**
   ▣ located in the parietal operculum and parainsular cortex.
   ▣ receives taste input from the VPM nucleus of the thalamus.

10. **Vestibular cortex (area 2)**
    ▣ located in the postcentral gyrus.
    ▣ receives input from the ventral posteroinferior and the VPL nuclei of the thalamus.

B. **Motor areas**
   1. **Primary motor cortex (area 4)**
      ▣ located in the **precentral gyrus** and in the anterior part of the **paracentral lobule**.
      ▣ contributes to the corticospinal tract.
      ▣ somatotopically organized as the **motor homunculus** (see Figure 22.2B).
      ▣ contains the giant cells of Betz in layer V.
      ▣ stimulation results in contralateral movements of voluntary muscles, especially distal muscles of the limbs; ablation results in a **contralateral upper motor neuron (UMN) lesion**.

contains UMNs of the somatic motor neuron nuclei of the brainstem and the anterior horn of the spinal cord.

bilateral lesions of the paracentral lobule (eg, parasagittal meningiomas) result in **urinary incontinence**, owing to the bilateral innervation of the sphincters.

2. **Premotor cortex (area 6)**

located anterior to the precentral gyrus.

contributes to the corticospinal tract.

plays a role in the **control of proximal** and **axial muscles**; prepares the motor cortex for specific movements in advance of their execution.

stimulation results in adversive movements of the head and trunk and flexion and extension of the limbs.

lesions in the dominant hemisphere may cause **sympathetic apraxia** (motor apraxia in the left hand).

3. **Supplementary motor cortex (area 6)**

located on the medial surface of the hemisphere anterior to the paracentral lobule.

contributes to the corticospinal tract.

plays a role in **programming complex motor sequences** and in **coordinating bilateral movements**; it regulates the somatosensory input into the motor cortex.

stimulation results in vocalization with associated facial movements and coordinated movements of the limbs.

ablation in human subjects has resulted in transient **speech deficits** or **aphasias**.

bilateral lesions result in **hypertonus of the flexor muscles** without paralysis.

4. **Frontal eye field (area 8)**

located in the posterior part of the middle frontal gyrus.

projects via the corticotectobulbar tract to the contralateral lateral gaze center of the pons (abducens nucleus).

stimulation (irritative lesion) results in conjugate deviation of the eyes to the opposite side.

destructive lesions result in conjugate deviation of the eyes toward the side of the lesion.

C. **Areas of higher cortical function**

1. **Prefrontal cortex (areas 9-12)**

Characteristics of the prefrontal cortex

a. extends from area 6 to the frontal pole (area 10).

b. has reciprocal connections with the dorsomedial nucleus of the thalamus.

Frontal lobe syndrome (Phineas Gage syndrome)

a. results from lesions of the prefrontal cortex.

b. results in the following signs:

inappropriate social behavior—lesions usually involve the fronto-orbital prefrontal cortex.

difficulty in adaptation and loss of initiative—lesions involve the dorsolateral prefrontal cortex.

sucking, groping, and grasping movements.

gait apraxia, incontinence, abulia (loss of the ability to perform voluntary actions), or akinetic mutism (a coma-like state called coma vigil)—these signs result from bilateral disease.

2. **Motor (Broca) speech area (areas 44 and 45)** (Figure 22.3)

Characteristics of the motor speech area

a. located in the posterior part of the inferior frontal gyrus in the dominant hemisphere.

b. connected to the sensory speech area by the arcuate fasciculus.

Motor (Broca) aphasia

a. results from lesions in the motor speech area.

b. also called **motor, expressive, nonfluent**, or **anterior aphasia**.

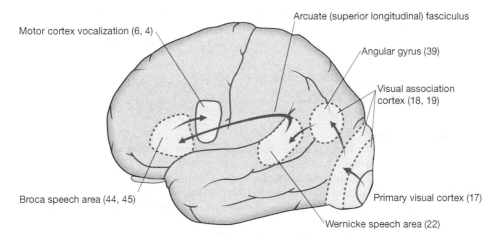

Motor cortex vocalization (6, 4)

Arcuate (superior longitudinal) fasciculus

Angular gyrus (39)

Visual association cortex (18, 19)

Broca speech area (44, 45)

Primary visual cortex (17)

Wernicke speech area (22)

FIGURE 22.3. Cortical areas of the dominant hemisphere that play an important role in language production. The visual image of a word is projected from the visual cortex (area 17) to the visual association cortices (areas 18 and 19) and then to the angular gyrus (area 39). Further processing occurs in the sensory speech area (area 22), where the auditory form of the word is recalled. Via the arcuate fasciculus, this information reaches the motor speech area (areas 44 and 45), where motor speech programs control the vocalization mechanisms of the precentral gyrus. Lesions of the motor or sensory speech areas or the arcuate fasciculus result in dysphasias.

    c. causes patients to speak slowly (nonfluent) and with effort; however, they have intact comprehension of spoken and written language.

    d. frequently accompanied by **contralateral weakness of the lower face and arm** and a **sympathetic apraxia** of the left hand (the inability to write with the nonparalyzed hand).

3. Sensory (Wernicke) speech area (area 22) (see Figure 22.3)

    ▦ Characteristics of the sensory speech area

      a. located in the posterior part of the superior temporal gyrus in the dominant hemisphere.

      b. connected to the motor speech area by the arcuate fasciculus.

    ▦ Sensory (Wernicke) aphasia

      a. results from lesions in the dominant hemisphere.

      b. also called **sensory, receptive, fluent,** or **posterior aphasia**.

      c. patients have poor comprehension of speech, speak faster than normal, and have difficulty in finding the right words to express themselves. They may be unaware of the deficit.

4. Arcuate fasciculus

    ▦ Characteristics of the arcuate fasciculus

      a. underlies the supramarginal gyrus (area 40) and the frontoparietal operculum.

      b. connects the audiovisual association areas (areas 22, 39, and 40) with the motor speech area (areas 44 and 45).

    ▦ Conduction aphasia

      a. results from transection of the arcuate fasciculus.

      b. a **fluent aphasia** associated with poor repetition of spoken language. Speech comprehension and expression are relatively intact.

      c. **paraphasic errors** (using incorrect words) are common, and **object naming is impaired** (nominal aphasia or amnestic aphasia). Patients are aware of the deficit.

5. Corpus callosum

    ▦ interconnects corresponding hemispheric areas.

    ▦ damage results in split-brain syndrome (see section on Split-Brain Syndrome and Figure 22.5)

- does not contain commissural fibers from the hand region of the motor or sensory strips, or from the striate cortex.
- receives its blood supply from the anterior and posterior cerebral arteries.

IV. CEREBRAL DOMINANCE

A. Dominant hemisphere

- responsible for propositional language consisting of grammar, syntax, and semantics.
- also responsible for speech and calculation.
- the left hemisphere is dominant in 95% of people.
  1. Lesions of the dominant superior parietal lobule (Figure 22.4A)
     - result in contralateral loss of sensory discrimination (**astereognosis**; ie, loss of posterior column modalities; area 5).
     - result in contralateral sensory neglect (area 7).
  2. Lesions of the dominant inferior parietal lobule (see Figure 22.4A)
     - involve the supramarginal and angular gyri (areas 40 and 39).
     - result in the following conditions:
       a. Receptive aphasia
       b. Gerstmann syndrome
       c. Alexia with agraphia (often coexists with Gerstmann syndrome)
       d. Tactile agnosia
       e. Ideomotor apraxia
       f. Ideational apraxia

B. Nondominant hemisphere

- primarily responsible for three-dimensional or spatial perception and nonverbal ideation (music and poetry).
  1. **Lesions of the nondominant superior parietal lobule** (see Figure 22.4B)
     - result in **contralateral loss of sensory discrimination** (ie, loss of posterior column modalities; area 5).
     - result in **contralateral neglect** (area 7).
  2. **Lesions of the nondominant inferior parietal lobule**
     - involve the supramarginal and angular gyri.
     - result in the following conditions:
       a. Left-sided hemineglect
          - results in a lack of awareness of the left half of space or the left half of the body.
          - results in hemi-inattention or extinction.
       b. Topographic memory loss
          - results in the inability to negotiate familiar surroundings.
       c. Anosognosia (denial of deficit)
          - results in indifference to the causal disease (eg, hemiparesis or hemianopia).
       d. Constructional apraxia
          - results in the inability to draw simple designs (eg, cross, star, or clock); the left side of the design is omitted.
          - may also occur in lesions of the dominant hemisphere.
       e. Dressing apraxia
          - results in the inability to dress oneself.
  3. **Lesions of the nondominant inferior frontal gyrus (areas 44 and 45)**
     - correspond to the motor speech area and result in **expressive dysprosody** (the inability to articulate the pitch and rhythm of speech).
  4. **Lesions of the nondominant superior temporal gyrus (area 22)**
     - correspond to the sensory speech area and result in **receptive dysprosody** (the inability to perceive pitch and rhythm of speech).

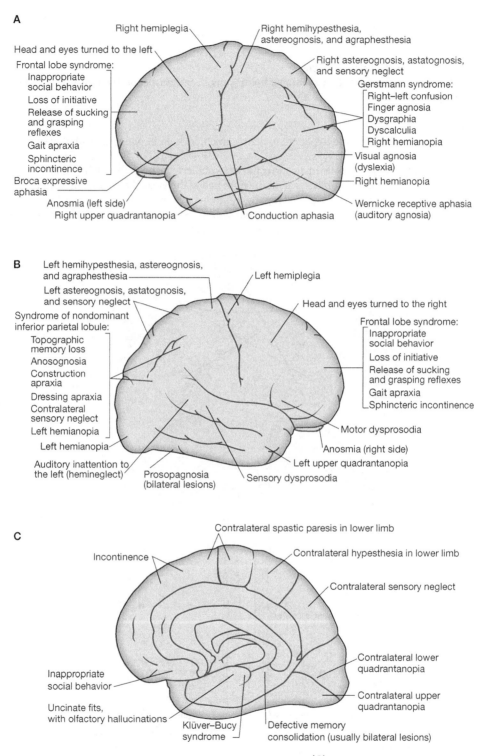

FIGURE 22.4. Focal destructive hemispheric lesions and resulting symptoms. **(A)** Lateral convex surface of the dominant left hemisphere. **(B)** Lateral convex surface of the nondominant right hemisphere. **(C)** Medial surface of the nondominant hemisphere. (Modified with permission from Fix JD. *High-Yield Neuroanatomy.* 3rd ed. Lippincott Williams & Wilkins; 2005:161.)

V. SPLIT-BRAIN SYNDROME (Figure 22.5)

A. Description of split-brain syndrome
- represents a **disconnection syndrome** that results from transection (commissurotomy) of the corpus callosum.

B. Deficits
1. inability of a blindfolded patient to match an object held in one hand with that held in the other hand.
2. inability, when blindfolded, to correctly name objects placed in the left hand (**anomia**).
3. inability to match an object seen in the right half of the visual field with one seen in the left half (the test must be performed rapidly to eliminate bilateral visual scanning).
4. **alexia** in the left visual fields (the verbal symbols seen in the right visual cortex have no access to the language centers of the left hemisphere).

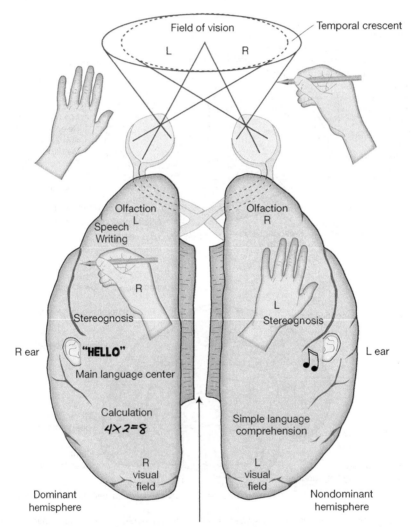

FIGURE 22.5. Functions of the split brain after transection of the corpus callosum. Tactile and visual perception is projected to the contralateral hemisphere, olfaction is perceived on the same side, and audition is perceived predominantly in the opposite hemisphere. The left hemisphere is dominant for language, and the right hemisphere is dominant for spatial construction and nonverbal ideation. (Modified 4th ed. with permission from Noback CR, Demarest RJ. *The Human Nervous System.* Williams & Wilkins; 1991:416.)

VI. BLOOD SUPPLY TO THE MAJOR FUNCTIONAL CORTICAL AREAS

▧ only **cortical branches** are discussed in this section.

A. **Anterior cerebral artery (see Figure 3.3)**
   1. **Territory of the anterior cerebral artery**
      ▧ supplies the medial aspect of the hemisphere.
   2. **Occlusion: affected areas and deficits**
      ▧ Paracentral lobule
      a. contralateral somatosensory loss in the lower limb with paresthesia, numbness, and apallesthesia (loss of vibratory sense).
      b. contralateral weakness and hyperreflexia in the lower limb with Babinski sign.
      c. urinary incontinence with bilateral infarction.
      ▧ Corpus callosum: infarction
      a. dyspraxia and tactile agnosia of the left limbs.

B. **Middle cerebral artery (see Figure 3.4)**
   1. **Territory of the middle cerebral artery**
      ▧ supplies the lateral surface of the hemisphere.
   2. **Occlusion: affected areas and deficits**
      ▧ Frontal lobe
      a. Precentral gyrus
         ▧ contralateral facial weakness and weakness in the upper limb.
      b. Frontal eye field
         ▧ conjugate deviation of the eyes to the affected side.
      c. Prefrontal cortex
         ▧ affects judgment, insight, and mood (frontal lobe syndrome).
      d. Inferior frontal gyrus of the dominant side
         ▧ motor aphasia and contralateral weakness of the lower face and arm.
         ▧ sympathetic apraxia of the left hand.
      ▧ Temporal lobe
      a. Transverse temporal gyri (of Heschl)
         ▧ deafness with bilateral destruction.
      b. Superior temporal gyrus of the dominant side
         ▧ sensory aphasia.
      c. Superior and middle temporal gyri (superolateral parts)
         ▧ auditory illusions and hallucinations.
      ▧ Parietal lobe
      a. Postcentral gyrus and superior parietal lobule
         ▧ loss of sensory discrimination and stereognosis.
         ▧ hemineglect (may occur with either left or right parietal lesions).
      b. Inferior parietal lobule of the dominant hemisphere
         ▧ ideomotor and ideational apraxia.
         ▧ Gerstmann syndrome.
      c. Inferior parietal lobule of the nondominant hemisphere
         ▧ hemineglect syndrome.
         ▧ topographic memory loss, anosognosia, and constructional and dressing apraxia.

C. **Posterior cerebral artery (see Figure 3.5)**
   1. **Territory of the posterior cerebral artery**
      ▧ supplies the occipital lobe, the inferior aspect of the temporal lobe (excluding the temporal pole), and the splenium of the corpus callosum.
   2. **Occlusion: affected areas and deficits**
      ▧ Occipital lobe: visual cortex (striate and extrastriate)
      a. if bilateral, cortical blindness (pupils are reactive to light).
      b. contralateral homonymous hemianopia with macular sparing.

    ◼ Temporal lobe (inferomedial aspect): hippocampal formation and amygdale
        a. also perfused by the anterior choroidal artery.
        b. if bilateral or in the dominant hemisphere, memory deficit (amnesia).
        c. incapacity to create and store new long-term memories; the patient retains and may recall long-term memories.
    ◼ Occipitotemporal region (inferomedial aspect)
        a. bilateral lesions may result in **prosopagnosia** (the inability to identify a familiar face) and **achromatopsia** (acquired color blindness).

D. Left posterior cerebral artery

1. Territory of the left posterior cerebral artery

    ◼ supplies the splenium of the corpus callosum and the left visual cortex.

2. Occlusion

    ◼ results in **infarction** of the splenium of the corpus callosum and the left visual cortex; visual input from the right visual cortex cannot reach the parietal language centers of the dominant hemisphere.
    ◼ may cause **alexia without agraphia and aphasia**; because the left inferior parietal lobule and the sensory speech area are intact, the patient can write and is not dysphasic.

E. Jacksonian seizures (Jacksonian march)

    ◼ unilateral simple partial motor seizures that start with a tonic contraction of the fingers on one hand, the face on one side, or one foot, and progress to clonic contractions of the entire half of the body; they may progress to grand mal seizures.
    ◼ can result from tumors, hematomas, and brain abscesses.
    ◼ can affect the opposite side via the corpus callosum.

VII. APRAXIA

◼ the inability to perform motor activities in the presence of intact motor and sensory systems and normal comprehension.

A. Ideomotor apraxia

    ◼ the loss of the ability to perform intransitive or imaginary gestures, resulting in the inability to perform complicated motor tasks (eg, saluting, blowing a kiss, or making the V-for-peace sign).
    ◼ may be typified by facial apraxia, which is also known as buccofacial or facial-oral apraxia, the most common type of apraxia.
    ◼ results from a lesion of the sensory speech area.

B. Ideational apraxia

    ◼ the inability to demonstrate the use of real objects (eg, brush your teeth [a multistep complex sequence]).
    ◼ a misuse of objects owing to a disturbance of identification (agnosia).
    ◼ results from a lesion in the sensory speech area.

C. Construction apraxia

    ◼ the inability to draw or construct a geometric figure (eg, the face of a clock).
    ◼ called hemineglect if the patient draws only the right half of the clock. The lesion is located in the right inferior parietal lobule (see Figure 22.4).

D. Gait apraxia

    ◼ characterized by diminished cadence, wide base, short steps, and shuffling progression; it is reminiscent of Parkinsonian gait.
    ◼ a frontal lobe sign seen in normal-pressure hydrocephalus with gait apraxia, dementia, and incontinence.

VIII. APHASIA

- impaired or absent communication by speech, writing, or signs (ie, loss of the capacity for spoken language).
- results from lesions in the dominant hemisphere.
- the following symptoms and signs are associated with certain aphasias (Figure 22.6).

A. Motor (Broca) aphasia

- characterized by good comprehension; effortful, dysarthric, telegraphic, and nonfluent speech; poor repetition; and contralateral lower facial and upper limb weakness.
- results from a lesion in the frontal lobe, in the inferior frontal gyrus (Brodmann areas 44 and 45).

B. Sensory (Wernicke) aphasia

- characterized by poor comprehension, fluent speech, poor repetition, and quadrantanopia.
- also marked by paraphasic errors such as non sequiturs (Latin—does not follow logically what is said previously), neologisms (words with no meaning), and driveling speech.
- results from a lesion in the posterior temporal lobe, in the superior temporal gyrus (Brodmann area 22).

C. Conduction aphasia

- involves the transection of the arcuate fasciculus; the arcuate fasciculus interconnects the motor speech area with the sensory speech area.
- characterized by good comprehension, poor repetition, and fluent speech.

D. Transcortical motor aphasia

- involves good comprehension, good repetition, and nonfluent speech.

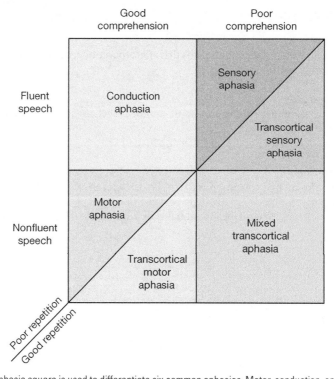

FIGURE 22.6. The aphasia square is used to differentiate six common aphasias. Motor, conduction, and sensory aphasias are all characterized by poor repetition. (Modified with permission from Miller J, Fountain N. *Neurology Recall*. 1st ed. Williams & Wilkins; 1997:35.)

E. Transcortical mixed aphasia
- involves poor comprehension, good repetition, and nonfluent speech.

F. Transcortical sensory aphasia
- involves poor comprehension, good repetition, and fluent speech.

G. Global aphasia
- results from a lesion of the perisylvian (ie, lateral fissure/sulcus) area, which contains the motor and sensory speech areas.
- combines all the symptoms of motor and sensory aphasias.

H. Thalamic aphasia
- a dominant thalamic syndrome that closely resembles a thought disorder of patients with schizophrenia and chronic drug-induced psychosis.
- involves fluent paraphasic speech with normal comprehension and repetition.

I. Basal nuclei
- diseases of the basal nuclei may cause aphasia.
- lesions of the anterior aspect of the basal nuclei result in nonfluent aphasia, and lesions of the more posterior aspects of the basal nuclei result in fluent aphasia.

J. Watershed infarcts
- areas of infarction in the boundary zones of the anterior, middle, and posterior cerebral arteries. Infarcts cause motor, mixed, and sensory transcortical aphasias.
- vulnerable to hypoperfusion and thus may separate the motor and sensory speech areas from the surrounding cortex.

IX. DYSPROSODIES

- nondominant hemispheric language deficits that affect the emotionality of speech (inflection, melody, emphasis, and gesturing).

A. Expressive dysprosody
- results from a lesion that corresponds to the motor speech area but is located in the nondominant hemisphere.
- patients cannot express emotion or inflection in their speech.

B. Receptive dysprosody
- results from a lesion that corresponds to the sensory speech area but is located in the nondominant hemisphere.
- patients cannot comprehend the emotionality or inflection in the speech they hear.

Review Test

1. A 50-year-old man presents to his primary care physician for a follow-up consultation regarding the diagnosis of hemineglect syndrome. The diagnosis was confirmed after imaging revealed a vascular lesion affecting what part of the brain?

(A) Inferior parietal lobule
(B) Primary sensory cortex
(C) Sensory speech area
(D) Superior frontal gyrus
(E) Transverse temporal gyrus

2. A 55-year-old right-handed veteran received a small shrapnel wound in the head. Within 1 year of receiving his wound, the man complained of seizures and was treated with seizure medication. The medication was not effective, and a section of the anterior corpus callosum was performed successfully. Which of the following neurologic deficits is most likely?

(A) Alexia
(B) Gait dystaxia
(C) Loss of binocular vision
(D) Sympathetic apraxia; right hand
(E) Dysnomia; left hand

3. A 70-year-old man, with previously diagnosed hypertension, suddenly experiences numbness on the right side of his body. When asked to raise his left hand, he raises his right hand. The lesion is most likely in the:

(A) left parietal lobe.
(B) left temporal lobe.
(C) right frontal lobe.
(D) right internal capsule.
(E) right parietal lobe.

4. A 45-year-old man presents to his primary care physician with a complaint of headaches. Neurologic examination reveals pronator drift and mild hemiparesis on the right side. The patient's eyes and head are turned to the left side, and papilledema is visible on the left side. The lesion is most likely in which of the following cortices?

(A) Frontal
(B) Insular
(C) Occipital
(D) Parietal
(E) Temporal

5. An 80-year-old woman presents to the emergency department in clear distress. Her speech is limited to expletives, she cannot write but does respond to questions by shaking her head, and she has lower facial weakness on the right side. Imaging reveals a cerebral infarction. The lesion is most likely in the:

(A) left frontal lobe.
(B) left parietal lobe.
(C) left temporal lobe.
(D) right frontal lobe.
(E) right parietal lobe.

6. A lesion resulting in a nonfluent expressive aphasia will be found most likely in the:

(A) frontal lobe.
(B) limbic lobe.
(C) occipital lobe.
(D) parietal lobe.
(E) temporal lobe.

7. Motor aphasia is frequently associated with:

(A) a UMN lesion.
(B) auditory hallucinations.
(C) construction apraxia.
(D) finger agnosia.
(E) visual field deficits.

8. Alexia without agraphia and aphasia will most likely result from occlusion of which artery:

(A) left anterior cerebral.
(B) left middle cerebral.
(C) left posterior cerebral.
(D) right anterior cerebral.
(E) right posterior cerebral.

9. Agraphia and dyscalculia will most likely result from a lesion in the:

(A) left frontal lobe.
(B) left parietal lobe.
(C) left temporal lobe.
(D) right occipital lobe.
(E) splenium of corpus callosum.

10. A 40-year-old woman presents to her neurologist for follow-up, after suffering a stroke the previous year. She is asked to bisect a horizontal line through the middle, to draw the face of a clock, and to copy a cross. The patient bisected the horizontal line to the left of the midline, placed all of the numerals of the clock on the right side, and did not complete the cross on the left side. The most likely lesion site for this deficit is the:

(A) left frontal lobe.
(B) left occipital lobe.
(C) left parietal lobe.
(D) right parietal lobe.
(E) right temporal lobe.

11. A 45-year-old man with previously diagnosed multiple sclerosis presents to his primary care physician for increasing concerns regarding his speech. Although he personally hasn't taken much notice, his wife and friends report that he seems to lack excitement and enthusiasm, even when discussing topics he is passionate about. Patient interview reveals a somewhat robotic rhythm to his speech, all other aspects of speech and comprehension are normal. Imaging reveals a sclerotic plaque in the posterior aspect of the inferior frontal gyrus of the right hemisphere. What is the most appropriate diagnosis in this patient?

(A) Expressive dysprosody
(B) Global aphasia
(C) Ideomotor apraxia
(D) Receptive dysprosody
(E) Transcortical mixed aphasia

Questions 12 to 17

Match the descriptions in items 12 to 17 with the appropriate lettered area shown in the figure.

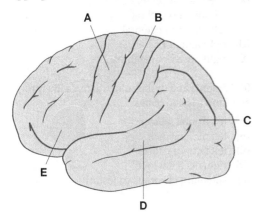

12. Motor speech area

13. Sensory speech area

14. Lesion in this area results in contralateral astereognosis.

15. Infarction in this area results in a UMN lesion.

16. Lesion in this area results in contralateral homonymous hemianopia.

17. Lesion in this area results in finger agnosia, agraphia, and dyscalculia.

Questions 18 to 22

Match the descriptions in items 18 to 22 with the appropriate lettered area shown in the figure.

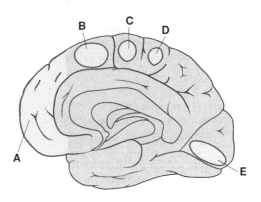

18. Supplementary motor area

19. Lesion in this area results in paresthesias and numbness in the contralateral foot.

20. Lesion in this area results in contralateral lower homonymous quadrantanopia.

21. Lesion in this area results in a contralateral Babinski sign.

22. Lesion in this area results in loss of initiative and inappropriate social behavior.

23. An occlusion of which of the following arteries may result in motor aphasia?

(A) Angular artery
(B) Anterior choroidal artery
(C) Anterior temporal artery
(D) Medial striate artery (of Heubner)
(E) Operculofrontal artery

24. A 50-year-old woman visits a physical therapist for increasing frustration over not being to accomplish simple tasks at home. As part of the examination, she is given a toothbrush and toothpaste and asked to demonstrate how they are used. She rubs the toothbrush along the outside of the tube of toothpaste. Which of the following neurologic diagnoses best describes this behavior?

(A) Construction apraxia
(B) Dysprosody
(C) Ideational apraxia
(D) Ideomotor apraxia
(E) Prosopagnosia

25. A 65-year-old man presents to the emergency department with a complaint of difficulty walking. He has a history of chronic subdural hematomas. Neurologic examination reveals psychomotor slowing, sphincter incontinence, and enlarged ventricles without convolutional atrophy. The most likely diagnosis is:

(A) Huntington disease.
(B) normal-pressure hydrocephalus.
(C) Parkinson disease.
(D) progressive supranuclear palsy.
(E) Wilson disease.

26. Neurologic examination indicates that a 50-year-old woman with hypertension has left homonymous hemianopia but is not aware of her deficit (anosognosia). When asked to copy a drawing of a clock face, she neglects to draw the numerals on the left side of the clock. Based on this examination, the lesion would most likely be in the:

(A) frontal lobe.
(B) insula.
(C) left parietal lobe.
(D) right parietal lobe.
(E) right temporal lobe.

27. A 48-year-old woman who has had a stroke complains of weakness of her right arm and weakness of her right lower face. Language assessment reveals the following speech deficits: slow, labored speech; dysarthric, telegraphic speech; usually good comprehension; and poor repetition. Which of the following types of aphasia do these neurologic findings describe best?

(A) Motor
(B) Conduction
(C) Transcortical motor
(D) Transcortical sensory
(E) Sensory

28. A 65-year-old man presents to the emergency department concerned about changes in his ability to speak. Language assessment reveals the following speech abnormalities: impaired comprehension; impaired repetition; and paraphasic speech, including non sequiturs and neologisms. Spontaneity and fluency are normal. Imaging reveals a cerebrovascular accident. Which of the following types of aphasia best fits this evaluation?

(A) Motor
(B) Conduction
(C) Mixed transcortical
(D) Transcortical motor
(E) Sensory

29. A 50-year-old man has a mass lesion underlying the left frontoparietal operculum. Language assessment reveals good comprehension, fluent speech, poor repetition, anomia, and agraphia. Which of the following types of aphasia best fits this case?

(A) Motor
(B) Conduction
(C) Global
(D) Transcortical sensory
(E) Sensory

30. A 45-year-old woman has a stroke. She exhibits weakness in her left arm, and she is unable to show emotion, inflection, and emphasis and gesturing in her propositional language. The lesion responsible for this language difficulty would most likely be in which lobe?

(A) Left frontal
(B) Left parietal
(C) Left temporal
(D) Right frontal
(E) Right temporal

Answers and Explanations

1. **A.** Lesions of the inferior parietal lobule may produce a variety of symptoms, including memory loss, constructional apraxia, anosognosia, and/or ideational apraxia. Hemineglect syndrome involves a combination of symptoms generally resulting in inattention to one side of the body or space. A lesion of the primary sensory cortex will primarily result in a deficit in the ability to localize sensations. Lesion of the sensory speech area will result in a deficit in the ability to comprehend speech. Lesion of the superior frontal gyrus will produce motor deficits. The transverse temporal gyrus (of Heschl) is primary auditory cortex.

2. **E.** Transection of corpus callosum results in the inability, when blindfolded, to identify verbally an object held in the left hand (dysnomia). The left hemisphere is dominant for language and naming objects. Alexia is found in lesions of the inferior parietal lobule. Gait dystaxia may result from normal-pressure hydrocephalus, which also involves dementia and incontinence. The man's visual pathways are not affected. Transection of callosal fibers adjacent to the left premotor cortex produces right hemiparesis, motor dysphasia, and sympathetic dyspraxia of the left, nonparalyzed, arm.

3. **A.** The right hemiparesis points to a lesion on the left side involving the corticospinal tract. Left-right confusion is seen in Gerstmann syndrome along with finger agnosia. This syndrome results from destruction of the left angular gyrus.

4. **A.** The cortical center for lateral conjugate gaze is located in area 8 of the frontal lobe. Destruction of this area results in turning of the head and eyes toward the side of the lesion. Stimulation of this area results in contralateral turning of the eyes and head; pronator drift and hemiparesis are frontal lobe signs.

5. **A.** Lower facial weakness is a localizing neighborhood sign. The motor speech area is located in the posterior part of the inferior frontal gyrus (Brodmann areas 44 and 45).

6. **A.** Nonfluent, expressive motor aphasia results from a lesion in the posterior inferior frontal gyrus (areas 44 and 45) of the dominant frontal lobe.

7. **A.** Motor aphasia is frequently associated with a UMN lesion of the contralateral face and upper limb and occasionally of the lower limb. The motor speech area lies just anterior to the motor strip; both are irrigated by the superior division of the middle cerebral artery (prerolandic and Rolandic arteries). Motor aphasia is frequently associated with sympathetic apraxia, an apraxia of the nonparalyzed left hand.

8. **C.** Alexia without agraphia and aphasia results from occlusion of the left posterior cerebral artery, which supplies the left visual cortex and callosal fibers (within the splenium) from the right visual association cortex. Interruption of bilateral visual association fibers en route to the left angular gyrus results in alexia. The patient will not be agraphic or dysphasic because the angular gyrus and the sensory speech area are spared.

9. **B.** Lesions of the angular gyrus of the dominant hemisphere may result in Gerstmann syndrome, which consists of agraphia, dyscalculia, finger agnosia, and left-right confusion.

10. **D.** The inability to draw a clock face or bisect a line through the middle is called construction apraxia. Lesions of the right (nondominant) parietal lobe result in construction apraxia, dressing apraxia, anosognosia, and sensory hemineglect.

11. **A.** Expressive dysprosody is characterized by monotone, robotic speech that lacks emotion. Expressive dysprosody is caused by a lesion of the motor speech are in the nondominant hemisphere. Global aphasia is both an inability to produce and comprehend speech (written or verbal). Ideomotor apraxia results from a lesion of the sensory speech areas and is not related to monotone speech production. Receptive dysprosody is the opposite of what this patient has; it is an inability to comprehend emotion and inflection in speech. Transcortical mixed aphasia does involve nonfluent speech, with the patient may demonstrate to a degree, but also involved poor comprehension.

12. **E.** Motor speech area (areas 44 and 45) is found in the posterior part of the inferior frontal gyrus of the dominant hemisphere, directly anterior to the premotor and motor cortices.

13. **D.** Sensory speech area is located in the posterior part of the superior temporal gyrus (part of Brodmann area 22) of the dominant hemisphere. A lesion of this area results in a fluent sensory (receptive) aphasia.

14. **B.** A lesion of the left postcentral gyrus results in a right astereognosis (tactile agnosia), the inability to identify objects by touch. Lesions of the superior parietal lobule result in contralateral astereognosis and in sensory neglect.

15. **A.** A lesion in the precentral gyrus is a UMN lesion. The precentral gyrus (motor strip) gives rise to 1/3 of the pyramidal tract (corticospinal tract) fibers.

16. **C.** A deep lesion of the angular gyrus can involve the visual radiation, resulting in a contralateral homonymous hemianopia.

17. **C.** The dominant angular gyrus is the neurologic substrate of Gerstmann syndrome, which consists of right-left confusion, finger agnosia, agraphia, and dyscalculia.

18. **B.** The supplementary motor cortex (area 6) lies on the medial aspect of the hemisphere, just anterior to the paracentral lobule.

19. **D.** A lesion in the posterior part of the paracentral lobule results in loss of joint and position sense (asomatognosia) and loss of tactile discrimination (astereognosis) in the contralateral foot.

20. **E.** A lesion of the superior bank of the calcarine sulcus (cuneus) results in a contralateral lower homonymous quadrantanopia. A lesion destroying both cunei produces a lower homonymous altitudinal hemianopia.

21. **C.** A lesion of the anterior part of the paracentral lobule results in a contralateral paresis of the foot muscles and in Babinski sign (ie, plantar reflex extensor or extensor toe sign).

22. **A.** Lesions of the prefrontal cortex can result in personality changes, with disorderly and inappropriate conduct and facetiousness and jocularity. Lesions interrupt fibers that interconnect the dorsomedial nucleus and the prefrontal cortex (eg, prefrontal lobotomy or leukotomy).

23. **E.** The motor speech area, located in the lower frontal gyrus of the left hemisphere, is supplied by the operculofrontal artery. This area may also be perfused by the prerolandic artery. Both arteries arise from the middle cerebral artery.

24. **C.** The patient, who is unable to demonstrate proper use of the toothbrush and toothpaste on command, has ideational or sensory apraxia, a disorder of a multistep action sequence. Construction apraxia is the inability to draw an entire clock face; patients with nondominant parietal lobe lesions cannot draw the left side of the clock (sensory neglect). Ideomotor apraxia is the inability to follow simple commands (ie, stick out your tongue or make a fist). Prosopagnosia is the inability to recognize faces. Dysprosody is the difficulty producing or understanding the normal pitch, rhythm, and variation in stress in speech.

25. **B.** Normal-pressure hydrocephalus is characterized by the triad of gait apraxia (frontal lobe ataxia), incontinence, and dementia. The ventricles are moderately dilated. Huntington disease is a neurodegenerative disorder characterized by choreoathetosis, tremor, and dementia. Parkinson disease is characterized by a pill-rolling resting tremor, cogwheel rigidity, and bradykinesia (slowness in movement). Progressive supranuclear palsy is a movement disorder characterized by paresis of downgaze. Wilson disease (hepatolenticular degeneration) is a disease of copper metabolism characterized by a coarse "wing-beating" tremor. The corneal Kayser-Fleischer ring is pathognomonic.

26. **D.** Lesions of the nondominant (right) parietal lobe have the following deficits: anosognosia, topographic memory loss, dressing apraxia, sensory neglect, sensory extinction, and left homonymous hemianopia. Frontal lobe signs may include motor abnormalities, impairment of cognitive function, personality changes (disinhibition of behavior), and incontinence. The insula receives olfactory and gustatory input. Temporal lobe signs may include sensory aphasia, auditory, visual, olfactory, and gustatory hallucinations, and loss of recent memory.

27. A. Key features that point to motor aphasia are slow, labored dysarthric telegraphic speech; relatively good speech comprehension; poor repetition; frequent depression; and frequent buccolingual dyspraxia. Motor aphasia is also called Broca, expressive, and anterior aphasia. See Figure 22.6.

28. E. Sensory aphasia is characterized by fluent speech, poor comprehension, poor repetition, and paraphasic errors (eg, driveling speech, non sequiturs, and neologisms).

29. B. Conduction aphasia results from a lesion that transects the arcuate fasciculus, thus separating the motor speech area from the sensory speech area. This condition is characterized by markedly impaired repetition, with preserved fluency and comprehension. Conduction aphasia is usually associated with agraphia.

30. D. The center for expressive prosody is located in the posterior part of the inferior frontal gyrus of the nondominant lobe. The center for receptive prosody is located in the posterior part of the superior temporal gyrus of the nondominant hemisphere.

Comprehensive Examination

1. The cuneus is separated from the lingual gyrus by the:

(A) calcarine sulcus.
(B) collateral sulcus.
(C) intraparietal sulcus.
(D) parieto-occipital sulcus.
(E) rhinal sulcus.

2. Which sinus receives drainage from the greatest number of arachnoid granulations?

(A) Cavernous sinus
(B) Sigmoid sinus
(C) Straight sinus
(D) Superior sagittal sinus
(E) Transverse sinus

3. Which one of the following statements concerning Rathke pouch is true? It

(A) is a mesodermal diverticulum.
(B) is derived from the neural tube.
(C) gives rise to the adenohypophysis.
(D) gives rise to the epiphysis.
(E) gives rise to the neurohypophysis.

4. Which of the following statements concerning the lateral horn of the spinal cord is true? It

(A) contains preganglionic parasympathetic neurons.
(B) gives rise to a spinocerebellar tract.
(C) gives rise to preganglionic sympathetic fibers.
(D) is most prominent at sacral levels.
(E) is present at all spinal cord levels.

5. Which of the following statements concerning the posterior thoracic nucleus (of Clarke) is true? It

(A) is found in the anterior horn.
(B) is homologous to the cuneate nucleus of the medulla.
(C) is most prominent at upper cervical levels.
(D) is present at all spinal levels.
(E) projects to the cerebellum.

6. Which one of the following groups of cranial nerves is closely related to the corticospinal tract? CN III and:

(A) CN IV and CN V
(B) CN V and CN VII
(C) CN V and CN VIII
(D) CN VI and CN XII
(E) CN IX and CN X

7. The primary auditory cortex is located in the:

(A) frontal operculum.
(B) inferior parietal lobule.
(C) postcentral gyrus.
(D) superior parietal lobule.
(E) transverse temporal gyri.

8. The neocerebellum projects to the motor cortex via the:

(A) anterior thalamic nucleus.
(B) lateral dorsal nucleus.
(C) lateral posterior nucleus.
(D) ventral anterior nucleus.
(E) ventral lateral nucleus.

9. The dentatorubrothalamic tract decussates in the:

(A) caudal midbrain.
(B) caudal pons.
(C) diencephalon.
(D) rostral midbrain.
(E) rostral pons.

10. A pituitary tumor is most frequently associated with:

(A) altitudinal hemianopia.
(B) binasal hemianopia.
(C) bitemporal hemianopia.
(D) homonymous hemianopia.
(E) homonymous quadrantanopia.

11. Resection of the anterior portion of the left temporal lobe is most frequently associated with:

(A) left homonymous hemianopia.
(B) left lower homonymous quadrantanopia.
(C) left upper homonymous quadrantanopia.
(D) right lower homonymous quadrantanopia.
(E) right upper homonymous quadrantanopia.

12. A 65-year-old farmer has had dull frontal headaches for the last 3 weeks. Neurologic examination reveals spastic hemiparesis on the right side and a pronator drift on the right side. What is the most likely diagnosis?

(A) Brain tumor
(B) Myasthenia gravis
(C) Progressive supranuclear palsy
(D) Pseudotumor cerebri
(E) Subacute combined degeneration

13. An 18-year-old high school student has a fractured cervical vertebra. Neurologic examination reveals hemiparesis on the right side, Babinski and Hoffman signs on the right side, loss of pain and temperature sensation on the left side, and normal pallesthesia in all limbs. The spinal cord lesion that will most likely explain the deficits involves the:

(A) anterior column, bilateral.
(B) lateral column, left side.
(C) lateral column, right side.
(D) posterior column, left side.
(E) posterior column, right side.

14. Light shone into the left eye elicits a direct pupillary reflex but no consensual reflex. A lesion in which of the following structures accounts for this deficit?

(A) Oculomotor nerve, right side
(B) Oculomotor nerve, left side
(C) Optic nerve, left eye
(D) Optic nerve, right eye
(E) Optic tract, right side

15. A 53-year-old woman has a normal corneal blink reflex on her left side but no consensual blink on her right side. Which of the following neurologic deficits or signs will you expect to find on the right side?

(A) Hemianesthesia
(B) Hemianhidrosis
(C) Hyperacusis
(D) Internal ophthalmoplegia
(E) Severe ptosis

16. A 49-year-old man has a loss of tactile sensation involving the anterior two-thirds of his tongue on the left side. Neurologic examination reveals paralysis of the masseter on the left side and loss of pain and temperature sensation from the teeth of the mandible on the left side. He has a lesion involving which one of the following nerves?

(A) Chorda tympani
(B) Facial

(C) Hypoglossal
(D) Trigeminal, mandibular division
(E) Trigeminal, ophthalmic division

17. A 62-year-old man has a stroke and falls while cutting his lawn. He does not lose consciousness. Neurologic examination reveals loss of pain sensation on the right side of the face and on the left side of the body, falling and past-pointing to the right side, difficulty in swallowing, horizontal nystagmus to the right side, deviation of the uvula to the left when asked to say "ah," and Horner syndrome on the right side. The most likely site of this man's lesion is the:

(A) internal capsule, left side.
(B) lateral medulla, right side.
(C) medial medulla, right side.
(D) midbrain, right side.
(E) pontine tegmentum.

18. A 64-year-old woman complains of weakness in her right leg and double vision, especially when moving her eyes to the left. Neurologic examination reveals a dilated pupil and ptosis on the left side and a Babinski sign (extensor plantar reflex) on the right side. The most likely site of this patient's lesion is the:

(A) internal capsule, right side.
(B) midbrain crus cerebri, left side.
(C) midbrain crus cerebri, right side.
(D) pontine base, left side.
(E) pontine tegmentum, right side.

19. While working in her shop, a 21-year-old machinist is struck by a penetrating metal fragment in the side of the head. Neurologic examination reveals the following language deficits: fluent speech, an inability to read aloud, an inability to repeat what is said, and an inability to communicate by writing. The patient understands the problem but cannot resolve it. Where would you expect to find the fragment?

(A) Between the supramarginal gyrus and the inferior frontal gyrus
(B) In the angular gyrus
(C) In the paracentral gyrus
(D) In the posterior third of the superior temporal gyrus
(E) In the transverse gyri

20. Norepinephrine is the primary neurotransmitter found in the:

(A) suprarenal cortex.
(B) preganglionic parasympathetic neurons.

(C) postganglionic parasympathetic neurons to the circular smooth muscle layer of the jejunum.
(D) postganglionic sympathetic neurons to the smooth muscle of the renal arterioles.
(E) postganglionic sympathetic neurons to the sweat glands.

21. A 30-year-old man sustains brain damage as the result of an automobile accident. Neurologic examination reveals incomplete retrograde amnesia, severe anterograde amnesia, and inappropriate social behavior, including hyperphagia, hypersexuality, and general disinhibition. The brain injury most likely involves the:

(A) frontal lobes, lateral convexity.
(B) frontal lobes, medial surface.
(C) temporal lobes, lateral convexity.
(D) temporal lobes, medial surface.
(E) thalami.

22. A 55-year-old woman has difficulty reading small print. She most likely has:

(A) astigmatism.
(B) cataracts.
(C) optic atrophy.
(D) macular degeneration.
(E) presbyopia.

23. The principal postnatal change in the pyramids is the result of:

(A) an increase in endoneural tubes to guide sprouting axons.
(B) an increase of corticospinal neurons from the paracentral lobule.
(C) an increase in the total number of corticospinal axons.
(D) a large increase of Schwann cells in the motor cortex.
(E) myelination of preexisting corticospinal axons.

24. Special visceral afferent neurons that innervate receptor cells in taste buds synapse in the:

(A) geniculate ganglion.
(B) inferior salivatory nucleus.
(C) nucleus of the solitary tract.
(D) spinal trigeminal nucleus.
(E) ventral posteromedial nucleus.

25. A woman receives an injection of a radioisotope to determine regional blood flow in the brain. She has a positron emission tomography scan to visualize variations in cortical blood flow. The examiner asks her to think about flexing her index finger without actually doing it. In which of the following cortical areas would you expect to see increased blood flow?

(A) Angular gyrus
(B) Broca area
(C) Motor strip
(D) S1 somatosensory cortex
(E) Supplementary motor cortex

26. Which of the following sensory deficits results from the destruction of the right cuneate nucleus?

(A) Analgesia, left hand
(B) Analgesia, right foot
(C) Apallesthesia, left foot
(D) Apallesthesia, left hand
(E) Apallesthesia, right hand

27. Which of the following postganglionic sympathetic responses results from the elaboration of acetylcholine?

(A) Constriction of cutaneous blood vessels
(B) Contraction of arrector pili muscles
(C) Decreased gastrointestinal motility
(D) Increased ventricular contractility
(E) Stimulation of eccrine sweat glands

28. Which of the following neural structures mediates nausea?

(A) Celiac ganglion
(B) Greater splanchnic nerve
(C) Inferior mesenteric ganglion
(D) Superior mesenteric ganglion
(E) Vagal nerves

29. Cerebrospinal fluid enters the bloodstream via the:

(A) arachnoid villi.
(B) choroid plexus.
(C) interventricular foramen (of Monro).
(D) lateral foramina (of Luschka).
(E) median foramen (of Magendie).

30. Computed tomography of the head of a newborn infant reveals enlargement of the lateral ventricles and the third ventricle.

Which of the following is the most likely cause of this hydrocephalus?

(A) Adhesive arachnoiditis
(B) Aqueductal stenosis
(C) Calcification of the arachnoid granulations
(D) Choroid plexus papilloma
(E) Stenosis of the median foramen

31. The cellular neuropathology of Alzheimer disease resembles most closely that seen in:

(A) Huntington disease.
(B) multi-infarct dementia.
(C) neurosyphilis.
(D) Pick disease.
(E) trisomy 21.

32. A 40-year-old man visits his primary care physician. He complains of shortness of breath and difficulty in performing his construction work. During the history taking, he tells his physician that he had an attack of gastroenteritis 3 weeks ago. The neurologic examination reveals ascending weakness and tingling in the legs and absence of muscle stretch reflexes in the legs. Cerebrospinal fluid analysis shows elevated protein without significant pleocytosis. The most likely diagnosis is:

(A) amyotrophic lateral sclerosis.
(B) Guillain-Barré syndrome.
(C) multiple sclerosis.
(D) myasthenia gravis.
(E) Werdnig-Hoffmann syndrome.

33. A 25-year-old woman has had difficulty walking. Five years ago, she experienced a loss of vision in her left eye that improved in 3 weeks. Neurologic examination reveals a right afferent pupillary defect, hyperreflexia in both legs, reduced proprioception in both feet, and extensor plantar reflexes. Cerebrospinal fluid analysis shows oligoclonal bands. The most likely diagnosis is:

(A) amyotrophic lateral sclerosis.
(B) Guillain-Barré syndrome.
(C) multiple sclerosis.
(D) subacute combined degeneration.
(E) syringobulbia.

34. A 48-year-old woman complains of a progressive loss of hearing and a buzzing noise in her right ear. Neurologic examination reveals an absent corneal reflex on the right side and sagging of the right corner of the mouth. Magnetic resonance imaging shows a mass in the right cerebellopontine angle. From which of the following cell type proliferation will the neoplasm most likely arise?

(A) Fibrous astrocytes
(B) Microglia
(C) Oligodendrocytes
(D) Protoplasmic astrocytes
(E) Schwann cells

35. A 50-year-old man complains of weakness in his left leg and loss of pain and temperature in his right leg. Neurologic examination reveals exaggerated muscle stretch reflexes in the left leg and an extensor plantar reflex on the left side. The lesion would most likely be located in the:

(A) crus cerebri.
(B) internal capsule.
(C) lateral medulla.
(D) medial medulla.
(E) spinal cord.

36. A 20-year-old comatose man has sustained massive head injuries in an automobile accident. Ice water injected into the external auditory meatus elicits no ocular response. Head rotation does not result in the doll's eye phenomenon. The lesion causing the injuries most likely affects the:

(A) cochlear nuclei.
(B) dentate nuclei.
(C) ossicles.
(D) utricles.
(E) vestibular nuclei.

37. Which of the following agents may be used as an alternative to L-DOPA to alleviate the chemical imbalance found in the striatum of a patient with Parkinson disease?

(A) Aspartate
(B) Anticholinergic agent
(C) Dopamine antagonist
(D) Glutamate
(E) Serotonin reuptake inhibitor

38. Which of the following antidepressants is the most selective inhibitor of serotonin reuptake?

(A) Amitriptyline
(B) Doxepin
(C) Fluoxetine
(D) Nortriptyline
(E) Tranylcypromine

39. A 20-year-old woman suddenly develops double vision. Neurologic examination reveals diplopia when she attempts to look to the left, the inability to adduct the right eye, nystagmus in the left eye on attempted lateral conjugate gaze to the left, and convergence of both eyes on a near point. These deficits would result from occlusion of a branch of:

(A) anterior cerebral artery.
(B) basilar artery.
(C) middle cerebral artery.
(D) ophthalmic artery.
(E) posterior cerebral artery.

40. A 50-year-old man had a stroke and developed ipsilateral paralysis and atrophy of the tongue, contralateral loss of vibratory sense, contralateral hemiplegia, and contralateral Babinski sign. The level of this vascular syndrome is in the:

(A) lateral medulla.
(B) medial medulla.
(C) midbrain.
(D) pontine base.
(E) pontine tegmentum.

41. Tritiated proline [(^{3}H)-proline] is injected into the left upper quadrant of the left retina for anterograde transport. Radioactive label would be found in the:

(A) cuneus, left side.
(B) cuneus, right side.
(C) lingual gyrus, left side.
(D) lingual gyrus, right side.
(E) optic nerve, left side.

42. Tritiated leucine [(^{3}H)-leucine] is injected into the left inferior olivary nucleus for anterograde transport. Radioactive label would be found in the:

(A) dorsal nucleus (of Clarke).
(B) dentate nucleus, right side.
(C) lateral cuneate nucleus, left side.
(D) nuclei of the lateral lemnisci.
(E) superior olivary nucleus, left side.

43. (^{3}H)-proline is injected into the right ventral posterolateral nucleus for retrograde transport. Radioactive label would be found in the:

(A) lateral cuneate nucleus, left side.
(B) nucleus gracilis, left side.
(C) nucleus gracilis, right side.
(D) nucleus ruber, right side.
(E) ventral lateral nucleus.

44. Horseradish peroxidase is injected into the nucleus of the inferior colliculus for retrograde transport. In which of the following nuclei will the label be found?

(A) Inferior olivary nucleus
(B) Medial geniculate nucleus
(C) Lateral geniculate nucleus
(D) Superior olivary nucleus
(E) Transverse gyrus of Heschl

45. A 30-year-old man complains of difficulty chewing and weakness in the contralateral limbs and loss of pain and temperature sensation from the ipsilateral face. In which of the following will the lesion most likely be found?

(A) Medulla, lateral
(B) Medulla, medial
(C) Midbrain, base
(D) Pons, base
(E) Pons, tegmentum

46. A 45-year-old woman has bilateral paralysis of the tongue. Fasciculations are seen on the tongue, and she has bilateral loss of proprioception in the trunk and limbs. The lesion would most likely be in the:

(A) medulla at the level of the pyramidal decussation.
(B) midbrain, tegmentum.
(C) medulla at the level of the medial lemniscus bilateral.
(D) pons, base.
(E) pons, tegmentum.

47. A 25-year-old woman has paralysis of the face and lateral rectus, medial rectus palsy on attempted lateral conjugate gaze, nystagmus, normal convergence, miosis, ptosis, and multiple sclerosis. Where will the lesion producing most of the symptoms be located?

(A) Lateral medulla
(B) Medial medulla
(C) Midbrain, tegmentum
(D) Pons, tegmentum
(E) Pons, base

48. A 40-year-old man had a stroke and developed ipsilateral paralysis and atrophy of the tongue, contralateral loss of vibratory sense, contralateral hemiplegia, and contralateral Babinski sign. Which artery's thrombosis will result in these neurologic deficits?

(A) Anterior inferior cerebellar artery
(B) Anterior spinal artery
(C) Labyrinthine artery
(D) Posterior inferior cerebellar artery
(E) Posterior spinal artery

49. A 55-year-old right-handed man had abnormal speech and language usage. The psychiatric interview revealed poor comprehension, fluent speech, and poor repetition. Which gyrus is most likely lesioned in this patient?

(A) Inferior frontal
(B) Inferior temporal
(C) Middle frontal
(D) Precentral
(E) Superior temporal

50. Which disease is preferentially found in the frontal lobe?

(A) Creutzfeldt-Jakob disease
(B) Down syndrome
(C) Pick disease
(D) Sturge-Weber syndrome
(E) Tuberous sclerosis

51. A 60-year-old right-handed man had abnormal speech and language usage. The psychiatric interview revealed the following speech and language findings: good comprehension of spoken and written language; spontaneous speech fluent but paraphasic; poor repetition; inability to repeat polysyllabic words. Which is the most likely site of the lesion?

(A) Arcuate fasciculus
(B) Arcuate nucleus
(C) Dorsal longitudinal fasciculus
(D) Indusium griseum
(E) Medial longitudinal fasciculus

52. Which of the following structures contains calcium concrements?

(A) Cerebral aqueduct
(B) Cerebral peduncle
(C) Inferior colliculus
(D) Oculomotor nerve
(E) Pineal gland

Questions 53 to 56

The response options for items 53 to 56 are the same. Select one answer for each nerve in the set.

(A) Abducens
(B) Accessory
(C) Facial
(D) Glossopharyngeal
(E) Hypoglossal
(F) Oculomotor
(G) Olfactory
(H) Optic
(I) Trigeminal
(J) Trochlear
(K) Vagal
(L) Vestibulocochlear

Match each description with the most appropriate cranial nerve.

53. Is derived from the walls of the diencephalic vesicle

54. Is often damaged in the process of transtentorial herniation

55. Mediates the sensory and motor innervation of pharyngeal arches 4 and 6

56. Innervates the muscle that depresses, intorts, and abducts the globe

Questions 57 and 58

The response options for items 57 and 58 are the same. Select one answer for each item in the set.

(A) Anterior horn
(B) Basal nuclei
(C) Cerebellum
(D) Frontal lobe
(E) Occipital lobe
(F) Parietal lobe
(G) Temporal lobe
(H) Subthalamic nucleus

For each patient described, select the structure or region most likely involved.

57. A 50-year-old man complains of tremor in both hands. This tremor is most obvious at rest. While the man is reaching for an object, the tremor disappears.

58. A 35-year-old tennis player is concerned about weakness in his arms and hands, and he notices a loss of muscle mass in the upper limbs. His muscle stretch reflexes are exaggerated in the lower limbs, and he has muscle twitches in the upper limbs.

Questions 59 to 65

The response options for items 59 to 65 are the same. Select one answer for each item in the set.

(A) Diencephalon
(B) Medulla
(C) Midbrain
(D) Pons
(E) Telencephalon

Match each of the following structures with the appropriate part of the brain.

59. Cerebral aqueduct

60. Cranial nerves III and IV

61. Caudate nucleus

62. Optic chiasm

63. Olive and the pyramid

64. Pineal gland

65. Cranial nerves IX, X, and XII

Questions 66 to 70

The response options for items 66 to 70 are the same. Select one answer for each item in the set.

(A) Astrocytes
(B) Ependymal cells
(C) Microglial cells
(D) Oligodendrocytes
(E) Schwann cells

Match each of the following descriptions with the most appropriate type of cell.

66. Are derived from the neural crest

67. May myelinate numerous axons

68. Have filaments that contain glial fibrillary acidic protein

69. Myelinate only one internode

70. Arise from monocytes

Questions 71 to 75

Match the descriptions in items 71 to 75 with the appropriate lettered lesion (shaded area) in the diagram of a cross-section of the spinal cord.

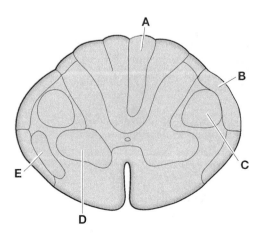

71. Ipsilateral lower limb dystaxia

72. Ipsilateral flaccid paralysis

73. Contralateral loss of pain and temperature sensation one segment below the lesion

74. Exaggerated muscle stretch reflexes below the lesion

75. Loss of two-point tactile discrimination in the ipsilateral foot

Questions 76 to 81

Match the descriptions in items 76 to 81 with the appropriate lettered lesion (shaded area) shown on one of the two cross-sections of the brainstem.

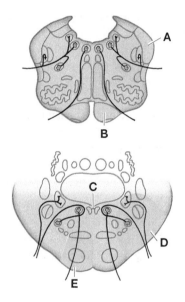

76. Medial rectus palsy on attempted lateral gaze

77. Lateral rectus paralysis; contralateral spastic hemiparesis

78. Occlusion of the posterior inferior cerebellar artery

79. Loss of the corneal blink reflex; contralateral loss of pain and temperature sensation from the body and limbs

80. Hemiatrophy of the tongue; contralateral hemiparesis; contralateral loss of vibration sensation

81. Hoarseness, Horner syndrome, singultus

Questions 82 to 87

The response options for items 82 to 87 are the same. Select one answer for each item in the set.

(A) Anterior thalamic nucleus
(B) Centromedian nucleus
(C) Mediodorsal nucleus
(D) Ventral lateral nucleus
(E) Ventral posteromedial nucleus

Match each of the following descriptions with the appropriate nucleus.

82. Receives input from the dentate nucleus

83. Receives input of taste sensation from the solitary nucleus

84. Receives input of pain and temperature sensation from the face

85. Receives the mammillothalamic tract

86. Projects to the putamen

87. Has reciprocal connections with the prefrontal cortex

Questions 88 to 93

The response options for items 88 to 93 are the same. Select one answer for each item in the set.

(A) Anterior nucleus
(B) Arcuate nucleus
(C) Mammillary nucleus
(D) Paraventricular nucleus
(E) Suprachiasmatic nucleus

Match each description with the most appropriate hypothalamic nucleus.

88. Receives input from the hippocampal formation

89. Destruction results in hyperthermia.

90. Receives input from the retina

91. Projects to the neurohypophysis

92. Regulates the activity of the adenohypophysis

93. Regulates water balance

Questions 94 to 98

The response options for items 94 to 98 are the same. Select one answer for each item in the set.

(A) Caudate nucleus
(B) Centromedian nucleus
(C) Globus pallidus
(D) Substantia nigra
(E) Subthalamic nucleus

Match each description with the most appropriate nucleus.

94. Destruction causes contralateral hemiballism.

95. Receives dopaminergic input from the midbrain

96. Gives rise to the ansa lenticularis and the lenticular fasciculus

97. Destruction causes hypokinetic rigidity.

98. A loss of cells in this structure causes greatly dilated lateral ventricles.

Questions 99 to 105

The response options for items 99 to 105 are the same. Select one answer for each item in the set.

(A) Acetylcholine
(B) Dopamine
(C) Gamma-aminobutyric acid
(D) Norepinephrine
(E) Serotonin

Match each of the following nuclei or cells with the appropriate neurotransmitter.

99. Raphe nuclei

100. Purkinje cells

101. Nucleus basalis (of Meynert)

102. Motor cranial nerve nuclei

103. Pars compacta of the substantia nigra

104. Locus ceruleus

105. Globus pallidus

Questions 106 to 110

The response options for items 106 to 110 are the same. Select one answer for each item in the set.

(A) Beta-endorphin
(B) Enkephalin
(C) Glutamate
(D) Glycine
(E) Substance P

Match each description with the appropriate neurotransmitter.

106. Neurotransmitter of afferent pain fibers

107. Major inhibitory neurotransmitter of the spinal cord

108. Major neurotransmitter of the corticospinal pathway

109. Located almost exclusively in the hypothalamus

110. Helps inhibit input from afferent pain fibers

Questions 111 to 117

The response options for items 111 to 117 are the same. Select one answer for each item in the set.

(A) Left frontal lobe
(B) Left parietal lobe
(C) Left temporal lobe
(D) Right occipital lobe
(E) Right parietal lobe

Match each of the following neurologic deficits with the most likely lesion site.

111. Left upper quadrantanopia

112. Muscle weakness and clumsiness in the right hand; slow, effortful speech

113. Inability to identify a key placed in the left hand with the eyes closed

114. Denial of hemiparesis: patient ignores stimuli from one side of the body.

115. Poor comprehension of speech; patient is unaware of the deficit.

116. Patient is unable to identify fingers touched by the examiner when eyes are closed; is unable to perform simple calculations

117. Babinski sign and ankle clonus

Questions 118 to 122

Match the descriptions in items 118 to 122 with the appropriate lettered structure shown in the MRI of the axial section of the brain.

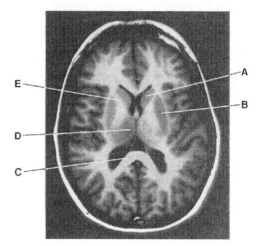

118. Thalamus

119. Internal capsule

120. Putamen

121. Caudate nucleus

122. Splenium

Questions 123 to 127

Match the descriptions in items 123 to 127 with the appropriate lettered structure shown in the MRI of the axial section of the brain.

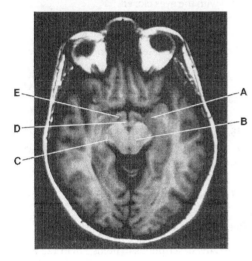

123. Medial geniculate body

124. Mesencephalon

125. Mammillary body

126. Optic tract

127. Amygdala

Questions 128 to 132

Match the descriptions in items 128 to 132 with the appropriate letter shown in the MRI of the midsagittal section of the brain.

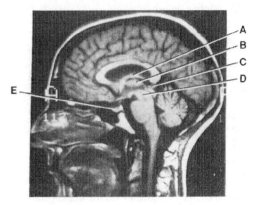

128. Pineal gland

129. Hypophysis

130. Mesencephalon

131. Thalamus

132. Fornix

Questions 133 to 142

Match the descriptions in items 133 to 142 with the appropriate diagnoses shown in the figure.

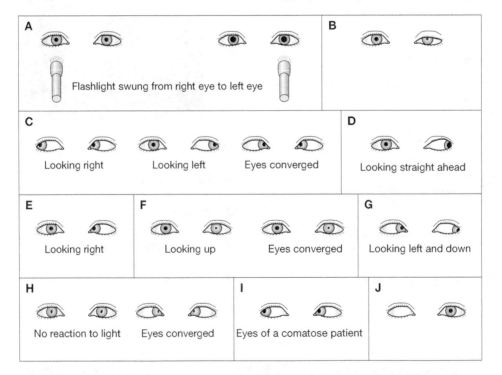

133. Right third nerve palsy

134. Destructive lesion of the right frontal lobe

135. Argyll Robertson pupil

136. Right fourth nerve palsy

137. Parinaud syndrome

138. Right sixth nerve palsy

139. Left third nerve palsy

140. Internuclear ophthalmoplegia

141. Horner syndrome

142. Retrobulbar neuritis

Questions 143 to 147

The response options for items 143 to 147 are the same. Select one answer for each item in the set.

(A) Anorexia
(B) Diabetes insipidus
(C) Hyperphagia and rage
(D) Hyperthermia
(E) Inability to thermoregulate

Match each defect below with the condition it best describes.

143. Bilateral lesions of the ventromedial hypothalamic nucleus

144. Bilateral lesions of the posterior hypothalamic nuclei

145. Lesions involving the supraoptic and paraventricular nuclei

146. Destruction of the anterior hypothalamic nuclei

147. Stimulation of the ventromedial nuclei

Questions 148 to 155

Match the descriptions in items 148 to 155 with the appropriate lettered structure in the figure.

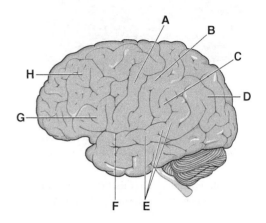

148. Stimulation of this area results in turning the eyes and head to the contralateral side.

149. A lesion here results in nonfluent, effortful, telegraphic speech.

150. Ablation in this area results in a contralateral upper homonymous quadrantanopia.

151. A lesion here results in fluent speech with paraphasic errors (eg, non sequiturs, neologisms, driveling speech).

152. A lesion of this area is characterized by finger agnosia, dyscalculia, dysgraphia, and dyslexia.

153. Destruction of this area results in aphasia characterized by fluent speech, good comprehension, and poor repetition.

154. Lesions in this gyrus result in contralateral astereognosis.

155. Lesions in this gyrus result in contralateral spasticity.

Questions 156 to 162

Match the descriptions in items 156 to 162 with the appropriate lettered structure in the figure.

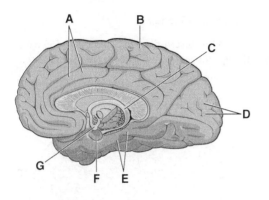

156. In thiamine (vitamin B$_1$) deficiency, hemorrhagic lesions are found in this structure.

157. Bilateral lesions in this structure result in hyperphagia, hypersexuality, and psychic blindness (visual agnosia).

158. Infarction (owing to cardiac arrest) of this area results in short-term memory loss.

159. Lesions of this area result in a lower homonymous quadrantanopia.

160. Bilateral transection of this structure may result in acute amnestic syndrome.

161. Lesion of this area results in a contralateral extensor plantar reflex and ankle clonus.

162. Ablation of this area may result in akinesia, mutism, apathy, and indifference to pain.

163. Which of the following arteries perfuses the medullary pyramid?

(A) Anterior communicating
(B) Anterior choroidal
(C) Anterior spinal
(D) Posterior inferior cerebellar
(E) Posterior spinal

164. Which artery supplies the intra-axial fibers of the hypoglossal nerve XII?

(A) Anterior inferior cerebellar
(B) Anterior spinal
(C) Basilar
(D) Posterior spinal
(E) Vertebral

165. A berry aneurysm puts pressure on the optic chiasm in the anteroposterior plane resulting in bitemporal hemianopia. On which one of the following arteries will aneurysm be most likely found?

(A) Anterior communicating
(B) Anterior spinal
(C) Basilar
(D) Ophthalmic
(E) Posterior communicating

166. A 10-year-old boy was struck on the side of the head with a golf ball. The middle meningeal artery was lacerated. In which space was blood found?

(A) Confluence of the sinuses
(B) Epidural
(C) Subarachnoid
(D) Subdural
(E) Subpial

167. A 25-year-old man was examined by an ophthalmologist, who observed headaches; ptosis; a fixed, dilated pupil; and an eye that looked down and out. An aneurysm was demonstrated with carotid angiogram anteroposterior projection. Which artery harbored the aneurysm?

(A) Anterior cerebral
(B) Anterior communicating
(C) Internal carotid
(D) Ophthalmic
(E) Posterior communicating

168. Which one of the following arteries irrigates the dentate nucleus?

(A) Anterior inferior cerebellar
(B) Posterior cerebral
(C) Posterior inferior cerebellar
(D) Superior cerebellar
(E) Vertebral

169. A glioma deep to the facial colliculus results in diplopia and horizontal nystagmus on attempted lateral conjugate gaze. Paralysis of which one of the following muscles will explain the neurologic deficits?

(A) Buccinator
(B) Lateral pterygoid
(C) Lateral rectus
(D) Orbicularis oculi
(E) Posterior belly of digastric

170. In adults, the choroid plexus of the lateral ventricle is calcified and can be visualized with plain film or computed tomography. Where, within the ventricular system, is the calcified glomus of the choroid plexus?

(A) Body
(B) Frontal horn
(C) Occipital horn
(D) Trigone
(E) Temporal horn

171. Which one of the following circumventricular organs has a blood-brain barrier?

(A) Area postrema
(B) Median eminence of the tuber cinereum
(C) Pineal body
(D) Subcommissural organ
(E) Subfornical organ

172. Which artery perfuses the leg area of the motor strip?

(A) Medial striate
(B) Middle cerebral
(C) Pericallosal
(D) Posterior cerebral
(E) Splenial

173. Which one of the following arteries, following bilateral hypoperfusion, results in Klüver-Bucy syndrome?

(A) Anterior choroidal
(B) Anterior communicating
(C) Medial striate
(D) Posterior cerebral
(E) Posterior choroidal

174. Which cranial nerve(s) exit(s) the brainstem from the pontomedullary junction?

(A) Abducens
(B) Abducens, facial, and vestibulocochlear
(C) Facial
(D) Intermediate
(E) Vestibulocochlear

175. Which is an abnormal quantity of white cells per microliter in the cerebrospinal fluid?

(A) 2
(B) 3
(C) 4
(D) 5
(E) 8

176. The normal value of cerebrospinal fluid protein in milligrams per deciliter is less than:

(A) 25.
(B) 35.
(C) 45.
(D) 55.
(E) 65.

177. Which is an example of a normal value for cerebrospinal fluid serum glucose in milligrams per deciliter?

(A) 40
(B) 50
(C) 60
(D) 70
(E) 80

178. A 20-year-old woman was evaluated by a neurologist. The neurologic examination reveals severe headaches, papilledema without mass, elevated cerebrospinal fluid pressure, and deteriorating vision. The diagnosis will most likely be:

(A) Arnold Chiari II.
(B) Dandy-Walker.
(C) hydrocephalus ex vacuo.
(D) normal pressure hydrocephalus.
(E) pseudotumor cerebri.

179. A 10-year-old boy presents with seizures, olfactory hallucinations, and a right upper quadrantanopia. The most likely causative lesion will be:

(A) aneurysm of the anterior communicating artery.
(B) Charcot-Bouchard aneurysm.
(C) frontal lobe astrocytoma.
(D) olfactory groove meningioma.
(E) temporal lobe astrocytoma.

180. A 60-year-old woman has upgoing toes and spastic paralysis of all limbs and intact sensibility. Where is the corresponding lesion site in this case?

(A) Base of pons, abducens nucleus
(B) Base of pons, trigeminal nucleus
(C) Caudal medulla
(D) Midbrain, inferior colliculus
(E) Rostral medulla

181. The optic cup is an evagination of which of the following?

(A) Diencephalon
(B) Mesencephalon
(C) Metencephalon
(D) Myelencephalon
(E) Telencephalon

182. General somatic afferent fibers are primarily concerned with conveying sensory input:

(A) from skin, muscle, bone, and joints.
(B) relating to information from visceral organs.
(C) relating to taste and smell.
(D) relating to vision.
(E) relating to vision, audition, and equilibrium.

183. From what part of the neural tube is the spinal cord derived?

(A) Anterior neuropore
(B) Caudal
(C) Cavity
(D) Cranial
(E) Posterior neuropore

184. Which one of the following basal nuclei is derived from the diencephalon?

(A) Amygdala
(B) Globus pallidus
(C) Head of the caudal nucleus
(D) Putamen
(E) Tail of the caudal nucleus

185. Which of the following represents general somatic efferent column of the pons?

(A) Abducens nucleus
(B) Hypoglossal nucleus
(C) Inferior olivary nucleus
(D) Inferior salivatory nucleus
(E) Nucleus ambiguus

186. Which of the following represents the general visceral efferent column of the pons?

(A) Cerebellum
(B) Chief trigeminal nucleus
(C) Pontine nuclei
(D) Spinal trigeminal nucleus
(E) Superior salivatory nucleus

187. When are the axons of the corticospinal tracts fully myelinated?

(A) At birth
(B) By the end of the first postnatal year
(C) By the end of the second postnatal year
(D) In the late embryonic period
(E) In the midfetal period

188. The cochlear duct contains the spiral organ of Corti and is derived from:

(A) both ectoderm and mesoderm.
(B) ectoderm.
(C) endoderm.
(D) mesoderm.
(E) neural crest.

189. The stapedius that moves the stapes is innervated by:

(A) cervical nerves C2 and C3.
(B) CN III.
(C) CN V.
(D) CN VII.
(E) CN XII.

190. Which one of the following is a classic cerebellar sign?

(A) Athetosis
(B) Chorea
(C) Cogwheel rigidity
(D) Hemiballismus
(E) Intention tremor

191. Which one of the following spinocerebellar tracts shows the phenomenon of doubling?

(A) Anterior spinocerebellar tract
(B) Cuneocerebellar tract
(C) Olivocerebellar tract
(D) Posterior spinocerebellar tract
(E) Trigeminocerebellar fibers

192. Which of the following triads of cranial nerves is damaged if the muscles attached to the styloid process are paralyzed?

(A) V, IX, and X
(B) VII, IX, and X
(C) VII, IX, and XII
(D) VII, X, and XII
(E) X, XI, and XII

193. A 25-year-old man was involved in a car accident. The emergency department physician noticed clear fluid dribbling from the nose. Rhinorrhea will most likely result from a fracture of which bone?

(A) Ethmoid
(B) Frontal
(C) Lacrimal
(D) Nasal
(E) Palatine

194. Horseradish peroxidase is injected into the circumvallate papillae on the anterior two-thirds of the tongue for retrograde transport labeling. In which of the following way stations will marker be found?

(A) Geniculate ganglion
(B) Medial dorsal nucleus of the thalamus
(C) Nodose ganglion
(D) Petrosal ganglion
(E) Ventroposterior lateral nucleus of the thalamus

195. To which one of the following nerves does trauma to the foramen rotundum cause damage?

(A) Mandibular
(B) Maxillary
(C) Ophthalmic
(D) Optic
(E) Trochlear

196. An optic glioma is found in the optic canal. Which structures will most likely be damaged by the invasive tumor?

(A) Ophthalmic artery and ophthalmic vein
(B) Ophthalmic nerve and optic nerve
(C) Ophthalmic vein and ophthalmic nerve
(D) Optic nerve and ophthalmic artery
(E) Optic nerve and ophthalmic vein

197. A 60-year-old hypertensive woman complained of facial numbness on the right side including the tongue. A cortical lesion was seen with MRI. Where will the lesion most likely be found?

(A) Anterior paracentral lobule
(B) Middle frontal gyrus
(C) Postcentral gyrus
(D) Posterior paracentral lobule
(E) Precentral gyrus

198. A 20-year-old woman is examined by a neurologist. The patient presents initially with spastic paresthesia and double vision; additional neurologic deficits and signs are optic neuritis, internuclear ophthalmoplegia, urinary urgency, scanning speech, and Lhermitte sign. Match the neurologic deficits and signs to the syndromes.

(A) Amyotrophic lateral sclerosis
(B) Brown-Séquard syndrome
(C) Multiple sclerosis
(D) Poliomyelitis
(E) Syringomyelia

Answers and Explanations

1. **A** [Chapter 1 II A 1 d, Figures 1.4 and 1.5]. The calcarine sulcus separates the cuneus from the lingual gyrus. The banks of the calcarine sulcus contain the primary visual cortex of the occipital lobe. The collateral and rhinal sulci are in the temporal lobe, the intraparietal sulcus is on the lateral surface of the parietal lobe, while the parieto-occipital sulcus separates the parietal and occipital lobes.

2. **D** [Chapter 2 I B 1 and Figure 2.3]. Most arachnoid granulations drain into the superior sagittal sinus.

3. **C** [Chapter 4 X C 1 and Figure 4.9]. The Rathke pouch is an ectodermal outpocketing of the stomodeum anterior to the buccopharyngeal membrane. It gives rise to the adenohypophysis (pars distalis, pars tuberalis, and pars intermedia).

4. **C** [Chapter 6 III A 2]. The lateral horn (T1-L2) gives rise to preganglionic sympathetic fibers.

5. **E** [Chapter 6 III A 1 d]. The posterior thoracic nucleus (of Clarke; T1-L2) gives rise to the posterior spinocerebellar tract that ascends and enters the cerebellum through the inferior cerebellar peduncle.

6. **D** [Chapter 9 II B 2; III B 2 and B 4; IV D 5]. In the midbrain, the pyramidal tract lies in the basis pedunculi; fibers of CN III pass through the medial part of the basis pedunculi. In the pons, the pyramidal tract lies in the base of the pons; abducens fibers pass through the lateral part of the pyramidal fasciculi. In the medulla, the pyramidal tracts form the medullary pyramids; hypoglossal fibers of CN XII lie just lateral to the pyramids.

7. **E** [Chapter 1 II A 1 c (1)]. The primary auditory cortex (areas 41 and 42) is located in the transverse temporal gyrus (of Heschl), part of the superior temporal gyrus.

8. **E** [Chapter 13 III E 2]. The neocerebellum sends input to the motor cortex through the ventral lateral nucleus of the thalamus. The pathway is the neocerebellar cortex, dentate nucleus, contralateral ventral lateral nucleus of the thalamus, and motor cortex (area 4).

9. **A** [Chapter 12 IV B 2]. The dentatorubrothalamic tract decussates in the caudal midbrain tegmentum at the level of the inferior colliculus. This massive decussation of the superior cerebellar peduncles is characteristic of this level.

10. **C** [Chapter 16 III C and Figure 16.2]. Pituitary tumors frequently compress the decussating fibers of the optic chiasm and produce a bitemporal hemianopia. Nasal retinal fibers decussate, and temporal retinal fibers remain ipsilateral.

11. **E** [Chapter 16 III F 2 and Figure 16.2]. Resection of the anterior portion of the temporal lobe transects the fibers of Meyer loop and results in a contralateral upper homonymous quadrantanopia. Inferior retinal quadrants are represented in the inferior banks of the calcarine sulcus.

12. **A** [Chapter 5 III F and Figure 5.3]. Headache and papilledema are signs of brain tumor, and pronator drift is a frontal lobe sign owing to weakness of the supinator. Tumor pressure on the corticospinal tract results in contralateral spastic hemiparesis. In progressive supranuclear palsy, the patient cannot look down. In myasthenia gravis, there is skeletal muscle weakness. In pseudotumor cerebri, there are no mass lesions but headache and papilledema. In subacute combined degeneration, the posterior columns and the corticospinal tracts are affected.

13. **C** [Chapter 8 VI A and Figure 8.3]. The lateral corticospinal tract and the lateral spinothalamic tract are both found in the lateral funiculus. Transection of the corticospinal tract results in ipsilateral paresis, and transection of the spinothalamic tract results in contralateral loss of pain and temperature sensation. Pallesthesia (vibration sense) is normal.

14. **A** [Chapter 16 IV and Figure 16.4]. The contralateral oculomotor nerve is responsible for the consensual reaction. The optic nerve on each side serves as the afferent limb of the reflex and the

oculomotor nerve conveys the parasympathetic fibers from the accessory oculomotor nucleus as the efferent limb of the reflex on each side.

15. **C** [Chapter 10 IX and Figure 10.6; Chapter 11 V B]. Hyperacusis is increased acuity of hearing and undue sensitivity to low tones. It results from paralysis of the stapedius (CN VII); CN VII is the nerve responsible for the afferent limb of the corneal blink reflex. The stapedius reduces the amplitude of sound vibrations of the stapes in the oval window.

16. **D** [Chapter 11 I A 3]. The mandibular division of the trigeminal nerve (CN V$_3$) innervates the muscles of mastication (eg, masseter) and mediates the tactile sensation of the anterior two-thirds of the tongue. The glossopharyngeal nerve (CN IX) provides the tactile, nociceptive, and taste innervation of the posterior third of the tongue. The facial nerve (CN VII) provides taste innervation to the anterior two-thirds of the tongue via the chorda tympani. The hypoglossal nerve provides motor innervation to the tongue musculature.

17. **B** [Chapter 12 II B and Figure 12.1]. This is the classic lateral medullary syndrome, which is also known as Wallenberg syndrome (see Figure 12.1B).

18. **B** [Chapter 12 II A and Figure 12.1]. This is a classic medial midbrain lesion characteristic of Weber syndrome. It includes the crus cerebri and the intra-axial fibers of the oculomotor nerve (see Figure 12.3C).

19. **A** [Chapter 22 III C 4 and Figure 22.3]. The metal fragment is found between the inferior frontal gyrus and the supramarginal gyrus. The two gyri are connected by the arcuate fasciculus; transection results in conduction aphasia. The arcuate fasciculus interconnects the Broca area and the Wernicke area. The key deficit is the inability to repeat (see Figure 22.6).

20. **D** [Chapter 21 VI]. Norepinephrine is the neurotransmitter of postganglionic sympathetic neurons, with the exception of sweat glands and some blood vessels that receive cholinergic sympathetic innervation. Epinephrine is produced by the chromaffin cells of the suprarenal medulla.

21. **D** [Chapter 17 III D]. Bilateral damage of the medial temporal gyri, including the amygdalae, can cause severe memory loss. Such damage to the amygdalae may lead to inappropriate social behavior (eg, hyperphagia, hypersexuality, general disinhibition). Bilateral destruction of the amygdalae results in Klüver-Bucy syndrome.

22. **E** [Chapter 16 VI B]. Presbyopia is progressive loss of the ability to accommodate the decreased ability to focus on near objects. Astigmatism is the difference in refracting power of the cornea and lens in different meridians. Cataracts are opacities that appear with aging. Optic atrophy is degeneration of the optic nerve and papillomacular bundle and loss of central vision.

23. **E** [Chapter 4 VI B; Chapter 8 II]. The corticospinal fibers are not completely myelinated at birth; this does not occur until 18 months to 2 years of age. During this time, the Babinski reflex can be elicited; later it is suppressed by descending inhibitory influences.

24. **C** [Chapter 17 II]. The nucleus of the solitary tract receives taste fibers from cranial nerves VII, IX, and X. Neurons of this tract project to the medial-most aspect of the ventral posteromedial nucleus of the thalamus. The geniculate ganglion contains primary afferent cell bodies associated with CN VII; there are no synapses there. The inferior salivatory nucleus contains preganglionic parasympathetic cell bodies associated with CN IX. The spinal trigeminal nucleus mediates somatosensation for the head/face. The ventral posteromedial nucleus of the thalamus does receive taste from the solitary nucleus, as a central projection from the solitary nucleus.

25. **E** [Chapter 22 III B]. The supplementary motor cortex plans for motor activity. Broca area is a language center. The angular gyrus is concerned with the visual perception of words. The motor strip gives rise to the corticospinal and corticobulbar tracts. The S1 somatosensory cortex subserves somatic sensibility.

26. **E** [Chapter 8 III A]. Destruction of the right cuneate nucleus results in apallesthesia (loss of vibration sensation) in the right hand. The cuneate nucleus, a way station in the posterior column-medial lemniscus pathway, mediates fine touch, conscious proprioception, and vibratory sense.

27. **E** [Chapter 20 II A]. Eccrine sweat glands are innervated by postganglionic sympathetic cholinergic fibers. Apocrine sweat glands are innervated by postganglionic sympathetic norepinephrinergic fibers.

28. **E** [Chapter 10 XII]. The vagal nerves mediate the feeling of nausea via general visceral afferent fibers. The celiac, superior and inferior mesenteric ganglia contain postganglionic sympathetic (visceral motor) cell bodies to the gut. The greater splanchnic nerve conveys pain, for example, feelings of distension from the gut, not nausea.

29. **A** [Chapter 2 I B, III and Figure 2.3]. Cerebrospinal fluid enters the bloodstream via the arachnoid villi. Hypertrophied arachnoid villi are called arachnoid granulations or pacchionian bodies. The choroid plexus is found in all four ventricles and is the site of cerebrospinal fluid formation and release. The interventricular foramen is the connection between the lateral and third ventricle. The lateral (2) and median foramina are the sites of cerebrospinal fluid exiting the ventricles to enter the subarachnoid space.

30. **B** [Chapter 2 IV]. Aqueductal stenosis results in enlargement of the third and lateral ventricles. The condition is strongly associated with prenatal infections (eg, cytomegalovirus infection). Congenital hydrocephalus occurs in 1 in 1,000 live births. Mental retardation, spasticity, and tremor are common. Shunting is the treatment of choice; cerebrospinal fluid is shunted from the distended ventricle to the peritoneal cavity.

31. **E** [Chapter 21 X D]. Alzheimer disease is commonly seen in trisomy 21, or Down syndrome, after 40 years of age. The neuropathology of Down syndrome is similar to that of Alzheimer disease: reduced choline acetyltransferase activity, cell loss in the nucleus basalis of Meynert, an increase of amyloid beta-protein, and Alzheimer neurofibrillary changes and neuritic plaques are found.

32. **B** [Chapter 8 IV B]. This describes classic Guillain-Barré syndrome, with prior infection, ascending paralysis, distal paresthesias, and albuminocytologic dissociation.

33. **C** [Chapter 8 VI J and Figure 8.1B]. This is a classic description of multiple sclerosis. Characteristics of the condition are exacerbations and remissions, involvement (demyelination) of long tracts, blurred vision, and an afferent pupillary defect. Cerebrospinal fluid contains electrophoretically detectable oligoclonal immunoglobulin (oligoclonal bands). In addition, rates of synthesis and concentration of intrathecally generated immunoglobulin G and immunoglobulin M in the cerebrospinal fluid are elevated. Oligoclonal bands are also found in syphilis, meningoencephalitis, subacute sclerosing panencephalitis, and Guillain-Barré syndrome.

34. **E** [Chapter 12 V and Figure 12.4]. Proliferating Schwann cells may give rise to schwannomas, which are also called acoustic neuromas or neurilemmomas.

35. **E** [Chapter 8 VI and Figure 8.1E]. Hemisection of the spinal cord would result in ipsilateral spastic paresis below the lesion and loss of pain and temperature on the contralateral side. The plantar response would be extensor and ipsilateral (Babinski sign).

36. **E** [Chapter 15 VI and Figure 15.3]. A lesion of the vestibular nuclei eliminates oculovestibular reflexes.

37. **B** [Chapter 21 III]. An anticholinergic agent (eg, trihexyphenidyl) may be used as an alternative to L-DOPA to alleviate the chemical imbalance found in the striatum of a patient with Parkinson disease.

38. **C** [Chapter 21 V]. Fluoxetine (Prozac) is the most selective inhibitor of serotonin reuptake.

39. **B** [Chapter 3 III C]. The paramedian (transverse pontine) branches of the basilar artery supply the medial longitudinal fasciculus of the pons. Destruction of this fasciculus results in medial longitudinal fasciculus syndrome or internuclear ophthalmoplegia. In addition, the superior cerebellar artery may irrigate the medial longitudinal fasciculus.

40. **A** [Chapter 12 II B and Figure 12.1]. Lateral medullary syndrome, also called Wallenberg syndrome; symptoms include contralateral loss of pain and temperature sensation from the face, loss of gag reflex, hemiataxia and hemiasynergia of cerebellar type, Horner syndrome, and ipsilateral nystagmus. The affected structures are the medial and inferior vestibular nuclei, inferior cerebellar peduncle, nucleus ambiguus, glossopharyngeal nerve roots, vagal nerve roots, spinothalamic tracts, the spinal trigeminal nucleus and tract, and the descending sympathetic tract.

41. **A** [Chapter 16 III]. A lesion of the upper left retinal quadrant in the left eye would show radioactive label in the left cuneus. Lesions of the cuneus result in lower field defects, and lesions of the

lingual gyrus result in upper field defects. Remember the upper retinal quadrants project to the upper banks of the calcarine fissure, whereas the lower retinal quadrants project to the lower banks of the calcarine fissure.

42. B [Chapter 19 IV]. The dentate nucleus receives massive input from the contralateral inferior olivary nucleus; it projects crossed fibers to the ventral lateral nucleus of the thalamus and red nucleus (parvocellular part). The lateral cuneate nucleus gives rise to the cuneocerebellar tract, and the lateral lemniscus and its nuclei are important way stations in the auditory pathway.

43. B [Chapter 13 III E]. The right ventral posterolateral nucleus receives posterior column modalities via the medial lemniscus from the left side of the body. The red nucleus is a midbrain motor nucleus: it plays a role in the control of flexor tone. The lateral cuneate nucleus projects unconscious proprioception to the cerebellum (eg, from muscles and tendons). The ventral lateral nucleus receives input from the cerebellum (dentate nucleus).

44. A [Chapter 9 II B 3]. The inferior olivary nucleus of the caudal pons projects to the nucleus of the inferior colliculus. The medial geniculate nucleus is an auditory way station, the inferior olivary nucleus is a cerebellar relay station, and the transverse gyrus of Heschl is a primary auditory center. Retrograde transport studies show that horseradish peroxidase is picked up by the axon terminals and transported to the perikarya; anterograde studies show that labeled amino acids are taken up by the perikarya and transported to distant nuclei.

45. D [Chapter 9 III]. The base of the pons contains intra-axial root fibers of CN V, corticobulbar fibers to the hypoglossal nucleus, and corticospinal fibers. Spinotrigeminal fibers mediate pain and temperature sensation from the ipsilateral face.

46. C [Chapter 9 II]. Near the medial lemniscus bilateral and root fibers of CN XII bilaterally. Deficits to the medial lemniscus will result in contralateral loss of conscious proprioception, fine touch, and vibratory sense from the trunk and lower limb. The medulla gives rise to CN IX, CN X, and CN XII; CN XII controls the movement of the tongue.

47. D [Chapter 9 III]. The pontine tegmentum contains CN VI and CN VII; the medial longitudinal fasciculus (MLF), medial lemniscus, spinotrigeminal nucleus and tract; spinothalamic tract; and the spinohypothalamic tract (Horner syndrome). Internuclear ophthalmoplegia, also known as MLF syndrome, results from a lesion of the MLF. Lesions occur in the dorsomedial pontine tegmentum and may affect one or both MLFs. This is a frequent sign of multiple sclerosis; it results in medial rectus palsy on attempted lateral gaze and monocular nystagmus in the abducting eye with normal convergence.

48. B [Chapter 12 II A and Figure 12.1]. Thrombosis of the anterior spinal artery results in medial medullary syndrome. Symptoms of medial medullary syndrome include contralateral hemiparesis of the trunk and limbs; contralateral loss of conscious proprioception, fine touch, and vibratory sense from the trunk and limbs; and ipsilateral flaccid paralysis of the tongue.

49. E [Chapter 22 III C 3 and Figure 22.3]. Wernicke speech area is in the posterior superior temporal gyrus (Brodmann area 22). Wernicke aphasia is characterized by faster-than-normal speech, difficulty finding the right words to express ideas, and poor comprehension of the speech of others. Patients appear unaware of the deficit.

50. C [Chapter 22 IV]. Pick disease—frontotemporal lobar degeneration—shows an extreme degree of atrophy in the temporal and frontal lobes. Creutzfeldt-Jakob is a human prion disease affecting the central nervous system. Down syndrome is a chromosomal anomaly characterized by trisomy 21. Tuberous sclerosis and Sturge-Weber syndrome are neurocutaneous diseases that result in lesions of the skin and neurologic problems (eg, mental retardation and seizures).

51. A [Chapter 22 III C 4 and Figure 22.3]. The arcuate fasciculus (superior longitudinal fasciculus) is a fiber bundle that interconnects the motor speech area (44 and 45) with the sensory speech area (22). Transection of this fiber bundle results in conduction aphasia with poor repetition of spoken language, relatively good speech comprehension and expression, paraphasic errors (using incorrect words), and impaired object naming. Patients are aware of the deficit. The arcuate nucleus is part of the hypothalamus and is unrelated to speech. The dorsal longitudinal fasciculus is a hypothalamic fiber tract, unrelated to speech, while the medial longitudinal fasciculus yolks cranial nerve motor nuclei together, primarily for conjugate movement of the eyes. Indusium griseum is a thin lamina of gray matter near the corpus callosum, it is primitive cortical tissue related to the hippocampal formation.

52. **E** [Chapter 2 VII E and Figure 2.9]. The pineal body is a midline diencephalic structure that contains calcium concrements; it is seen in computed tomographic images. The cerebral peduncles, the superior and inferior colliculi, the oculomotor nerves, and the cerebral aqueduct are found in the midbrain. Stenosis of the cerebral aqueduct results in noncommunicating hydrocephalus.

53. **H** [Chapter 4 X C]. The optic nerve is derived from the wall of the diencephalic vesicle.

54. **F** [Chapter 10 V B]. The oculomotor nerve is often damaged in the process of transtentorial herniation.

55. **K** [Chapter 10 XII A]. The vagus nerve mediates the sensory and motor innervation of the pharyngeal arches 4 and 6.

56. **J** [Chapter 10 VI]. The trochlear nerve innervates the superior oblique, which depresses, intorts, and abducts the globe.

57. **B** [Chapter 18 II E]. Parkinson disease is characterized by a triad of symptoms: pill-rolling tremor, rigidity, and hypokinesia. The substantia nigra bears the brunt of the cell loss. Cerebellar disease is characterized by intention tremor, ataxia, and hypotonia. Destruction of the subthalamic nucleus results in contralateral hemiballismus.

58. **A** [Chapter 8 V B]. In amyotrophic lateral sclerosis, there is loss of both anterior horn cells and cortical pyramidal cells that give rise to the pyramidal tract. This motor system disease consists of an upper motor neuron component and a lower motor neuron component. There are no sensory deficits in amyotrophic lateral sclerosis.

59. **C** [Chapter 2 II C and Figure 2.4A and B]. The cerebral aqueduct is in the midbrain (mesencephalon). It interconnects the third and fourth ventricles.

60. **C** [Chapter 9 IV]. The tegmentum of the midbrain contains the nuclei of the oculomotor (CN III) and trochlear (CN IV) nerves. The midbrain also contains the mesencephalic nucleus of the trigeminal sensory system.

61. **E** [Chapter 18 II and Figure 18.1]. The caudate nucleus, a basal nucleus, is located in the white matter of the telencephalon. It forms the lateral wall of the frontal horn of the lateral ventricle.

62. **A** [Chapter 16 III C and Figure 16.4]. The optic chiasm is in the diencephalon between the anterior commissure and the infundibulum of the pituitary gland (hypophysis).

63. **B** [Chapter 9 II]. The olive and the pyramid are prominent structures on the ventral surface of the medulla. The olive contains the inferior olivary nucleus. The pyramid contains the corticospinal tract.

64. **A** [Chapter 2 VII E and Figure 2.9]. The pineal gland is part of the epithalamus—a subdivision of the diencephalon.

65. **B** [Chapter 9 II, Figures 9.3 and 9.5]. Cranial nerves IX, X, and XII are located in the medulla.

66. **E** [Chapter 4 III]. Schwann cells of the peripheral nervous system are neural crest derivatives.

67. **D** [Chapter 5 III B]. Oligodendrocytes of the central nervous system can myelinate numerous axons. Schwann cells myelinate only one internode.

68. **A** [Chapter 5 III A]. The filaments of astrocytes contain fibrillary glial acidic protein, a marker for astrocytes and astrocytic tumor cells. Another biochemical marker is glutamine synthetase found exclusively in astrocytes.

69. **E** [Chapter 5 III E]. Schwann cells are myelin-forming cells of the peripheral nervous system. They myelinate only one internode and are derived from the neural crest. Schwann cells function in regeneration and remyelination of severed axons in the peripheral nervous system but may proliferate to form schwannomas, benign tumors of peripheral nerves (eg, acoustic neuromas of CN VIII).

70. **C** [Chapter 5 III C]. Microglial cells arise from monocytes. They are phagocytes of the central nervous system.

71. **B** [Chapter 7 I C; Chapter 8 III D and Figure 8.2]. Interruption of the posterior spinocerebellar tract results in ipsilateral lower limb dystaxia (ie, incoordination). The cerebellum is deprived of its muscle spindle input from the lower limb.

72. **D** [Chapter 8 I A and Figure 8.2]. Destruction of anterior horn cells (lower motor neurons) results in ipsilateral flaccid paralysis with muscle atrophy and loss of muscle stretch reflexes (areflexia).

73. **E** [Chapter 8 III B and Figure 8.2]. Interruption of the lateral spinothalamic tract results in a contralateral loss of pain and temperature sensation one segment below the lesion. The decussation occurs in the anterior white commissure in the spinal cord.

74. **C** [Chapter 8 II A and Figure 8.2]. Interruption of the lateral corticospinal tract results in an ipsilateral upper motor neuron lesion. It is characterized by exaggerated muscle stretch reflexes (hyperreflexia), spastic paresis, muscle weakness, loss or diminution of superficial reflexes (ie, abdominal and cremaster reflexes), and Babinski sign. The deficits are below the lesion on the same side. The lateral corticospinal tract decussates in the caudal medulla.

75. **A** [Chapter 8 III A and Figure 8.2]. A lesion of the gracile fasciculus results in a loss of two-point tactile discrimination in the ipsilateral foot. The posterior column-medial lemniscus pathway decussates in the caudal medulla.

76. **C** [Chapter 12 VI]. This lesion includes the two medial longitudinal fasciculi. The patient has medial longitudinal fasciculus syndrome and medial rectus palsy on attempted lateral gaze to either side. Convergence remains intact.

77. **E** [Chapter 12 III A and Figure 12.2]. This lesion includes three major structures: the medial lemniscus, corticospinal fibers, and exiting abducens root fibers (CN VI) traversing the corticospinal fibers. Interruption of the abducens fibers causes ipsilateral lateral rectus paralysis with medial strabismus. Damage to the uncrossed corticospinal fibers results in contralateral spastic hemiparesis.

78. **A** [Chapter 12 II B and Figure 12.1]. Occlusion of the posterior inferior cerebellar artery (PICA) infarcts the lateral zone of the medulla, causing PICA (lateral medullary) syndrome. The major structures involved are the inferior cerebellar peduncle, spinal trigeminal tract and nucleus, spinal lemniscus, nucleus ambiguus, and exiting fibers of CN X.

79. **D** [Chapter 12 III B and Figure 12.2]. This lesion includes the facial motor nucleus and its intra-axial fibers, hence the loss of the corneal blink reflex (efferent limb). The spinal trigeminal tract and nucleus and the spinal lemniscus are also damaged by this lesion. Damage to the spinal trigeminal tract and nucleus causes ipsilateral facial anesthesia, including loss of the corneal blink reflex (afferent limb). Damage to the spinal lemniscus (lateral spinothalamic tract) causes a contralateral loss of pain and temperature sensation from the body and limbs.

80. **B** [Chapter 12 II A and Figure 12.1]. This lesion damages the hypoglossal nucleus and exiting root fibers, the medial lemniscus, and the corticospinal tract. Damage to the hypoglossal nerve results in an ipsilateral flaccid paralysis of the tongue, a lower motor neuron lesion. Damage to the medial lemniscus results in a contralateral loss of tactile discrimination and vibration sensation. Damage to the corticospinal (pyramid) tracts results in contralateral spastic hemiparesis. This symptom complex is known as medial medullary syndrome.

81. **A** [Chapter 12 II B and Figure 12.1]. Lateral medullary syndrome (posterior inferior cerebellar artery syndrome) usually includes hoarseness, Horner syndrome, and singultus (hiccups). Damage to the nucleus ambiguus causes flaccid paralysis of the muscle of the larynx with hoarseness (dysphonia and dysarthria). Interruption of descending autonomic fibers to the ciliospinal center at T1 causes sympathetic paralysis of the eye (Horner syndrome).

82. **D** [Chapter 13 III E 2 and Figure 13.2]. The ventral lateral nucleus receives input from the dentate nucleus of the cerebellum and projects to the motor cortex (area 4).

83. **E** [Chapter 13 III E and Figure 13.2]. The ventral posteromedial nucleus receives input of taste sensation from the solitary nucleus of the medulla and pons and projects this input to the gustatory cortex of the parietal operculum (area 43).

84. **E** [Chapter 13 III E and Figure 13.2]. The ventral posteromedial nucleus receives general somatic afferent input from the face, including pain and temperature sensation. It also receives special visceral afferent taste sensation input from the tongue, palate, and epiglottis.

85. A [Chapter 13 III A and Figure 13.2]. The anterior thalamic nucleus receives input from the mammillary nucleus via the mammillothalamic tract and direct input from the hippocampal formation via the fornix. The anterior nucleus projects, via the anterior limb of the internal capsule, to the cingulate gyrus (areas 23, 24, and 32).

86. B [Chapter 13 III C and Figure 13.2]. The centromedian nucleus, the largest of the intralaminar nuclei, projects to the putamen and to the motor cortex. The centromedian nucleus receives input from the globus pallidus and the motor cortex (area 4).

87. C [Chapter 13 III B and Figure 13.2]. The dorsomedial nucleus of the thalamus, or the mediodorsal nucleus, has reciprocal connections with the prefrontal cortex (areas 9-12).

88. C [Chapter 13 X B 4 and Figure 13.5]. The mammillary nucleus receives input from the hippocampal formation (ie, subiculum) via the fornix.

89. A [Chapter 13 X B 2 and Figure 13.5]. The anterior nucleus of the hypothalamus helps prevent a rise in body temperature by activating processes that favor heat loss (eg, vasodilation of cutaneous blood vessels, and sweating). Lesions of this nucleus result in hyperthermia (hyperpyrexia).

90. E [Chapter 13 X B 2 and Figure 13.5]. The suprachiasmatic nucleus receives direct input from the retina; it plays a role in the maintenance of circadian rhythms.

91. D [Chapter 13 X B 2 and Figure 13.5]. The neurons of the paraventricular and supraoptic nuclei of the hypothalamus produce antidiuretic hormone (vasopressin) and oxytocin. These peptides are transported via the supraopticohypophyseal tract to the neurohypophysis. Lesions of the nuclei or the hypophyseal tract result in diabetes insipidus.

92. B [Chapter 13 X B 3 and Figure 13.5]. The neurons of the arcuate nucleus (infundibular nucleus) produce hypothalamic-releasing and release-inhibiting hormones, which are conveyed to the adenohypophysis through the hypophyseal portal system. These hormones regulate the production of adenohypophyseal hormones and their release into the systemic circulation.

93. D [Chapter 13 X B 2 and Figure 13.5]. The paraventricular and supraoptic nuclei produce antidiuretic hormone, which helps regulate water balance in the body.

94. E [Chapter 18 II E]. Hemiballism results from lesions of the subthalamic nucleus.

95. A [Chapter 18 II B]. The caudate nucleus and the putamen (neostriatum) receive dopaminergic input from the pars compacta of the substantia nigra—via the nigrostriatal tract.

96. C [Chapter 18 II B]. Neurons of the globus pallidus give rise to the ansa lenticularis and the lenticular fasciculus, two pathways that project to the ventral anterior, ventral lateral, and centromedian nuclei of the thalamus.

97. D [Chapter 18 II E]. Destruction or degeneration of the substantia nigra results in parkinsonism, a symptom of which is rigidity.

98. A [Chapter 18 II E]. In Huntington chorea, there is a loss of neurons in the striatum. Cell loss in the head of the caudate nucleus causes dilation of the frontal horn of the lateral ventricle (hydrocephalus ex vacuo), which is visible on CT and MRI.

99. E [Chapter 21 V and Figure 21.5]. Serotonin (5-HT) is produced by neurons located in the raphe nuclei. This paramidline column of cells extends from the caudal medulla to the rostral midbrain.

100. C [Chapter 21 VIII and Figure 21.10]. Purkinje neurons are GABAergic. GABAergic neurons are also found in the striatum, globus pallidus, and pars reticularis of the substantia nigra.

101. A [Chapter 22 III and Figure 21.3]. The nucleus basalis (of Meynert) contains cholinergic neurons that project to the entire neocortex.

102. A [Chapter 22 III and Figure 21.3]. Acetylcholine is the neurotransmitter of motor cranial nerves (general somatic efferent, special visceral efferent, and general visceral efferent) and anterior horn cells of the spinal cord.

103. B [Chapter 21 III and Figure 21.3]. Neurons of the pars compacta of the substantia nigra contain dopamine. Dopamine is present also in the ventral tegmental area of the midbrain, the superior colliculus, and the arcuate nucleus of the hypothalamus.

104. D [Chapter 21 IV and Figure 21.4]. The locus ceruleus is the largest assembly of noradrenergic (norepinephrinergic) neurons in the brain. It is located in the lateral pontine and midbrain tegmenta. Locus ceruleus neurons project to the entire neocortex and cerebellar cortex.

105. C [Chapter 21 VIII and Figure 21.10]. The globus pallidus contains GABAergic neurons that project to the thalamus and subthalamic nucleus.

106. E [Chapter 21 VII and Figure 21.8]. Substance P is contained in spinal ganglion cells and is the neurotransmitter of afferent pain fibers. Substance P is also produced by striatal neurons, which project to the globus pallidus and substantia nigra.

107. D [Chapter 21 VIII]. Glycine is the major inhibitory neurotransmitter of the spinal cord. The Renshaw interneurons of the spinal cord are glycinergic.

108. C [Chapter 21 VIII and Figure 21.11]. Glutamate is the major excitatory neurotransmitter of the brain; neocortical glutamatergic neurons project to the caudate nucleus and the putamen (striatum).

109. A [Chapter 21 VI and Figure 21.6]. Beta-endorphinergic neurons are located almost exclusively in the hypothalamus (arcuate and premammillary nuclei).

110. B [Chapter 21 VI and Figure 21.7]. Enkephalinergic neurons in the posterior horn of the spinal cord presynaptically inhibit the spinal ganglion cells that mediate pain impulses.

111. D [Chapter 16 III G and Figure 16.3; Chapter 22 III A]. A lesion of the lingual gyrus of the right occipital lobe can cause a left upper homonymous quadrantanopia. Lower retinal quadrants are represented in the lower banks of the calcarine sulcus.

112. A [Chapter 22 III C, VIII, and Figure 22.6]. A lesion of the motor (Broca) speech area (areas 44 and 45) and the adjacent motor cortex of the precentral gyrus (area 4) can cause expressive aphasia and an upper motor neuron lesion involving the hand area of the motor strip. This territory is supplied by the superior division of the middle cerebral artery (prerolandic and rolandic arteries).

113. E [Chapter 22 III A, VI A, and VI B]. A parietal lesion in the right postcentral gyrus (areas 3, 1, and 2) or in the right superior parietal lobule (areas 5 and 7) can cause astereognosis, the deficit in which a patient with eyes closed cannot identify a familiar object placed in the left hand. This territory is supplied by the superior division of the middle cerebral artery (the rolandic and anterior parietal arteries). The dorsal aspect of the superior parietal lobule on the convex surface is also supplied by the anterior cerebral artery.

114. E [Chapter 22 IV and Figure 22.5]. Characteristic signs of damage to the nondominant hemisphere include hemineglect, topographic memory loss, denial of deficit (anosognosia), and construction and dressing apraxia. A lesion in the right inferior parietal lobule could account for these deficits. This territory is supplied by the inferior division of the middle cerebral artery (posterior parietal and angular arteries).

115. C [Chapter 22 VIII B and Figure 22.6]. Receptive (Wernicke) aphasia is characterized by poor comprehension of speech, unawareness of the deficit, and difficulty finding the correct words to express a thought. The sensory speech area is found in the posterior part of the left superior temporal gyrus (area 22). This territory is supplied by the inferior division of the middle cerebral artery (posterior temporal branches).

116. B [Chapter 22 III A 6]. Gerstmann syndrome includes left-right confusion, finger agnosia, dysgraphia, and dyscalculia. This syndrome results from a lesion of the left angular gyrus of the inferior parietal lobule. This territory is supplied by branches from the inferior division of the middle cerebral artery (angular and posterior parietal arteries).

117. A [Chapter 22 III B]. A lesion of the anterior paracentral lobule results in an upper motor neuron lesion (spastic paresis) involving the contralateral foot. Ankle clonus, exaggerated muscle stretch reflexes, and Babinski sign are common.

118. D [Chapter 1 Figure 1.12]. The thalamus.

119. E [Chapter 1 Figure 1.12]. The anterior limb of the internal capsule.

120. B [Chapter 1 Figure 1.12]. The putamen.

121. A [Chapter 1 Figure 1.12]. The head of the caudate nucleus.

122. C [Chapter 1 Figure 1.12]. The splenium of the corpus callosum.

123. C [Chapter 1 Figure 1.2; Chapter 13 Figure 13.1]. The medial geniculate body.

124. B [Chapter 1 Figures 1.6 and 1.8]. The mesencephalon.

125. D [Chapter 1 Figure 1.8]. The mammillary body.

126. E [Chapter 1 Figures 1.2 and 1.7]. The optic tract.

127. A [Chapter 1 Figure 1.10]. The amygdala (amygdaloid nuclear complex).

128. C [Chapter 1 Figures 1.6 and 1.8]. The pineal gland (epiphysis).

129. E [Chapter 1 Figure 1.5; Chapter 13 Figure 13.8]. The hypophysis (pituitary gland).

130. D [Chapter 1 Figures 1.6 and 1.8]. The mesencephalon (midbrain).

131. B [Chapter 1 Figure 1.8]. The thalamus.

132. A [Chapter 1 Figure 1.8]. The fornix.

133. J [Chapter 16 Figure 16.7]. A right third nerve palsy with complete ptosis. The ptosis results from paralysis of the levator palpebrae superioris.

134. I [Chapter 16 Figure 16.7]. A destructive lesion of the frontal eye fields results in a deviation of the eyes toward the lesion. An irritative lesion results in deviation of the eyes away from the lesion.

135. H [Chapter 16 Figure 16.7]. The Argyll Robertson pupil is characterized by irregular miotic pupils that do not respond to light but do converge in response to accommodation. It is a sign of tertiary syphilis.

136. G [Chapter 16 Figure 16.7]. A right fourth nerve palsy is characterized by the inability of the patient to depress the globe from the adducted position.

137. F [Chapter 16 Figure 16.7]. Parinaud syndrome is characterized by an inability to perform upward or downward conjugate gaze and may be associated with ptosis and pupillary abnormalities.

138. E [Chapter 16 Figure 16.7]. A right sixth nerve palsy is characterized by inability to abduct the eye.

139. D [Chapter 16 Figure 16.7]. A third nerve palsy is characterized by a down-and-out eye, complete ptosis, and a dilated (blown) pupil. The lid was retracted to view the pupil.

140. C [Chapter 16 Figure 16.7]. Internuclear ophthalmoplegia results from a lesion of one or both medial longitudinal fasciculi. Transection of the right medial longitudinal fasciculus results in medial rectus palsy on attempted lateral gaze to the left. Convergence is normal, and nystagmus is seen in the abducting eye.

141. B [Chapter 16 Figure 16.7]. Horner syndrome consists of miosis, mild ptosis, hemianhidrosis, and enophthalmos. It results from loss of sympathetic input to the head.

142. A [Chapter 16 Figure 16.7]. Retrobulbar neuritis is an inflammation of the optic nerve that reduces the light-carrying ability of the nerve. This condition can be diagnosed by the swinging flashlight test. Light shown into the normal eye results in constriction of both pupils. Swinging the flashlight to the affected eye results in a dilated pupil in both eyes. This pupil is called an afferent, or Marcus Gunn, pupil.

143. C [Chapter 13 XIII D]. A bilateral lesion of the ventromedial hypothalamic nucleus results in hyperphagia and savage behavior.

144. E [Chapter 13 XIII B]. A bilateral lesion of the posterior hypothalamic nucleus results in the inability to thermoregulate (poikilothermia). Bilateral destruction of only the posterior aspect of the lateral hypothalamic nucleus results in anorexia and emaciation.

145. B [Chapter 13 X B and XII H]. Lesions involving the supraoptic and paraventricular nuclei or the supraopticohypophyseal tract result in diabetes insipidus with polydipsia and polyuria.

146. D [Chapter 13 XIII B]. Destruction of the anterior hypothalamic nuclei results in hyperthermia.

147. A [Chapter 13 XIII D]. Stimulation of the ventromedial nuclei inhibits the urge to eat, resulting in emaciation (cachexia), whereas destruction of the ventromedial nuclei results in hyperphagia and savage behavior.

148. H [Chapter 16 II A]. Stimulation of the frontal eye field (Brodmann area 8) results in turning of the eyes and head to the contralateral side.

149. G [Chapter 22 III C and Figure 22.3]. A lesion of the motor (Broca) speech area (Brodmann areas 44 and 45) results in nonfluent, effortful, and telegraphic speech as well as motor (expressive) aphasia.

150. F [Chapter 16 III F and Figure 16.3]. Ablation of the anterior third of the temporal lobe interrupts Meyer loop, which projects to the lingual gyrus (the lower bank of the calcarine fissure). The lower bank of the calcarine fissure represents the upper visual field. This lesion results in a contralateral upper homonymous quadrantanopia.

151. E [Chapter 22 III C and Figure 22.3]. A lesion destroying the sensory speech (Wernicke) area (Brodmann 22) results in sensory aphasia—characterized by poor comprehension, fluent speech, poor repetition, and paraphasic errors (non sequiturs, neologisms, and driveling speech [meaningless double talk]).

152. D [Chapter 22 III A and Figure 22.4A]. This constellation of dominant hemispheric deficits results from destruction of the angular gyrus (Brodmann area 39). Called Gerstmann syndrome, it is characterized by left-right confusion, finger agnosia, dyslexia, dysgraphia, dyscalculia, and a homonymous contralateral lower quadrantanopia.

153. C [Chapter 22 III C and Figure 22.3]. A lesion of the supramarginal gyrus (Brodmann area 40) or of the arcuate fasciculus results in conduction aphasia characterized by fluent speech, good comprehension, poor repetition, and paraphasic speech (fluently spoken jargon-like sensory aphasia) and writing.

154. B [Chapter 22 III A, IV A, and Figure 22.4A]. Lesions of the postcentral gyrus, sensory strip (Brodmann areas 3, 1, and 2) result in contralateral astereognosia, hemihypesthesia, and agraphesthesia.

155. A [Chapter 22 III B and Figure 22.4]. Lesions of the precentral gyrus, motor strip (Brodmann area 4) result in contralateral spastic hemiparesis with pyramidal signs.

156. G [Chapter 13 X B; Chapter 17 III D]. In thiamine (vitamin B_1) deficiency, hemorrhagic lesions are found in the mammillary bodies.

157. F [Chapter 17 III D]. Bilateral lesions of the amygdala result in Klüver-Bucy syndrome, with hyperphagia, hypersexuality, and psychic blindness (visual agnosia).

158. E [Chapter 17 III D]. Bilateral damage to the parahippocampal gyri and the underlying hippocampal formation results in severe loss of short-term memory (eg, hypoxia, hypoxemia, and herpes simplex virus encephalitis).

159. D [Chapter 16 III F and Figure 16.3]. Lesions of the cuneus interrupt the visual radiations en route to the upper bank of the calcarine fissure, which represents the inferior visual field quadrants.

160. C [Chapter 17 III B]. The fornix (a limbic structure) interconnects the septal area and the hippocampal formation. Bilateral transection of this structure may result in an acute amnestic syndrome.

161. B [Chapter 22 III B and Figure 22.2]. The motor strip for the foot is in the anterior paracentral lobule on the medial aspect of the hemisphere. A lesion here results in a contralateral hemiparesis of the foot and leg with pyramidal signs.

162. A [Chapter 17 III D]. Ablation of the cingulate gyrus (cingulectomies) has been used to treat patients with psychosis and neurosis. The cingulate gyrus is part of the limbic lobe; lesions can result in akinesia, mutism, apathy, and indifference to pain.

163. C [Chapter 3 I A and Figure 3.1]. The anterior spinal artery supplies the pyramids, medial lemniscus, and intra-axial fibers of the hypoglossal nerve (CN XII) in the medulla. The anterior communicating artery connects the two anterior cerebral arteries and is a common site for berry (saccular) aneurysms. The anterior choroidal artery supplies the choroid plexus of the temporal horn, the hippocampus, amygdala, optic tract, lateral geniculate body, and globus pallidus. The posterior spinal artery supplies the gracile and cuneate fasciculi and their posterior relay nuclei. The posterior inferior cerebellar artery supplies the dorsolateral zone of the medulla.

164. B [Chapter 3 I A and Figure 3.1]. The anterior spinal artery perfuses the intra-axial fibers of the anterior aspect of the caudal medulla and spinal cord. The basilar artery gives rise to the pontine arteries. The posterior spinal artery irrigates the posterior columns. The vertebral artery is a branch of the subclavian artery. The anterior inferior cerebellar artery supplies the facial and trigeminal nuclei as well as the vestibular and cochlear nuclei.

165. A [Chapter 3 III A and Figure 3.2]. The anterior communicating artery is a common site for berry aneurysms; berry aneurysms of the anterior communicating artery frequently pressure the optic chiasm and cause a bitemporal lower quadrantanopia. The basilar artery gives rise to the pontine arteries. The ophthalmic artery gives rise to the central artery of the retina. The anterior cerebral artery supplies the anterior limb of the internal capsule via the medial striate artery (Heubner artery). The posterior communicating artery irrigates the optic chiasm, optic tract, hypothalamus, subthalamus, and anterior half of the ventral portion of the thalamus. Berry aneurysms of the posterior communicating artery frequently cause third nerve palsy.

166. B [Chapter 3 III A and Figure 3.4]. Laceration of the middle meningeal artery results in epidural hemorrhage. It supplies most of the dura mater and calvaria.

167. E [Chapter 3 III A and Figure 3.2]. The aneurysm was on the posterior communicating artery; pressure on the oculomotor nerve results in a complete third nerve palsy with the following signs: dilated fixed pupil, ptosis, and eye looking down and out. The anterior cerebral artery supplies part of the caudate nucleus, putamen, and anterior limb of the internal capsule via the medial striate artery (of Heubner). The anterior communicating artery supplies the leg and foot areas of the motor and sensory cortices (paracentral lobule). The internal carotid artery provides direct branches to the optic nerve, optic chiasm, hypothalamus, and genu of the internal capsule. The ophthalmic artery branches into the central artery of the retina.

168. D [Chapter 3 III C and Figure 3.2]. The superior cerebellar artery supplies the dentate nucleus, the largest efferent nucleus of the cerebellum. Damage to this nucleus results in cerebellar signs: dystaxia, dysmetria, and intention tremor. The vertebral artery gives rise to the posterior inferior cerebellar artery, which supplies the medial and inferior vestibular nuclei, inferior cerebellar peduncle, nucleus ambiguus, intra-axial fibers of the glossopharyngeal nerve (CN IX) and vagus nerve (CN X), spinothalamic tract of the anterolateral system, and spinal trigeminal nucleus and tract. The anterior inferior cerebellar artery irrigates the dorsal lateral pons, CN V, CN VII, and CN VIII. The posterior cerebral artery supplies the posterior half of the thalamus, the medial and lateral geniculate bodies, the occipital lobe, visual cortex, and inferior surface of the temporal lobe, including the hippocampal formation.

169. C [Chapter 1 II D; Chapter 10 VIII]. A lesion of the lateral rectus results in diplopia and horizontal nystagmus on attempted lateral conjugated gaze. It is innervated by CN VI. The buccinator (facial expression), the posterior belly of the digastric (facial expression), and the orbicularis oculi (corneal blink reflex) are innervated by the facial nerve (CN VII). The pterygoids (mouth movement) are innervated by the mandibular division of the trigeminal nerve (CN V_3).

170. D [Chapter 2 II A and Figure 2.8]. The trigone contains a calcified globus of choroid plexus. In axial CT sections, the adult calcified pineal body is also visualized lying halfway between the two trigona.

171. D [Chapter 2 VII]. The subcommissural organ lies on the roof of the cerebral aqueduct near the posterior commissure; it has a blood-brain barrier. All circumventricular organs except the subcommissural organ have fenestrated capillaries and thus lack a blood-brain barrier.

172. C [Chapter 3 III A and Figure 3.3]. The pericallosal artery, a branch of the anterior cerebral artery, irrigates the lower limb area of the paracentral lobule. The middle cerebral artery supplies the trunk, upper limb, and face areas of the motor and sensory cortices. The posterior cerebral artery supplies the occipital lobe, visual cortex, and inferior surface of the temporal lobe, including the hippocampal formation. The splenial (posterior pericallosal) artery supplies the splenium of the corpus callosum. The medial striate artery irrigates the anterior limb of the internal capsule.

173. **A** [Chapter 3 III A; Chapter 17 III D]. The anterior choroidal artery is a branch of the middle cerebral artery. It supplies the amygdala, the posterior limb of the internal capsule, the globus pallidus, and the optic tract. Klüver-Bucy syndrome results in placidity, hypersexuality, hyperphagia, and psychic blindness (visual agnosia).

174. **B** [Chapter 1 Figure 1.7]. Three cranial nerves—the abducens, facial, and vestibulocochlear nerves—exit from the pontomedullary sulcus. The facial nerve has two divisions, the cranial nerve proper (motor) and the intermediate division (sensory). The intermediate division contains general somatic afferent and special visceral afferent fibers.

175. **E** [Chapter 2 III]. Cerebrospinal fluid typically contains no more than 5 lymphocytes/μL (see Table 2.1).

176. **C** [Chapter 2 III]. The normal total protein value for cerebrospinal fluid is <45 mg/dL in the lumbar cistern (see Table 2.1).

177. **E** [Chapter 2 III]. Normal serum glucose level in cerebrospinal fluid is 66% of blood, which is 80 to 120 mg/dL.

178. **E** [Chapter 2 IV E]. Pseudotumor cerebri, or benign intracranial hypertension, is characterized by papilledema without mass, elevated cerebrospinal fluid pressure, and deteriorating vision. Normal pressure hydrocephalus is characterized clinically by the triad of progressive dementia, ataxic gait, and urinary incontinence (wacky, wobbly, and wet). Hydrocephalus ex vacuo results from a loss of neurons in the caudate nucleus (eg, Huntington disease). Chiari malformation is a cerebellomedullary malformation in which the caudal vermis, cerebellar tonsils, and medulla herniate through the foramen magnum, resulting in an obstructive hydrocephalus. Dandy-Walker consists of a large cyst of the posterior fossa associated with atresia of the outlet foramina (of Luschka and Magendie).

179. **E** [Chapter 5 Figure 5.3; Chapter 16 III F]. Seizures have the highest incidence in the temporal lobe. Astrocytoma is the most common glioma in the temporal lobe. Charcot-Bouchard microaneurysms are found in the lenticulostriate arteries. They rupture most frequently in the basal nuclei. They are the most common cause of nontraumatic intraparenchymal hemorrhage. The olfactory groove meningioma impinges on the olfactory tract and optic nerve, causing ipsilateral anosmia, ipsilateral optic atrophy, and contralateral papilledema. The astrocytoma transected Meyer loop and produced contralateral quadrantanopia.

180. **C** [Chapter 9 Figures 9.2 and 9.3]. The lesion is found in the caudal medulla at the spinomedullary junction. A lesion of the decussation of the pyramids results in spastic paralysis of all limbs and intact sensibility. The location of the cranial nerve nuclei of the brainstem reveals where the lesion is in the neuraxis: midbrain, CN III, and CN IV; pons, CN V, CN VI, CN VII, and CN VIII; medulla, CN VIII, CN IX, and CN X.

181. **A** [Chapter 4 X B]. The optic cup and its derivatives, the retina and optic nerve, develop from the diencephalon.

182. **A** [Chapter 6 II D and Figure 6.3]. General somatic afferent fibers are one of four functional components of spinal nerves (see Figure 6.3). They convey sensory input from skin, muscle, bone, and joints to the central nervous system. General visceral afferent fibers convey sensory input from visceral organs to the central nervous system. Special somatic afferent fibers convey sensory information related to vision, audition, and equilibrium, whereas special visceral afferent fibers convey sensory information related to taste and smell.

183. **B** [Chapter 4 VI and Figure 4.4]. The spinal cord derives from the caudal part of the neural tube. The cranial part becomes the brain. The cavity gives rise to the central canal of the spinal cord and ventricles of the brain. The anterior neuropore is an opening in the neural tube that in the

fourth week becomes the lamina terminalis. The posterior neuropore is a second opening in the neural tube that closes in the fourth week.

184. B [Chapter 4 X A]. The globus pallidus originates in the diencephalon. Neuroblasts from the subthalamus migrate into the telencephalic white matter to form the globus pallidus.

185. A [Chapter 9 III B]. The abducens nucleus is the general somatic efferent column of the pons.

186. E [Chapter 9 III B]. The superior salivatory nucleus is the general visceral efferent column of the pons. All somatic and visceral motor nuclei are derived from the basal plate. The cerebellum and pontine nuclei and the sensory nuclei of cranial nerves are derivatives of the alar plate.

187. C [Chapter 4 VI B]. Axons of the corticospinal tracts are not fully myelinated until the end of the second postnatal year. Babinski sign (extensor plantar reflex) can be elicited in infants for this reason.

188. B [Chapter 14 II C]. The cochlear duct is derived from a thickening of the surface ectoderm called the otic placode.

189. D [Chapter 10 IX A]. The stapedius is innervated by CN VII.

190. E [Chapter 19 V C]. Intention tremor is a deficit in coordination of voluntary movements caused by lesions in the lateral cerebellum (eg, finger-to-nose test). Athetosis is slow, writhing movements representative of basal nuclei damage. Chorea is involuntary movements caused by overactivity of dopamine and is a classic symptom of Huntington disease. Cogwheel rigidity is a classic rigidity seen in Parkinson disease owing to lack of dopamine. Hemiballismus is large, flinging movements of the limbs owing to a lesion in the subthalamic nucleus.

191. A [Chapter 7 I C]. The anterior spinocerebellar tract crosses the midline via the anterior commissure and crosses the dorsal aspect of the superior cerebellar peduncle to terminate in the anterior cerebellar vermis.

192. C [Chapter 10 IX, XI, and XIV]. The stylohyoid, stylopharyngeus, and styloglossus are attached to the styloid process. The stylohyoid is innervated by CN VII. The stylopharyngeus is innervated by CN IX. The styloglossus is innervated by CN XII.

193. A [Chapter 10 III]. Rhinorrhea will most likely result from a fracture of the cribriform plate of the ethmoid bone, which can tear the arachnoid membrane and result in a leakage of cerebrospinal fluid into the nasal cavity.

194. A [Chapter 10 IX]. The facial nerve (CN VII) innervates the taste buds from the anterior two-thirds of the tongue, providing input to the solitary tract and solitary nucleus via the geniculate ganglion (see Figure 17.2).

195. B [Chapter 10 VII]. The maxillary nerve passes through the foramen rotundum; the mandibular nerve passes through the foramen ovale; the ophthalmic nerve passes through the superior orbital fissure; the optic nerve passes through the optic canal; and the trochlear nerve passes through the cavernous sinus. A fracture of the foramen rotundum causes damage to the maxillary nerve.

196. D [Chapter 10 IV]. The optic canal transmits the optic nerve (CN II) and the ophthalmic artery.

197. C [Chapter 22 III A and Figure 22.2]. The postcentral gyrus is the sensory strip, the somatosensory cortex (areas 3, 1, and 2). Sensation to the face and tongue areas is on the inferior aspect of the postcentral gyrus (see the sensory homunculus, Chapter 22). The anterior paracentral lobule subserves motor innervation to the feet. The posterior paracentral lobule subserves sensory innervation to the feet. The precentral gyrus is the motor cortex. The middle frontal gyrus contains the frontal eye field (area 8).

198. C [Chapter 8 VI J and Figure 8.1B; Chapter 16 VIII E]. Multiple sclerosis is a demyelinating disease characterized by exacerbations and remissions. In patients with multiple sclerosis, cerebrospinal fluid contains oligoclonal immunoglobulin G bands, indicating chronic inflammation. Amyotrophic lateral sclerosis is a motor neuron disease. Poliomyelitis is an enterovirus. Brown-Séquard syndrome is spinal cord hemisection. Syringomyelia is the central cavitation of the cervical spinal cord.

Appendix

Table of Cranial Nerves

Cranial Nerve	Type	Origin	Function	Course
I—Olfactory	SVA	Bipolar olfactory neurons (in olfactory epithelium in roof of nasal cavity)	Smell (olfaction)	Central axons project to the olfactory bulb via the cribriform plate of the ethmoid bone.
II—Optic	SSA	Retinal ganglion cells	Vision	Central axons converge at the optic disk and form the optic nerve, which enters the skull via the optic canal. Optic nerve axons terminate primarily in the lateral geniculate bodies.
III—Oculomotor Parasympathetic	GVE	Accessory oculomotor nucleus (rostral midbrain)	Sphincter pupillae, ciliaris	Axons exit the midbrain into the interpeduncular fossa, traverse the cavernous sinus, and enter the orbit via the superior orbital fissure.
Motor	GSE	Oculomotor nucleus (rostral midbrain)	Superior, inferior, and medial recti; inferior oblique; levator palpebrae superioris	
IV—Trochlear	GSE	Trochlear nucleus (caudal midbrain)	Superior oblique	Axons decussate in superior medullary velum, exit posteriorly inferior to the inferior colliculi, encircle the midbrain, traverse the cavernous sinus, and enter the orbit via the superior orbital fissure.
V—Trigeminal Motor	SVE	Trigeminal motor nucleus (mid pons)	Muscles of mastication, tensor tympani, anterior belly of the digastric, mylohyoid, and tensor veli palatini	Ophthalmic nerve exits via the superior orbital fissure; maxillary nerve exits via the foramen rotundum; mandibular nerve exits via the foramen ovale; ophthalmic and maxillary nerves traverse the cavernous sinus; GSA fibers enter the spinal trigeminal tract of CN V.
Sensory	GSA	Trigeminal ganglion and mesencephalic nucleus CN V (rostral pons and midbrain)	Tactile, pain, and thermal sensation from the face; the oral and nasal cavities and the supratentorial dura	
VI—Abducens	GSE	Abducens nucleus (caudal pons)	Lateral rectus	Axons exit the pons from the inferior pontine sulcus, traverse the cavernous sinus, and enter the orbit via the superior orbital fissure.
VII—Facial Parasympathetic	GVE	Superior salivatory nucleus (caudal pons)	Lacrimal gland (via pterygopalatine ganglion); submandibular and sublingual glands (via submandibular ganglion)	Axons exit the pons in the cerebellar pontine angle and enter the internal auditory meatus; motor fibers traverse the facial canal of the temporal bone and exit via the stylomastoid foramen; taste fibers traverse the chorda tympani and lingual nerve; GSA fibers enter the spinal trigeminal tract of CN V; SVA fibers enter the solitary tract.
Motor	SVE	Facial motor nucleus (caudal pons)	Muscles of facial expression; stapedius	
Sensory	GSA	Geniculate ganglion (temporal bone)	Tactile sensation to skin of ear	
Sensory	SVA	Geniculate ganglion	Taste sensation from the anterior two-thirds of tongue (via chorda tympani)	

(continued)

| table | A-1 | Table of Cranial Nerves (*continued*) |

Cranial Nerve	Type	Origin	Function	Course
VIII—Vestibulocochlear Vestibular nerve	SSA	Vestibular ganglion (internal auditory meatus)	Equilibrium (innervates hair cells of semicircular ducts, saccule, and utricle)	Vestibular and cochlear nerves join in the internal auditory meatus and enter the brain stem in the cerebellopontine angle; vestibular nerve projects to the vestibular nuclei and the flocculonodular lobe of the cerebellum; cochlear nerve projects to the cochlear nuclei.
Cochlear nerve	SSA	Spiral ganglion (modiolus of temporal bone)	Hearing (innervates hair cells of the organ of Corti)	
IX—Glossopharyngeal Parasympathetic	GVE	Inferior salivatory nucleus (rostral medulla)	Parotid gland (via the otic ganglion)	Axons exit (motor) and enter (sensory) medulla from the postolivary sulcus; axons exit and enter the skull via jugular foramen; GSA fibers enter the spinal trigeminal tract of CN V; GVA and SVA fibers enter the solitary tract.
Motor	SVE	Nucleus ambiguus (rostral medulla)	Stylopharyngeus	
Sensory	GSA	Superior ganglion (jugular foramen)	Tactile sensation to middle ear cavity	
Sensory	GVA	Inferior (petrosal) ganglion (in jugular foramen)	Tactile sensation to posterior third of tongue, pharynx, middle ear, and auditory tube; input from carotid sinus and carotid body	
Sensory	SVA	Inferior (petrosal) ganglion (in jugular foramen)	Taste from posterior third of the tongue	
X—Vagus Parasympathetic	GVE	Dorsal motor nucleus of CN X (medulla)	Viscera of the thoracic and abdominal cavities to the midtransverse colon (via terminal [intramural] ganglia)	Axons exit (motor) and enter (sensory) medulla from the postolivary sulcus; axons exit and enter the skull via the jugular foramen; GSA fibers enter the spinal trigeminal tract of CN V; GVA and SVA fibers enter the solitary tract.
Motor	SVE	Nucleus ambiguus (midmedulla)	Muscles of the larynx and pharynx	
Sensory	GSA	Superior ganglion (jugular foramen)	Tactile sensation to the external ear	
Sensory	GVA	Inferior (nodose) ganglion (in jugular foramen)	Mucous membranes of the pharynx, larynx, esophagus, trachea, and thoracic and abdominal viscera to the midtransverse colon	
Sensory	SVA	Inferior (nodose) ganglion (in jugular foramen)	Taste from the epiglottis	
XI—Accessory Motor	SVE	Anterior horn neurons C1–C6	Sternocleidomastoid and trapezius	Axons exit the spinal cord, ascend through the foramen magnum, and exit the skull via the jugular foramen.
XII—Hypoglossal	GSE	Hypoglossal nucleus (medulla)	Intrinsic and extrinsic muscles of the tongue (except the palatoglossus)	Axons exit from the preolivary sulcus of the medulla and exit the skull via the hypoglossal canal.

CN, cranial nerve; GSA, general somatic afferent; GSE, general somatic efferent; GVA, general visceral afferent; GVE, general visceral efferent; SSA, special somatic afferent; SVA, special visceral afferent; SVE, special visceral efferent.

Glossary

abasia—Inability to walk.

abulia—Inability to perform voluntary actions or to make decisions; seen in bilateral frontal lobe disease.

accommodation—Increase in thickness of the lens needed to focus a near object on the retina; mediated by the contraction of ciliaris.

adenohypophysis—Anterior lobe of the pituitary gland, derived from Rathke pouch.

adenoma sebaceum—Cutaneous lesion seen in tuberous sclerosis.

Adie pupil—Myotonic pupil; a tonic pupil, usually large, that constricts very slowly to light and convergence; generally unilateral and frequently occurs in young women with diminished deep tendon reflexes.

afferent pupil (Marcus Gunn pupil)—A pupil that reacts sluggishly to direct light stimulation; caused by a lesion of the afferent pathway (eg, multiple sclerosis involving the optic nerve).

agenesis—Failure of a structure to develop (eg, agenesis of the corpus callosum).

ageusia—Loss of the sensation of taste (gustation).

agnosia—Lack of the sensory-perceptional ability to recognize objects: visual, auditory, or tactile.

agraphesthesia—Inability to recognize figures written on the skin.

agraphia—Inability to write; seen in Gerstmann syndrome.

akathisia—Acathisia; the inability to remain in a sitting position; motor restlessness; may appear after the withdrawal of neuroleptic drugs.

akinesia—Absence or loss of the power of voluntary motion; seen in Parkinson disease.

akinetic mutism—State in which the patient can move and speak but cannot be prompted to do so; results from bilateral occlusion of the anterior cerebral artery or midbrain lesions.

alar plate—Division of the mantle zone of the developing spinal cord that gives rise to sensory neurons; receives sensory input from spinal ganglia.

albuminocytologic dissociation—Elevated cerebrospinal fluid (CSF) protein with a normal CSF cell count; seen in Guillain-Barré syndrome.

alexia—Visual aphasia; word or text blindness; loss of the ability to grasp the meaning of written or printed words; seen in Gerstmann syndrome.

alternating hemianesthesia—Ipsilateral facial anesthesia and a contralateral body anesthesia; results from a pontine or medullary lesion involving the spinal trigeminal tract and the anterolateral system.

alternating hemiparesis—Ipsilateral cranial nerve palsy and contralateral hemiparesis (eg, alternating abducens hemiparesis).

altitudinal hemianopia—Defect in which the upper or the lower half of the visual field is lost.

Alzheimer disease—Condition characterized pathologically by the presence of neuritic plaques, neurofibrillary degeneration—tangles, and amyloid beta-deposits; patients are demented with severe memory loss.

amaurosis fugax—Transient monocular blindness usually related to carotid artery stenosis or less often to embolism of retinal arterioles.

amnesia—Disturbance or loss of memory; seen with bilateral medial temporal lobe lesions.

amusia—Form of aphasia characterized by the loss of ability to express or recognize simple musical tones.

amyotrophic lateral sclerosis (ALS)—A nonhereditary motor neuron disease affecting both upper and lower motor neurons; characterized by muscle weakness, fasciculations, and fibrillations. There are no sensory deficits in ALS. Also called Lou Gehrig disease.

amyotrophy—Muscle wasting or atrophy.

analgesia—Insensibility to painful stimuli.

anencephaly—Failure of the cerebral and cerebellar hemispheres to develop; results from failure of the anterior neuropore to close.

anesthesia—Loss of sensation.

aneurysm—Circumscribed dilation of an artery (eg, berry aneurysm).

anhidrosis—Absence of sweating; found in Horner syndrome.

anisocoria—Pupils that are unequal in size; found in third nerve palsy and Horner syndrome.

anomia—Anomic aphasia; the inability to name objects; may result from a lesion of the angular gyrus.

anosmia—Olfactory anesthesia; loss of the sense of smell.

anosognosia—Ignorance of the presence of disease.

Anton syndrome (visual anosognosia)—Lack of awareness of being cortically blind; may result from bilateral occipital lobe lesions affecting the visual association cortex.

aphasia—Impaired or absent communication by speech, writing, or signs; loss of the capacity for spoken language.

aphonia—Loss of the voice.

apparent enophthalmos—Ptosis seen in Horner syndrome that makes the eye appear as if it is sunk back into the orbit.

apraxia—Disorder of voluntary movement; the inability to execute purposeful movements; the inability to properly use an object (eg, a tool).

aprosodia (aprosody)—Absence of normal pitch, rhythm, and the variation of stress in speech.

area postrema—Chemoreceptor zone in the medulla that responds to circulating emetic substances; it has no blood-brain barrier.

areflexia—Absence of reflexes.

Argyll Robertson pupil—Pupil that responds to convergence but not to light; seen in neurosyphilis and lesions of the pineal region.

arrhinencephaly—Characterized by agenesis of the olfactory bulbs; results from malformation of the forebrain; associated with trisomy 13 to 15 and holoprosencephaly.

ash-leaf spots—Hypopigmented patches typically seen in tuberous sclerosis.

asomatognosia—Position agnosia; the inability to recognize the position or disposition of a limb or digit in space.

astasia-abasia—Inability to stand or walk.

astereognosis (stereoanesthesia)—Tactile amnesia; the inability to judge the form of an object by touch.

asterixis—Flapping tremor of the outstretched arms seen in hepatic encephalopathy and Wilson disease.

ataxia (incoordination)—Inability to coordinate muscles during the execution of voluntary movement (eg, cerebellar and posterior column ataxia).

athetosis—Slow, writhing, involuntary purposeless movements seen with basal nuclei damage.

atresia—Absence of one or more normal openings (eg, atresia of the outlet foramina of the fourth ventricle, which results in Dandy-Walker syndrome).

atrophy—Muscle wasting; seen in lower motor neuron disease.

auditory agnosia—Inability to interpret the significance of sound; seen in sensory dysphasia/aphasia.

autotopagnosia (somatotopagnosia)—Inability to recognize parts of the body; seen with parietal lobe lesions.

Babinski sign—Extension of the great toe in response to plantar stimulation; indicates corticospinal (pyramidal) tract involvement.

ballism—Dyskinesia resulting from damage to the subthalamic nucleus; characterized by violent flailing and flinging of the contralateral limbs.

basal plate—Division of the mantle zone that gives rise to lower motor neurons.

Bell palsy—Idiopathic facial nerve paralysis.

Benedikt syndrome—Condition characterized by a lesion of the midbrain affecting the intra-axial oculomotor fibers, medial lemniscus, and cerebellothalamic fibers.

berry aneurysm—Small saccular dilation of a cerebral artery; ruptured berry aneurysms are the commonest cause of nontraumatic subarachnoid hemorrhage.

blepharospasm—Involuntary recurrent spasm of both eyelids; effective treatment is injections of botulinum toxin into the orbicularis oculi.

blood-brain barrier—Tight junctions (zonula occludens) of the capillary endothelial cells.

blood-cerebrospinal fluid barrier—Tight junctions (zonula occludens) of the choroid plexus.

bradykinesia—Slowness in movement; seen in Parkinson disease.

bulbar palsy—Progressive bulbar palsy; a lower motor neuron paralysis affecting primarily the motor nuclei of the medulla; the prototypic disease is amyotrophic lateral sclerosis, characterized by dysphagia, dysarthria, and dysphonia.

caloric nystagmus—Nystagmus induced by irrigating the external auditory meatus with either cold or warm water; remember **COWS** mnemonic: **C**old, **O**pposite; **W**arm, **S**ame.

cauda equina—Sensory and motor nerve rootlets found below the L2 vertebral level in the dural sac; lesions of the cauda equina result in motor and sensory defects of the lower limb.

central hypoventilation syndrome (Ondine curse)—Inability of patient to breathe while sleeping; results from damage to the respiratory centers of the medulla.

cerebral edema—Abnormal accumulation of fluid in the brain; associated with volumetric enlargement of brain tissue and ventricles; may be vasogenic, cytotoxic, or both.

cerebral palsy—A nonprogressive defect of motor function and coordination resulting from brain damage; prevalent contributing factors include premature birth.

Charcot-Bouchard aneurysm—Miliary aneurysm; microaneurysm; rupture of this type of aneurysm is the commonest cause of intraparenchymal hemorrhage; most commonly found in the basal nuclei.

Charcot-Marie-Tooth disease—Most commonly inherited peripheral neuropathy affecting lower motor neurons and spinal ganglion cells; characterized by distal muscle weakness and atrophy.

cherry-red spot (macula)—Seen in Tay-Sachs disease; resembles a normal-looking retina; the retinal ganglion cells surrounding the fovea are packed with lysosomes and no longer appear red.

Chiari malformation—Characterized by herniation of the caudal cerebellar vermis and cerebellar tonsils through the foramen magnum; associated with lumbar myelomeningocele, dysgenesis of the corpus callosum, and obstructive hydrocephalus.

chorea—Irregular, spasmodic, purposeless, involuntary movements of the limbs and facial muscles; seen in Huntington disease.

choreiform—Resembling chorea.

choreoathetosis—Abnormal body movements of combined choreic and athetoid patterns.

chromatolysis—Disintegration of Nissl substance following transection of an axon (axotomy).

clasp-knife spasticity—When a joint is moved briskly, resistance is felt initially and then fades like the opening of a pocket knife; seen with corticospinal lesions.

clonus—Rhythmic, reflexive contraction and relaxation of a muscle; seen with upper motor neuron lesions.

cogwheel rigidity—Rigidity characteristic of Parkinson disease. Bending a limb results in ratchet-like movements.

conduction aphasia—Aphasia in which the patient has relatively normal comprehension and spontaneous speech but difficulty with repetition; results from a lesion of the arcuate fasciculus, which interconnects the motor and sensory speech areas.

confabulation—Making bizarre and incorrect responses; seen in Wernicke-Korsakoff psychosis.

construction apraxia—Inability to draw or construct geometric figures; frequently seen in nondominant parietal lobe lesions.

conus medullaris syndrome—Condition characterized by paralytic bladder, fecal incontinence, impotence, and perianogenital sensory loss; involves segments S3-Co.

Creutzfeldt-Jakob disease—Rapidly progressing dementia, likely caused by an infectious prion; histologic picture is that of a spongiform encephalopathy; classic triad is dementia, myoclonic jerks, and typical electroencephalograph findings.

crocodile tears syndrome—Lacrimation during eating; results from a facial nerve injury proximal to the geniculate ganglion; regenerating preganglionic salivatory fibers are misdirected to the pterygopalatine ganglion, which projects to the lacrimal gland.

cupulolithiasis—Dislocation of the otoliths of the utricular macula that causes benign positional vertigo.

cycloplegia—Paralysis of accommodation (CN III) (ie, paralysis of the ciliaris).

Dandy-Walker malformation—Characterized by congenital atresia of the foramina of Luschka and Magendie, hydrocephalus, posterior fossa cyst, and dilation of the fourth ventricle; associated with agenesis of the corpus callosum.

decerebrate posture (rigidity)—Posture in comatose patients where the upper and lower limbs are extended, the hands are flexed, and the head is extended; the causal lesion is inferior to the level of the red nucleus.

decorticate posture (rigidity)—Posture in comatose patients where the upper limbs are flexed and the lower limbs are extended; the causal lesion superior to the level of the red nucleus.

dementia pugilistica (punch-drunk syndrome)—Condition characterized by dysarthria, parkinsonism, and dementia; ventricular enlargement and fenestration of the septum pellucidum are common; the commonest cause of death is subdural hematoma.

diabetes insipidus—Condition characterized by excretion of large amounts of pale urine; results from inadequate output of the antidiuretic hormone from the hypothalamus.

diplegia—Paralysis of the corresponding parts on both sides of the body.

diplopia—Double vision.

Down syndrome—Condition that results from a chromosomal abnormality (trisomy 21); Alzheimer disease is common in Down syndrome in persons older than 40 years.

dressing apraxia—Loss of the ability to dress oneself; frequently seen in nondominant parietal lobe lesions.

Duret hemorrhages—Midbrain and pontine hemorrhages resulting from transtentorial (uncal) herniation.

dysarthria—Disturbance of articulation (eg, vagal nerve paralysis).

dyscalculia—Difficulty in performing calculations; seen in lesions of the dominant parietal lobule.

dysdiadochokinesia—Inability to perform rapid alternating movements (eg, supination and pronation of the hand); seen in cerebellar disease.

dysesthesia—Impairment of sensation; disagreeable sensation produced by normal stimulation.

dyskinesias—Movement disorders attributed to pathologic states of the striatal (extrapyramidal) system; movements are generally characterized as insuppressible, stereotyped, and automatic.

dysmetria—Past-pointing; a form of dystaxia seen in cerebellar disease.

dysnomia—Dysnomic (nominal) aphasia; difficulty in naming objects or persons; seen to some degree in all aphasias.

dysphagia—Difficulty in swallowing; dysaglutition.

dysphonia—Difficulty in speaking; hoarseness.

dyspnea—Difficulty in breathing.

dysprosodia—Dysprosody; difficulty of speech in producing or understanding the normal pitch, rhythm, and variation in stress; lesions are found in the nondominant hemisphere.

dyssynergia—Incoordination of motor acts; seen in cerebellar disease.

dystaxia—Difficulty in coordinating voluntary muscle activity; seen in posterior column and cerebellar disease.

dystonia (torsion dystonia)—Sustained involuntary contractions of agonists and antagonists (eg, torticollis); may be caused by the use of neuroleptics.

dystrophy—Progressive changes possibly related to nutrition. When applied to muscle disease, it implies abnormal development and genetic determination.

edrophonium (Tensilon)—Diagnostic test for myasthenia gravis.

embolus—Plug formed by a detached thrombus.

emetic—Agent that causes vomiting; see **area postrema**.

encephalocele—Result of herniation of meninges and brain tissue through an osseous defect in the cranial vault.

encephalopathy—Any disease of the brain.

enophthalmos—Recession of the eye within the orbit.

epicritic sensation—Discriminative sensation; posterior column-medial lemniscus modalities.

epilepsy—Chronic disorder characterized by paroxysmal brain dysfunction caused by excessive neuronal discharge (seizure); usually associated with some alteration of consciousness; can be associated with a reduction of gamma-aminobutyric acid.

epiloia—Tuberous sclerosis, a neurocutaneous disorder; characterized by dementia, seizures, and adenoma sebaceum.

epiphora—Tear flow owing to lower eyelid palsy (CN VII).

exencephaly—Congenital condition in which the skull is defective, thus exposing the brain; seen in anencephaly.

extrapyramidal (motor) system—Motor system including the striatum (caudate nucleus and putamen), globus pallidus, subthalamic nucleus, and substantia nigra; also called the striatal (motor) system.

facial apraxia—Inability to perform facial movements on command.

fasciculations—Visible twitching of muscle fibers seen in lower motor neuron disease.

festination—Acceleration of a shuffling gait seen in Parkinson disease.

fibrillations—Nonvisible contractions of muscle fibers found in lower motor neuron disease.

flaccid paralysis—Complete loss of muscle power or tone resulting from lower motor neuron disease.

folic acid deficiency—Common cause of megaloblastic anemia; may also cause fetal neural tube defects (eg, spina bifida).

gait apraxia—Diminished capacity to walk or stand; frequently seen with bilateral frontal lobe disease.

Gerstmann syndrome—Condition characterized by right-left confusion, finger agnosia, dysgraphia, and dyscalculia; results from a lesion of the dominant inferior parietal lobule.

glioma—Tumor (neoplasm) derived from glial cells.

global aphasia—Difficulty with comprehension, repetition, and speech.

graphesthesia—Ability to recognize figures written on the skin.

hallucination—False sensory perception with localizing value.

hematoma—Localized mass of extravasated blood; a contained hemorrhage (eg, subdural or epidural).

hemianhidrosis—Absence of sweating on half of the body or face; seen in Horner syndrome.

hemianopia—Loss of vision in one half of the visual field of one or both eyes.

hemiballism—Dyskinesia resulting from damage to the subthalamic nucleus; characterized by violent flinging and flailing movements of the contralateral extremities.

hemiparesis—Slight paralysis affecting one side of the body; seen in stroke involving the internal capsule.

hemiplegia—Paralysis of one side of the body.

herniation—Pressure-induced protrusion of brain tissue into an adjacent compartment; may be transtentorial (uncal), subfalcine (subfalcial), or transforaminal (tonsillar).

herpes simplex encephalitis—Disorder characterized by headache, behavioral changes (memory), and seizures; herpes simplex is the commonest cause of encephalitis.

heteronymous—Referring to noncorresponding halves or quadrants of the visual fields (eg, binasal heteronymous hemianopia).

hidrosis—Sweating, perspiration, and diaphoresis.

Hirano bodies—Eosinophilic rodlike structures (inclusions) found in the hippocampus in Alzheimer disease.

holoprosencephaly—Failure of the prosencephalon to diverticulate and form two hemispheres.

homonymous—Referring to corresponding halves or quadrants of the visual fields (eg, left homonymous hemianopia).

Horner syndrome—Oculosympathetic paralysis consisting of miosis, hemianhidrosis, mild ptosis, and apparent enophthalmos.

hydranencephaly—Condition in which the cerebral cortex and white matter are replaced by membranous sacs; believed to be the result of circulatory disease.

hydrocephalus—Condition marked by excessive accumulation of cerebrospinal fluid and dilated ventricles.

hygroma—Collection of cerebrospinal fluid in the subdural space.

hypoacusis—Hearing impairment.

hypalgesia—Decreased sensibility to pain.

hyperacusis—Abnormal acuteness of hearing; the result of a facial nerve paralysis (eg, Bell palsy).

hyperphagia—Gluttony; overeating as seen in hypothalamic lesions.

hyperpyrexia—High fever as seen in hypothalamic lesions.

hyperreflexia—An exaggeration of muscle stretch reflexes as seen with upper motor neuron lesions; a sign of spasticity.

hyperthermia—Increased body temperature; seen with hypothalamic lesions.

hypertonia—Increased muscle tone; seen with upper motor neuron lesions.

hypesthesia—Hypoesthesia; diminished sensitivity to stimulation.

hypokinesia—Diminished or slow movement; seen in Parkinson disease.

hypophysis—Pituitary gland.

hypothermia—Reduced body temperature; seen in hypothalamic lesions.

hypotonia—Reduced muscle tone; seen in cerebellar disease.

ideational or sensory apraxia—Characterized by the inability to formulate the ideational plan for executing several components of a complex multistep act; the patient cannot go through the steps of boiling an egg when asked to; occurs most frequently in diffuse cerebral degenerating disease (eg, Alzheimer disease, multi-infarct dementia).

ideomotor or "classic" apraxia (ideokinetic apraxia)—Inability to button one's clothes when asked, to comb one's hair when asked, or to manipulate tools (eg, hammer or screwdriver), although the patient can explain their use.

idiopathic—Denoting a condition of an unknown cause (eg, idiopathic Parkinson disease).

infarction—Sudden insufficiency of blood supply caused by vascular occlusion (eg, emboli or thrombi), resulting in tissue necrosis (death).

intention tremor—Tremor that occurs when a voluntary movement is made; a cerebellar tremor.

internal ophthalmoplegia—Paralysis of the sphincter pupillae and ciliaris caused by a lesion of the oculomotor nerve.

internuclear ophthalmoplegia (INO)—Medial rectus palsy on attempted conjugate lateral gaze caused by a lesion of the medial longitudinal fasciculus.

intra-axial—Refers to structures found within the neuraxis; within the brain or spinal cord.

ischemia—Local anemia caused by mechanical obstruction of the blood supply.

junctional scotoma—results from a lesion of the decussating fibers from the inferior nasal retinal quadrant, where the optic nerve joins the optic chiasm; deficit seen in the contralateral upper temporal quadrant.

Kayser-Fleischer ring—Visible deposition of copper in the Descemet membrane of the corneoscleral margin; seen in Wilson disease (hepatolenticular degeneration).

Kernig sign—Test for meningitis. Subject lies on back with thigh flexed to a right angle, then tries to extend the leg; this movement is not possible with meningitis.

kinesthesia—Sensory perception of movement, muscle sense; mediated by the posterior column-medial lemniscus system.

Klüver-Bucy syndrome—Characterized by psychic blindness, hyperphagia, and hypersexuality; results from bilateral temporal lobe ablation including the amygdala.

labyrinthine hydrops—Excess of endolymphatic fluid in the membranous labyrinth; cause of Ménière disease.

lacunar infarct—Small infarcts of larger cerebral vessels, associated with hypertensive vascular disease.

Lambert-Eaton myasthenic syndrome—Condition that results from a defect in presynaptic acetylcholine release; 50% of the patients have a malignancy.

lead-pipe rigidity—Rigidity throughout the range of motion, characteristic of Parkinson disease.

Lewy bodies—Eosinophilic, intracytoplasmic inclusions found in the neurons of the substantia nigra in Parkinson disease.

Lhermitte sign—Electric-like shocks extending down the spine caused by flexing the head; results from damage of the posterior columns.

lipofuscin (ceroid)—Normal inclusion of many neurons and glial cells; increases as the brain ages.

Lisch nodules—Pigmented lesions of the iris seen in neurofibromatosis type 1.

lissencephaly—Agyria: results from failure of the germinal matrix neuroblasts to reach the cortical mantle and form the gyri; the surface of the brain remains smooth.

locked-in syndrome—Results from infarction of the base of the pons; infarcted structures include the corticobulbar and corticospinal tracts, leading to quadriplegia and paralysis of the lower cranial nerves; patients can communicate only by blinking or moving their eyes vertically.

locus ceruleus—Pigmented (neuromelanin) nucleus found in the pons and midbrain; contains the largest collection of norepinephrinergic neurons in the brain.

macrographia (megalographia)—Large handwriting seen in cerebellar disease.

magnetic gait—Patient walks as if feet were stuck to the floor; seen in normal-pressure hydrocephalus.

medial longitudinal fasciculus (MLF)—Fiber bundle found in the dorsomedial tegmentum of the brainstem just under the fourth ventricle; it carries vestibular and ocular motor axons, which mediate vestibulo-ocular reflexes; severance of this tract results in internuclear ophthalmoplegia.

Mees lines—Transverse lines on fingernails and toenails; results from arsenic poisoning.

megalencephaly—Large brain weighing more than 1,800 g.

meningocele—Protrusion of the meninges of the brain or spinal cord through an osseous defect in the skull or vertebral canal.

meningoencephalocele—Protrusion of the meninges and the brain through a defect in the skull.

meroanencephaly—Less severe form of anencephaly in which the brain is present in rudimentary form.

microencephaly—A small brain weighing more than 900 g; the adult brain weighs about 1,400 g.

micrographia—Small handwriting; seen in Parkinson disease.

microgyria (polymicrogyria)—Small gyri; the cortical lamination pattern is not normal; seen in Chiari syndrome.

Millard-Gubler syndrome—Alternating abducens and facial hemiparesis; an ipsilateral sixth and seventh nerve palsy and a contralateral hemiparesis.

mimetic muscles—Muscles of facial expression; innervated by facial nerve (CN VII).

miosis—Constriction of the pupil; seen in Horner syndrome.

Möbius syndrome—Congenital oculofacial palsy; consists of a congenital facial diplegia (CN VII) and a convergent strabismus (CN VI).

mononeuritis multiplex—Vasculitic inflammation of several different nerves (eg, polyarteritis nodosa).

motor (Broca; expressive) aphasia—Difficulty in articulating or speaking language; found in the dominant inferior frontal gyrus; also called anterior or nonfluent aphasia.

MPTP (1-methyl-4-phenyl-1,3,3,6-tetrahydropyridine) poisoning—Toxic destruction of the dopaminergic neurons in the substantia nigra, resulting in parkinsonism.

multi-infarct dementia—Dementia owing to the cumulative effect of repetitive infarcts; strokes characterized by cortical sensory, pyramidal, and bulbar and cerebellar signs, resulting in permanent damage; primarily seen in patients who are hypertensive.

multiple sclerosis—Myelinoclastic disease in which the myelin sheath is destroyed, with the axon remaining intact; characterized by exacerbations and remissions with paresthesias, double vision, ataxia, and incontinence; cerebrospinal fluid findings include increased gamma-globulin, increased beta-globulin, presence of oligoclonal bands, and increased myelin basic protein.

muscular dystrophy—X-linked myopathy characterized by progressive weakness, fiber necrosis, and loss of muscle cells; two commonest types are Duchenne and myotonic muscular dystrophy.

mydriasis—Dilation of the pupil; seen in oculomotor paralysis.

myelopathy—Disease of the spinal cord.

myeloschisis—Cleft spinal cord resulting from failure of the neural folds to close or from failure of the posterior neuropore to close.

myoclonus—Clonic spasm or twitching of a muscle or a group of muscles as seen in juvenile myoclonic epilepsy.

myopathy—Disease of the muscle.

myotatic reflex—Monosynaptic muscle stretch reflex.

neglect syndrome—Result of unilateral parietal lobe lesion; neglect of one-half of the body and of extracorporeal space; simultaneous stimulation results in extinction of one of the stimuli and there is loss of optokinetic nystagmus on one side.

Negri bodies—Intracytoplasmic inclusions observed in rabies; commonly found in the hippocampus and cerebellum.

neuraxis—Unpaired part of the central nervous system: spinal cord, rhombencephalon, and diencephalon.

neurilemma—Neurolemma; the sheath of Schwann cells; Schwann cells (neurilemmal cells) produce the myelin sheath in the peripheral nervous system.

neurofibrillary tangles—Abnormal double-helical structures found in the neurons of patients with Alzheimer disease.

neurofibromatosis (von Recklinghausen disease)—A neurocutaneous disorder. Neurofibromatosis type 1 consists predominantly of peripheral lesions (eg, café au lait spots, neurofibromas, Lisch nodules, schwannomas). Type 2 consists primarily of intracranial lesions (eg, bilateral acoustic schwannomas and gliomas).

neurohypophysis—Posterior lobe of the pituitary gland; derived from the downward extension of the hypothalamus, the infundibulum.

neuropathy—Disorder of the nervous system.

Nissl bodies/substance—Rough endoplasmic reticulum found in the nerve cell body and dendrites but not in the axon.

nociceptive—Capable of appreciation or transmission of pain.

normal-pressure hydrocephalus—Hydrocephalus characterized by normal cerebrospinal fluid pressure and the clinical triad of dementia, gait dystaxia (magnetic gait), and urinary incontinence; shunting is an effective treatment; mnemonic is **W**acky, **W**obbly, **W**et.

nucleus basalis of Meynert—Contains the largest collection of cholinergic neurons in the brain; located in the forebrain between the anterior perforated substance and the globus pallidus; neurons degenerate in Alzheimer disease.

nystagmus—Oscillations of the eyes; named after the fast component; seen in vestibular and cerebellar disease.

obex—Caudal apex of the rhomboid fossa.

oculocephalic reflex (doll's eye)—Moving the head of a comatose patient with intact brainstem; results in a deviation of the eyes to the opposite direction.

oppositional paratonia (gegenhalten)—Involuntary resistance to passive stretching of muscles; seen with frontal lobe disease.

optic ataxia (Balint syndrome)—Condition characterized by a failure to direct oculomotor function in the exploration of space; failure to follow a moving object in all quadrants of the field once the eyes are fixed on the object.

optokinetic nystagmus—Nystagmus induced by looking at moving stimuli (targets).

organ of Corti (spiral organ)—Structure containing hair cells that respond to vibrations of the basilar membrane, which stimulate the cochlear division of CN VIII.

otitis media—Infection of the middle ear, which can cause conduction deafness; can also cause Horner syndrome.

otorrhea—Discharge of cerebrospinal fluid via the ear canal.

otosclerosis—New bone formation in the middle ear resulting in fixation of the stapes; the most frequent cause of progressive conduction deafness.

palsy—Paralysis; often used to connote partial paralysis or paresis.

papilledema—Choked disk; edema of the optic disk; caused by increased intracranial pressure (eg, tumor, epidural or subdural hematoma).

paracusis—Impaired hearing; an auditory illusion or hallucination.

paralysis—Loss of muscle power owing to denervation; results from a lower motor neuron lesion.

paraphrasia (paraphasia)—A form of aphasia in which a person substitutes one word for another, resulting in unintelligible speech.

paraplegia—Paralysis of both lower limbs.

paresis—Partial or incomplete paralysis.

paresthesia—Abnormal sensation such as tingling, pricking, or numbness; seen with posterior column disease (eg, tabes dorsalis).

Parinaud syndrome—Lesion of the midbrain tegmentum resulting from pressure of a germinoma, a tumor of the pineal region; the patient has a paralysis of upward gaze.

Pick disease—Dementia affecting primarily the frontal lobes; spares the posterior third of the superior temporal gyrus; clinically indistinguishable from Alzheimer disease.

pill-rolling tremor—Tremor at rest; seen in Parkinson disease.

planum temporale—Auditory association cortex found posterior to the transverse gyri (of Heschl) on the inferior bank of the lateral sulcus; part of the sensory speech area.

poikilothermia—Inability to thermoregulate; seen with lesions of the posterior hypothalamus.

polydipsia—Frequent drinking; seen in lesions of the hypothalamus.

polyuria—Frequent micturition; seen with hypothalamic lesions.

porencephaly—Cerebral cavitation caused by localized agenesis of the cortical mantle; cysts are lined with ependyma.

presbycusis (presbyacusia)—The inability to perceive or discriminate sounds as part of the aging process; results from atrophy of the organ of Corti.

progressive supranuclear palsy—Characterized by supranuclear ophthalmoplegia, primarily a downward-gaze paresis followed by paresis of other eye movements; as the disease progresses, the remaining motor cranial nerves become involved.

proprioception—Reception of stimuli originating from muscles, tendons, and other internal tissues; conscious proprioception is mediated by the posterior column-medial lemniscus system. Reflex or unconscious proprioception is mediated by the spinocerebellar (body) and trigeminomesencephalic system (head).

prosopagnosia—Difficulty in recognizing familiar faces.

protopathic sensation—Pain, temperature, and light (crude) touch sensation; the modalities mediated by the anterolateral system.

pseudobulbar palsy (pseudobulbar supranuclear palsy)—Upper motor neuron syndrome resulting from bilateral lesions that interrupt the corticobulbar tracts; symptoms include difficulties with articulation, mastication, and deglutition; results from repeated bilateral vascular lesions.

psychic blindness—Type of visual agnosia seen in Klüver-Bucy syndrome.

psychosis—Severe mental thought disorder.

ptosis—Drooping of the upper eyelid; seen in Horner syndrome and oculomotor nerve paralysis (CN III).

pyramidal (motor) system—Voluntary motor system consisting of upper motor neurons in the corticobulbar and corticospinal tracts.

quadrantanopia—Loss of vision in one quadrant of the visual field in one or both eyes.

quadriplegia—Tetraplegia; paralysis of all four limbs.

rachischisis—Failure of the vertebral arches to develop and fuse and form the neural tube.

raphe nuclei—Paramedian nuclei of the brainstem that contain serotonergic neurons.

Rathke pouch—Ectodermal outpocketing of the stomodeum; gives rise to the adenohypophysis (anterior lobe of the pituitary gland).

retrobulbar neuritis—Optic neuritis frequently caused by multiple sclerosis.

rhinorrhea—Leakage of cerebrospinal fluid via the nose.

rigidity—Increased muscle tone in both extensors and flexors; seen in Parkinson disease; examples: cogwheel rigidity and lead-pipe rigidity.

Romberg sign—Loss of balance when the subject stands with feet together and closes the eyes; a sign of posterior column ataxia.

saccadic movement—Quick jump of the eyes from one fixation point to another; impaired saccades are seen in Huntington disease.

scanning speech—Scanning dysarthria; words are broken up into syllables; typical of cerebellar disease and multiple sclerosis; example: I DID not GIVE any TOYS TO my CHILDren for their BIRTHDAYS.

schizophrenia—Psychosis characterized by a disorder in the thinking processes (eg, delusions and hallucinations); associated with dopaminergic hyperactivity.

scotoma—Blind spot in the visual field.

senile (neuritic) plaques—Swollen dendrites and axons, neurofibrillary tangles, and a core of amyloid; found in Alzheimer disease.

sensory (Wernicke) aphasia—Difficulty in comprehending spoken language; also called receptive, posterior, sensory, or fluent aphasia.

shagreen spots—Cutaneous lesions found in tuberous sclerosis.

shaken baby syndrome—Syndrome with three major physical findings: retinal hemorrhages, large head circumference, and bulging fontanelle.

sialorrhea (ptyalism)—Excess of saliva (eg, drooling); seen in Parkinson disease.

simultanagnosia—Inability to understand the meaning of an entire picture even though some parts may be recognized; the inability to perceive more than one stimulus at a time.

singultus—Hiccups; frequently seen in posterior inferior cerebellar artery syndrome.

somatesthesia—Somesthesia; bodily sensations that include touch, pain, and temperature.

spastic paresis—Partial paralysis with hyperreflexia resulting from transection of the corticospinal tract.

spasticity—Increased muscle tone (hypertonia) and hyperreflexia (exaggerated muscle stretch reflexes); seen in upper motor neuron lesions.

spina bifida—Neural tube defect with the variants: spina bifida occulta, spina bifida with meningocele, spina bifida with meningomyelocele, and rachischisis; results from failure of the embryonic vertebral laminae to close in the midline.

status marmoratus—Hypermyelination in the putamen and thalamus; results from perinatal asphyxia; clinically presents as double athetosis.

stereoanesthesia—Astereognosis; inability to judge the form of an object by touch.

Stiff-person syndrome—Myopathy characterized by progressive and permanent stiffness of the muscles of the back, neck, and spreading to involve the proximal muscles of the limbs; caused by a disturbance of the inhibitory action of Renshaw cells in the spinal cord.

strabismus—Lack of parallelism of the visual axes of the eyes; heterotropia.

stria medullaris (of the thalamus)—Fiber bundle extending from the septal area to the habenular nuclei.

stria terminalis—Semicircular fiber bundle extending from the amygdala to the hypothalamus and septal area.

striae medullares (of the rhombencephalon)—Fiber bundles that divide the rhomboid fossa into a rostral pontine part and a caudal medullary part.

Sturge-Weber syndrome—Neurocutaneous congenital disorder including a port wine stain (venous angioma) and calcified leptomeningeal angiomatoses (railroad track images seen on plain film); seizures occur in up to 90% of patients.

subclavian steal syndrome—Occlusion of the subclavian artery, proximal to the vertebral artery, resulting in a shunting of blood down the vertebral and into the ipsilateral subclavian artery; physical activity of the ipsilateral upper limb may cause signs of vertebrobasilar insufficiency (dizziness or vertigo).

sulcus limitans—Groove separating the sensory alar plate from the motor basal plate; extends from the spinal cord to the mesencephalon.

sunset sign—Downward look by eyes; the sclerae are above the irides and the upper eyelids are retracted; seen in congenital hydrocephalus and in progressive supranuclear palsy.

swinging flashlight test—Test to diagnose a relevant afferent pupil; light shone into the afferent pupil results in a small change in pupil size bilaterally, and light shone into the normal pupil results in a decrease in pupil size in both eyes.

sympathetic apraxia—Motor apraxia (in the left hand); seen in lesions of the dominant frontal lobe.

syringomyelia—Cavitation, especially of the cervical spinal cord, resulting in bilateral loss of pain and temperature sensation and wasting of the intrinsic muscles of the hands; syrinxes may be found in the medulla (syringobulbia) and pons (syringopontia) and in Chiari malformation.

tabes dorsalis—Locomotor ataxia; progressive demyelination and sclerosis of the posterior columns and roots; seen in neurosyphilis.

tactile agnosia—Inability to recognize objects by touch.

tardive dyskinesia—Syndrome of repetitive, choreoathetoid movements frequently affecting the face; results from treatment with antipsychotic agents.

Tay-Sachs disease (GM2 gangliosidosis)—Inherited metabolic disease of the central nervous system; characterized by seizures, dementia, and blindness; a cherry-red spot occurs in 90% of cases; caused by a deficiency of hexosaminidase A.

tethered cord syndrome (filum terminale syndrome)—Syndrome characterized by numbness of the legs and feet, foot drop, loss of bladder control, and impotence.

thrombus—Clot in an artery that is formed from blood constituents; gives rise to an embolus.

tic douloureux—Trigeminal neuralgia.

tinnitus—Ringing in the ear(s); seen with irritative lesions of the cochlear nerve (eg, acoustic neuroma).

titubation—A head tremor in the anterior-posterior direction, often accompanying midline cerebellar lesions; also a staggering gait.

tremor—Involuntary, rhythmic, oscillatory movement.

tuberous sclerosis (Bourneville disease)—Neurocutaneous disorder characterized by the trilogy of mental retardation, seizures, and adenoma sebaceum; cutaneous lesions include periungual fibromas, shagreen patches, and ash-leaf spots.

uncinate fit—Form of psychomotor epilepsy, including hallucinations of smell and taste; results from lesions of the parahippocampal gyrus (uncus).

upper motor neurons (UMNs)—Cortical neurons that give rise to the corticospinal and corticobulbar tracts; destruction of UMNs or their axons results in spastic paresis; some authorities include brainstem neurons that synapse on lower motor neurons (ie, neurons from the red nucleus).

vertigo—Sensation of movement owing to vestibular disease.

visual agnosia—Inability to recognize objects by sight.

von Hippel-Lindau disease—Disorder characterized by lesions of the retina and cerebellum; retinal and cerebellar hemangioblastoma; non-central nervous system lesions may include renal, epididymal, and pancreatic cysts as well as renal carcinoma.

Wallenberg syndrome—Condition characterized by hoarseness, cerebellar ataxia, anesthesia of the ipsilateral face and contralateral body, and cranial nerve signs of dysarthria, dysphagia, dysphonia, vertigo, and nystagmus; results from infarction of the lateral medulla owing to occlusion of the vertebral artery or its major branch, the posterior inferior cerebellar artery; Horner syndrome is frequently found on the ipsilateral side.

Wallerian degeneration—Anterograde degeneration of an axon and its myelin sheath after axonal transection.

Weber syndrome—Lesion of the midbrain basis pedunculi involving the root fibers of the oculomotor nerve and the corticobulbar and the corticospinal tracts.

Werdnig-Hoffmann syndrome (spinal muscular atrophy)—Early childhood disease of the anterior horn cells (lower motor neuron disease).

Index

Note: Page numbers followed by f indicate illustrations; those followed by t indicate tables; and those followed by Q indicate end-of-chapter Question and Answer sections.

A

Abdomen, autonomic plexuses of, 93, 94f
Abducens nerve, 182
    anatomy of, 148f
Abducens nucleus, 134f, 136, 143Q, 148f, 178f
Abducens nerve, 7f, 9, 151, 351t
    anatomy of, 146f, 151
    clinical correlations for, 151
Abscess, brain, 80f
Abulia, 308
Accessory cuneate nucleus, 131f, 132
    medulla, 97
Accessory nerve, 2f, 7f, 10, 157, 161Q, 352t
    anatomy of, 148f, 157
    clinical correlations for, 157
Accessory nucleus, 148f
Accessory oculomotor nucleus, 62, 140, 148f, 149, 280, 282
Accommodation, visual, 232, 232f
Acervulus, 28
Acetylcholine (ACh), 279, 289, 291–292, 291f, 302Q
    in striatal system, 258
Achilles reflex, 100Q
Achromatopsia, 314
Acoustic neuroma, 171, 181–182, 181f, 211, 222Q
Acoustic schwannoma, 221
Acute idiopathic polyneuritis, 118, 125Q
Adenohypophysis, 63, 196, 199, 200f
Adie pupil, 234
Afferent limb, 99, 170
Afferent pupil, 233f, 234
Agenesis, 66
Ageusia, 153, 243
Agnosia
    finger, 307
    tactile, 306, 318Q
Agraphesthesia, 311f
Agraphia, 307, 314
Akinetic mutism, 308
Alar plate, 57–58, 59–62f, 61, 71Q
Albuminocytologic dissociation, 125Q
Alcohol, fetal injury from, 66
Alexia, 310, 312, 314, 317Q
Allocortex, 64, 304
Altitudinal hemianopia, 230
Alzheimer disease, 292, 299, 301Q
Amacrine cells, 227
Ambient cistern, 22, 31Q
Amino acid transmitters, 296–297
    excitatory, 297, 298f
    inhibitory, 296–297, 297f
Ampullae, 60f
Amygdala, 12f, 39f, 254f, 290f, 292–296f
    anatomy of, 245–246, 246f, 249Q
    lesions of, 247–248, 249Q
Amygdaloid nuclear complex, 198, 203Q, 244, 246f, 247
Amyotrophic lateral sclerosis, 117f, 119, 124Q

Amyotrophy, 116
Anencephaly, 65–66, 71Q
Anesthesia, 120f, 156, 194
Aneurysms
    aortic, 156
    berry, 45, 46f, 48Q
    Charcot-Bouchard, 45
    definition of, 45
    oculomotor nerve compression by, 149
Angiography
    carotid, 39f
    cerebral veins, 45f
    dural sinuses, 45f
    vertebral, 44f
Angular gyrus, 3f, 5, 307
Anhidrosis, 121
Anisocoria, 234, 236Q
Ankle jerk reflex, 100Q
Annulus fibrosus, herniation through, 123
Anomia, 312
Anosmia, 146, 161Q, 241
Anosognosia, 310
Anterior, 198f
Anterior aphasia, 308
Anterior cerebral artery, 13f, 26f, 36, 37f, 39f, 45f, 48Q
    occlusion of, 313
Anterior choroidal artery, 36, 37f, 39f
Anterior commissure, 4f, 8, 11f
    development of, 64
Anterior communicating artery, 36, 37f, 39f
Anterior cord syndrome, 34–35, 121, 121f
Anterior corticospinal tract, 107, 108f, 109f, 112Q, 118, 120, 125Q
    lesions of, 117f, 118, 120f
    transection of, 120, 121f
Anterior funiculus, 97f
Anterior horn, 22, 23f, 57f, 58, 97f, 130f
    destruction of, 121, 121f, 125Q
    motor neurons of, 219
Anterior hypothalamus and preoptic area, 296f
Anterior inferior cerebellar artery (AICA), 37f, 41, 48Q, 177, 178f, 184Q
Anterior internal frontal artery, 37f
Anterior lateral sulcus, 95
Anterior limb of internal capsule, 13f
Anterior lobe, 63f
    of cerebellum, 10, 264, 265f, 265t
Anterior median fissure, 57f, 95, 97f
Anterior medullary velum, 6f
Anterior meningeal artery, 42
Anterior neuropore, 53, 53f
Anterior nucleus, 6f, 190
    hypothalamic, 196f, 197, 203Q
    olfactory, 243
    thalamic, 188, 189f, 190f, 202Q, 243, 247
Anterior paracentral lobule, 5
Anterior parietal artery, 38f